APOMORPHINE AND OTHER DOPAMINOMIMETICS

Volume 2: Clinical Pharmacology

APOMORPHINE AND OTHER DOPAMINOMIMETICS

Volume 1: Basic Pharmacology
Volume 2: Clinical Pharmacology

Apomorphine and Other Dopaminomimetics

Volume 2
Clinical Pharmacology

Editors

Giovanni Umberto Corsini, M.D.
Gian Luigi Gessa, M.D.
Institute of Pharmacology
University of Cagliari
Cagliari, Italy

Raven Press ■ New York

Raven Press, 1140 Avenue of the Americas, New York, New York 10036

Made in the United States of America

International Standard Book Number 0–89004–667–0
Library of Congress Catalog Number 81–40610

Great care has been taken to maintain the accuracy of the information contained in the volume. However, Raven Press cannot be held responsible for errors or for any consequences arising from the use of the information contained herein.

Preface

Apomorphine was discovered in 1869 as a by-product of morphine, and has for many years been considered primarily for its emetic properties—in spite of its ability to produce other peripheral and central actions. In addition to its morphine-like actions, apomorphine exerts cardiovascular and hypotensive effects, selectively alters gastric motility, and induces a variety of stereotyped behaviors. Increased attention was given to apomorphine when it was found to have sedative properties, which made it a valuable aid in treating agitated patients, and in 1951 when Schwab described its usefulness in the treatment of Parkinson's disease.

The popularity of apomorphine, however, is linked to that of dopamine, which has also been considered a "cinderella" drug among neurotransmitters. The relationship of apomorphine to dopamine was clarified significantly by Ernst in 1967, whose studies indicated the existence of structural similarities between the two drugs, thus explaining the dopaminergic nature of apomorphine's effects. Apomorphine has since been known as a specific tool for the study of dopamine function in animals and humans. Research focusing in this direction has led to the development of several analogs with dopaminergic properties and of newly synthesized agonists, which have proven to be valuable pharmacological agents with a myriad of useful therapeutic applications.

Apomorphine and Other Dopaminomimetics is a two-volume set which organizes the material in this field into basic and clinical research. *Volume 1: Basic Pharmacology* is a comprehensive treatise on various aspects of the use of apomorphine and related dopaminomimetics to disclose central and peripheral roles of dopamine in regulating physiological functions such as motor activity, sleep, wakefulness, food intake, hormonal control, blood pressure, and diuresis. *Volume 2: Clinical Pharmacology* deals with the clinical aspects of dopamine agonists in relation to schizophrenic and affective disorders, Parkinson's disease and dyskinesias, sleep, pituitary hormone interactions, aging, and arterial pressure control.

These two volumes represent the establishment of apomorphine as an invaluable tool in basic and clinical research in the neurosciences, and will be of interest to pharmacologists as well as neuroscientists.

Acknowledgments

This volume is based on presentations from a symposium entitled "Clinical Pharmacology of Apomorphine and Other Dopaminomimetics," held in Villasimius, Italy in September 1980. We would like to thank the Fidia Research Laboratories of Abano Terme (Italy), who were the principal sponsors of the congress, and also Sandoz Ltd. of Basel (Switzerland) and Milan (Italy) for their contribution. Further, for the expert organization and smooth running of the symposium we wish to thank Dr. Cristina Schirato of Fidia Research Laboratories, and Miss Anne Farmer, whose assistance was also greatly appreciated in the publishing of this book.

Contents

Volume 2: Clinical Pharmacology

Clinical Aspects of Dopamine Agonists

Schizophrenia and Affective Disorders

Parkinson's Disease and Dyskinesias

Dopamine in Sleep Mechanisms

Dopamine and Pituitary Hormone Interactions

Aging and Neuronal Transmission

Peripheral Actions of Dopamine Agonists

Contents

Volume 1: Basic Pharmacology

Modulation of Dopamine Receptor Function

Pharmacology of Dopamine Agonists

Contributors

M. Ackenheil
Psychiatrische Klinik der Universität München
Nussbaumstrasse 7
8000 München, Germany

C. Adani
Department of Human Physiology
University of Modena
Via Campi 287
41100 Modena, Italy

Y. Agid
Clinique de Neurologie et Neuropsychologie
Hôpital de la Salpêtriere
91, Boulevard de l'Hôpital
75634 Paris, Cedex 13 France

L. F. Agnati
Department of Human Physiology
University of Modena
Via Campi 287
41100 Modena, Italy

A. Agnoli
I Neurologic Clinica
University of Roma
00100 Rome, Italy

M. G. Albizzati
Department of Neurology and Pharmacology
University of Milan
Bassini Hospital
20092 Cinisello Balsamo, Italy

C. Aldinio
Department of Biochemistry
Fidia Research Laboratories
35031 Abano Terme, Italy

S. Algeri
Mario Negri Institute for Pharmacological Research
Via Eritrea 62
20156 Milan, Italy

B. Angrist
Department of Psychiatry
New York University School of Medicine
550 First Avenue
New York, New York 10016

Gill Anzelark
Department of Neurology
Institute of Psychiatry
London SE5 8AF, United Kingdom

T. Asano
Department of Neurochem.
New York University Medical Center
550 First Avenue
New York, New York 10016

M. Baldassare
Neurologic Clinic
University Institute of Medicine
67100 L'Aquila, Italy

C. Barale
Institute of Pharmacology
Faculty of Medicine
University of Catania
V. le A. Doria 6
95125 Catania, Italy

S. Bassi
Department of Neurology and Pharmacology
University of Milan
Bassini Hospital
20092 Cinisello Balsamo, Italy

Judith E. Beach
Department of Obstetrics, Gynecology, and Reproductive Sciences
University of California School of Medicine
San Francisco, California 94143

F. Benfenati
Department of Human Physiology
University of Modena
Via Campi 287
41100 Modena, Italy

F. Bernardi
Department of Clinical Pharmacology
University of Cagliari
Via Porcell 4
09100 Cagliari, Italy

P. Bernardi
Department of Human Physiology
University of Modena
Via Campi 287
41100 Modena, Italy

A. Bocchetta
Department of Clinical Pharmacology
University of Cagliari
Via Porcell 4
09100 Cagliari, Italy

M. Boccuni
Department of Clinical Pharmacology
University of Florence
V. le Morgagni 85
50134 Florence, Italy

Jacques R. Boissier
Centre de Recherches Roussel-Uclaf 102
111 route de Noisy
93230 Romainville, France

C. L. E. Broekkamp
Biology Department
LERS
Synthélabo
58, rue de la Glacière
F75013 Paris, France

William E. Bunney, Jr.
Section on Psychobiology
Biological Psychiatry Branch
National Institute of Mental Health
Building 10, Room 3s239
9000 Rockvill Pike
Bethesda, Maryland 20205

Richard S. Burns
Experimental Therapeutics Branch
National Institute of Neurological and Commu-
  nicative Disorders and Stroke
Room 6D20, Clinical Center
National Institutes of Health
Bethesda, Maryland 20205

Donald B. Calne
Experimental Therapeutics Branch
National Institute of Neurological and Commu-
  nicative Disorders and Stroke
Room 6D20, Clinical Center
National Institutes of Health
Bethesda, Maryland 20205

G. Calderini
Department of Biochemistry
Fidia Research Laboratories
35031 Abano Terme, Italy

M. Capelli
Centralized Laboratory
St. Orsola Hospital
Bologna, Italy

P. L. Canonico
Institute of Pharmacology
Faculty of Medicine
University of Catania
V. le A. Doria 6
95125 Catania, Italy

F. Cathala
Biology Department
LERS
Synthélabo
58, rue de la Glacière
F75013 Paris, France

T. N. Chase
Experimental Therapeutics Branch
National Institute of Neurological and Commu-
  nicative Disorders and Stroke
National Institutes of Health
Bethesda, Maryland 20205

Jin K. Chun
University of Virginia School of Medicine
Charlottesville, Virginia 22908

C. Cianchetti
Department of Child Neurology and Psychiatry
University of Cagliari
Cagliari 09100, Italy

G. Clementi
Institute of Pharmacology
Faculty of Medicine
University of Catania
V. le A. Doria 6
95125 Catania, Italy

V. Cocchi
Centralized Laboratory
St. Orsola Hospital
Bologna, Italy

G. U. Corsini
Department of Clinical Pharmacology
University of Cagliari
Via Porcell 4
09100 Cagliari, Italy

F. Crews
Department of Pharmacology
University of Florida College of Medicine
Gainesville, Florida 32610

Michael Cronin
University of Virginia School of Medicine
Charlottesville, Virginia 22908

Neal R. Cutler
Section on Psychobiology
Biological Psychiatry Branch
National Institute of Mental Health
Building 10, Room 3S239
9000 Rockville Pike
Bethesda, Maryland 20205

John M. Davis
Illinois State Psychiatric Institute
1601 West Taylor Street
Chicago, Illinois 60612

E. G. DeFraites
Department of Psychiatry
Maryland Psychiatric Research Center
University of Maryland
Baltimore, Maryland 21228

S. Del Roscio
Neurologic Clinic
University Institute of Medicine
67100 L'Aquila, Italy

M. Del Zompo
Department of Clinical Pharmacology
University of Cagliari
Via Porcell 4
09100 Cagliari, Italy

A. Destee
Clinique de Neurologie
CHU
Lille, France

F. Drago
Institute of Pharmacology
Faculty of Medicine
University of Catania
V. le A. Doria 6
95125 Catania, Italy

Catherine Euvrard
Centre de Recerches Roussel-
Uclaf 102
111 route de Noisy
93230 Romainville, France

M. Fanciullacci
Department of Clinical Pharmacology
University of Florence
V. le Morgagni 85
50134 Florence, Italy

L. Frattola
Department of Neurology and Pharmacology
University of Milan
Bassini Hospital
20092 Cinisello Balsamo, Italy

P. Fresia
Ravizza Research Laboratories
Muggiò
20100 Milan, Italy

A. Gaiti
Department of Biochemistry
University of Perugia
06100 Perugia, Italy

G. L. Gessa
Institute of Pharmacology
University of Cagliari
Via Porcell 4
09100 Cagliari, Italy

J. Christian Gillin
Biological Psychiatry Branch
IRP, National Institute of Mental Health
Bethesda, Maryland 20205

M. D. Gotts
Department of Psychiatry
Maryland Psychiatric Research Center
University of Maryland
Baltimore, Maryland 21228

C. G. Gottfries
Department of Psychiatry and Neurochemistry
St. Jorgens Hospital
University of Goteborg
422 03 Hisings Backa, Sweden

M. Goldstein
Department of Neurochemistry
New York University Medical Center
550 First Avenue
New York, New York 10016

Leo E. Hollister
Department of Psychiatry and Pharmacology
Stanford University School of Medicine
Palo Alto, California 94304

A. Illas
Department of Neurology
Faculty of Medicine
Athens, Greece

David C. Jimerson
Section on Psychobiology
Biological Psychiatry Branch
National Institute of Mental Health
9000 Rockville Pile
Building 10, Room 3S239
Bethesda, Maryland 20205

Michel Jouvet
Department of Experimental Medicine
Université Claude-Bernard
Lyon, France

Farouk Karoum
Adult Psychiatry Branch
Division of Special Mental Health Research
Intramural Research Program
National Institute of Mental Health
St. Elizabeth's Hospital
Washington, D.C. 20032

Bernard Kerdelhue
Laboratoire Hormones Polypeptidiques
CNRS
91190 Gif-sur-Yvette, France

Joel E. Kleinman
Adult Psychiatry Branch
Division of Special Mental Health Research
Intramural Research Program
National Institute of Mental Health
St. Elizabeth's Hospital
Washington, D.C. 20032

S. Lal
Department of Psychiatry
Montreal General Hospital
Montreal, Quebec, Canada HG3 1A4

F. Lhermitte
Clinique de Neurologie et Neuropsychologie
Hôpital de la Salpêtriere
91, Boulevard de l'Hôpital
75634 Paris, Cedex 13, France

K. G. Lloyd
Biology Department
LERS
Synthélabo
58, rue de la Glacière
F75013 Paris, France

Ivan S. Login
University of Virginia School of Medicine
Charlottesville, Virginia 22908

G. Lomuscio
Mario Negri Institute for Pharmacological
  Research
Via Eritrea 62
20156 Milan, Italy

Robert M. MacLeod
University of Virginia School of Medicine
Charlottesville, Virginia 22908

G. Marrosu
Department of Child Neurology and Psychiatry
University of Cagliari
Via Ospedale
09100 Cagliari, Italy

C. D. Marsden
University Department of Neurology
Institute of Psychiatry
Denmark Hill
London SE5, United Kingdom

C. Masala
Clinic of Neurology
University of Cagliari
Via Ospedale
09100 Cagliari, Italy

Brian Meldrum
Department of Neurology
Institute of Psychiatry
London SE5 8AF, United Kingdom

S. Michelacci
Department of Clinical Pharmacology
University of Florence
V. le Morgagni 85
50134 Florence, Italy

Egidio A. Moja
Institute of Neurology
University of Cagiari
09100 Cagliari, Italy

F. Nicoletti
Institute of Pharmacology
Faculty of Medicine
University of Catania
V. le A. Doria 6
95125 Catania, Italy

P. Olivari
Department of Child Neurology and Psychiatry
University of Cagliari
Via Ospedale
09100 Cagliari, Italy

N. Palesse
Neurologic Clinic
University Institute of Medicine
67100 L'Aquila, Italy

P. Passouant
Service de Physiopathologie des Maladies Ner-
  veuses
Université de Montpellier
Boulevard Henri IV
Montpellier, France

Richard L. Perryman
University of Virginia School of Medicine
Charlottesville, Virginia 22908

M. P. Piccardi
Department of Clinical Pharmacology
University of Cagliari
Via Porcell 4
09100 Cagliari, Italy

G. F. Pitzalis
Department of Clinical Pharmacology
University of Cagliari
Via Porcell 4
09100 Cagliari, Italy

P. Pollak
Clinique de Neurologie
CHU
Grenoble, France

F. Ponzio
Mario Negri Institute for Pharmacological
*   Research*
Via Eritrea 62
20156 Milan, Italy

Robert M. Post
Section on Psychobiology
Biological Psychiatry Branch
National Institute of Mental Health
Building 10, Room 3S239
9000 Rockville Pike
Bethesda, Maryland 20205

Steven G. Potkin
Adult Psychiatry Branch
Division of Special Mental Health Research
*   Program*
Intramural Research Program
National Institute of Mental Health
St. Elizabeth's Hospital
Washington, D.C. 20032

A. Prato
Institute of Pharmacology
Faculty of Medicine
University of Catani
V. le A. Doria 6
95125 Catania, Italy

N. Quinn
Department of Neurology
Institute of Psychiatry
De Crespigny Park
London SE5 8AF, United Kingdom

J. Rotrosen
Department of Psychiatry
New York University School of Medicine
550 First Avenue
New York, New York 10016

S. Ruggieri
Neurologic Clinic
University Institute of Medicine
67100 L'Aquila, Italy

U. Scapagnini
Institute of Pharmacology
University of Catania
V. le A. Doria 6
95125 Catania, Italy

Martin H. Schaeffer
Department of Psychiatry
University of Chicago
Chicago, Illinois 60601

F. Sicuteri
Department of Clinical Pharmacology
University of Florence
V. le Morgagni 85
50134 Florence, Italy

J. L. Signoret
Clinique de Neurologie et Neuropsychologie
Hôpital de la Salpêtriere
91, Boulevard de l'Hôpital
75634 Paris, Cedex 13, France

Robert C. Smith
Texas Research Institute for Mental Sciences
Houston, Texas 77025

N. Sitaram
Biological Psychiatry Branch
IRP, National Institute of Mental Health
Bethesda, Maryland 20205

David M. Stoff
Adult Psychiatry Branch
Division of Special Mental Health Research
Intramural Research Program
National Institute of Mental Health
St. Elizabeth's Hospital
Washington, D.C. 20032

Carol A. Tamminga
Department of Psychiatry
Maryland Psychiatric Research Center
University of Maryland
Baltimore, Maryland 21228

Michael O. Thorner
University of Virginia School of Medicine
Charlottesville, Virginia 22908

G. Toffano
Department of Biochemistry
Fidia Research Laboratories
35031 Abano Terme, Italy

M. Trabucchi
Department of Neurology and Pharmacology
University of Milan
Bassini Hospital
20092 Cinisello Balsamo, Italy

D. P. van Kammen
Biological Psychiatry Branch
IRP, National Institute of Mental Health
Bethesda, Maryland 20205

Richard I. Weiner
Department of Obstetrics, Gynecology and
*   Reproductive Sciences*
University of California School of Medicine
San Francisco, California 94143

P. Worms
Biology Department

LERS
Synthélabo
58, rue del la Glacière
F75013 Paris, France

Richard J. Wyatt
Adult Psychiatry Branch
Division of Special Mental Health Research
Intramural Research Program
National Institute of Mental Health
St. Elizabeth's Hospital
Washington, D.C. 20032

I. Zini
Department of Human Physiology
University of Modena
Via Campi 287
41100 Modena, Italy

Apomorphine and Other Dopaminomimetics,
Vol. 2: Clinical Pharmacology, edited by
G. U. Corsini and G. L. Gessa, Raven Press,
New York © 1981.

Clinical Studies with Apomorphine

S. Lal

Department of Psychiatry, Montreal General Hospital, Montreal, Quebec, Canada H3G 1A4

Three reviews on the pharmacology of apomorphine (Apo) have appeared in recent years (13, 21, 69). Apo is a dopamine (DA) receptor agonist in animals and man. In keeping with the latter, Apo binds to DA receptors (51) and stimulates DA-sensitive adenylate cyclase in human brain (82). The relatively selective action of this aporphine alkaloid together with its short half-life (72, 84), have led to the use of this compound to evaluate DA mechanisms in physiological processes and to assess changes in DA function in neurological, psychiatric and other disorders in man. The present paper reviews some of these findings.

APOMORPHINE AND MOVEMENT DISORDERS

The effect of Apo has been assessed in a variety of movement disorders (Table 1). Apo improves Parkinson's disease (PD), a condition of striatal DA hypofunction, as well as Huntington's chorea (HC), tardive dyskinesia (TD) and Gilles de la Tourette's syndrome, conditions with presumed striatal DA hyperactivity. Improvement of the latter three pathologies has been explained on the basis of a preferential stimulation of presynaptic inhibitory DA receptors by low doses (1-4 mg) of Apo (16, 25, 79). However, doses as low as 0.5-2 mg Apo also improve PD (5, 18). This apparent paradox has been explained as follows: in PD there is degeneration of the nigrostriatal pathway which results in loss of presynaptic DA receptors and denervation supersensitivity of postsynaptic DA receptors. This combination of factors results in Apo-induced amelioration of PD by stimulation of postsynaptic DA receptors. Less easy to embrace in this concept is Apo-induced improvement in TD, a condition in which postsynaptic DA receptors are rendered supersensitive by chemical denervation. It is of course possible that Apo still preferentially stimulates the presynaptic DA receptors, which are intact, despite the presence of supersensitivity of postsynaptic DA receptors.

The therapeutic effect of Apo in PD is blocked by haloperidol whereas metoclopramide, sulpiride (14) and domperidone (17) block the emetic action without affecting the ameliorative effect on PD. Apo is also effective in PD when given orally (19, 67) in doses of 160-600 mg per day (19, 20). Many of the side effects usually associated with Apo are absent or rare when given by mouth. N-n-propylnorapomorphine (NPA) is effective orally but tolerance to the anti-Parkinsonian effects occurs after three weeks (20). The 'on-off' phenomenon as well as intermittent dyskinesias continue on oral Apo or NPA in patients who have previously manifested similar symptoms when on chronic L-dopa therapy.

Apo-induced improvement in HC is blocked by haloperidol or sulpiride which further points to the beneficial effect of Apo as acting via a DA mechanism (16) rather than by a nonspecific sedative action. However,

TABLE 1.   Apomorphine and movement disorders

Diagnosis	Response	Reference
Parkinson's disease	Improves	(5, 10, 14, 17, 18, 19, 20[a], 22, 67, 70, 71, 86, 87)
Huntington's chorea	No change	(37)
" " "	Improves	(16, 80)
Sydenham's chorea	Improves	(26)
Tardive dyskinesia	Improves	(9, 79, 81)
" " "	Improves or no change	(68)
" " "	No change	(24)
Spasmodic torticollis	Improves	(29)
" " " "	Improves or no change	(45[b], 81)
Torsion dystonia	Improves	(4)
" "	No change	(40)
Gilles de la Tourette's syndrome	No change	(40)
" " " " " "	Improves	(25)
Intention myoclonus	Little or no change	(85)
Spontaneous & photosensitive myoclonus	Improves	(1)
L-Dopa-induced choreoathetosis	Improves	(22[c])
Haloperidol-induced dyskinesia	Improves	(28)
Schizophrenic catalepsy	No change	(11)
Unipolar depressive psychomotor retardation	No change	(31)

[a]Oral Apo or N-n-propylnorapomorphine induced intermittent dyskinesia in patients previously developing dyskinesias on chronic L-dopa therapy. [b]Worsening in some patients.   [c]Choreoathetoid movements induced in some patients.

none of the studies on movement disorders have compared Apo with an active placebo having sedative properties. Such a control is important as it is well known that anxiety worsens and sedation or sleep improve involuntary movements.

Apo improves some patients with spasmodic torticollis (ST). In an extension of earlier work (45) we have now examined the effect of Apo in 18 subjects. Seven improved (25% or more), 2 worsened (25% or more) and 9 showed no change. Changes with Apo pointed to a trend towards predicting response to L-dopa therapy (Fig. 1). Thus, in 4 subjects who improved with Apo and then received L-dopa (max 2-3G per day for 16 weeks), two improved and two showed no change. Two of the patients who worsened also received L-dopa; one worsened and the other showed no change.

In animals, impairment of DA function induces catalepsy which is reversed by Apo. A relationship of catalepsy in animals to clinical catalepsy is often implied. In two patients with catalepsy associated with schizophrenia, Apo failed to reverse the symptom whereas rapid improvement followed sodium amytal (11). This observation together with the finding that naloxone has no effect on schizophrenic catalepsy (46) suggest that catalepsy induced by various drugs in animals has question-able relevance to clinical catalepsy.

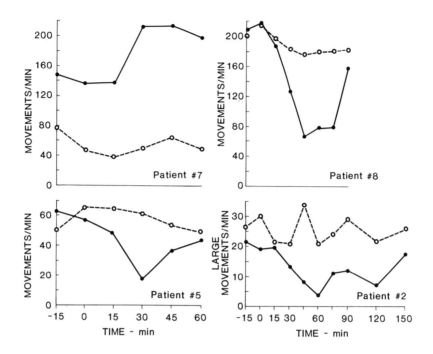

Figure 1: Effect of apomorphine on spasmodic torticollis. Subjects were injected with Apo HCl (1.5 mg sc) (closed circles) or saline placebo (open circles) at times 0 min. Subjects #2 and #5 improved, subject #7 worsened, and subject #8 showed no change with L-dopa. Based on (45).

It has been proposed that a deficiency of DA may subserve the symptom of psychomotor retardation in depressed patients. Apo has no effect on this symptom (31).

APOMORPHINE AND PHOTOSENSITIVE EPILEPSY

Apo abolishes photosensitive epilepsy in the Senegalese baboon, Papio papio (2). Following the observation that Apo antagonized extreme photo-sensitivity in a patient with Kuf's disease (1), we investigated the effect of Apo in 11 patients with primary generalized corticoreticular epilepsy in whom generalized epileptic discharges were regularly induced by photic stimulation (62). Apo HCl (1.25-1.5 mg sc) induced a transient total blockade in the photosensitive response in 9 out of 11 cases commencing 15±1.8 min after injection and lasting 45±5.5 min. The block-ade was independent of side effects of Apo and was not associated with EEG or clinical evidence of drowsiness. Saline control injections were without effect. Visual evoked potentials were unaffected by Apo.

DA exerts an inhibitory effect on neocortical neurones in animals and in the cat photic stimulation (15 flashes/second) reduces the release of endogenous DA in the visual cortex (63). In human cerebral cortex, Apo increases cyclic AMP and this effect is blocked by the selective DA blocker, pimozide (82). Thus, our data suggest the role of DA in the pathophysiology of photically-induced seizures in man and that Apo exerts its beneficial effect by stimulating postsynaptic DA receptors. Whether spontaneously occurring epileptic activity is also antagonized by DA agonists requires investigation.

APOMORPHINE AND PSYCHOPATHOLOGY

Commencing in 1961, Tesarová and colleagues (in uncontrolled studies) reported that Apo (0.5-1.0 mg sc three times a day for 12-14 days) induced a depressive state resembling an endogenous depression in mentally healthy and neurotic individuals (77). In a double blind replication study we found that none of the subjects (mainly alcoholics) developed a clinical picture of endogenous depression. There were no differences in the Hamilton Rating Scale or Zung Self-Rating Scale between Apo-treated and placebo-treated subjects (31).

Overactivity of DA function has been implicated in the pathophysiology of schizophrenia. Strian et al. (70) noted the development of an exogenous psychosis with sexual colouring and paranoid symptoms in a Parkinsonian patient after oral Apo (max 150 mg/day in 4 divided doses). However, the patient was also on L-dopa. Further, the patient exhibited disorientation which suggests more a picture of organic confusional state than a schizophrenic picture. Cotzias et al. (20) reported a 'transient mental aberration' with NPA in 7 out of 20 Parkinsonian patients. In only one patient was the aberration described. The symptoms were agitation, garrulity, hallucinations and confusion which point to an organic disorder rather than schizophrenia. Interestingly, the same symptoms had emerged on L-dopa treatment. In our study with subcutaneously administered Apo, none developed schizophrenic symptoms. Scores on the Brief Psychiatric Rating Scale improved in both placebo and Apo treated individuals (31). In an earlier study with chronic alcoholics based on Dent's treatment (66), we administered repeated large doses of oral Apo (Table 2). None of the subjects developed schizophrenic symptoms even though in 13 subjects maximal oral doses of more than 600 mg over a single 24 hour period were administered and of these 6 received between 1-2 G and one received 3 G. The failure of Apo to induce significant psychopathology is in keeping with the paucity of such reports in the literature. In fact prior to the neuroleptic era Apo was used in the management of schizophrenic excitement, mania and agitation associated with involutional melancholia (26).

Recently, Apo has been reported to induce transient improvement in schizophrenia following a single dose of 3 mg sc (in patients under neuroleptic therapy) (75) or 1 mg sc (15). This improvement has been attributed to the stimulation of presynaptic inhibitory DA receptors with a subsequent decrease in DA mediated neurotransmission. In catatonic patients, however, Corsini et al. (15) found no improvement which is in keeping with our finding that catalepsy and other catatonic symptoms are not altered by Apo (11). Changes in the latter symptoms are more accessible to observation and easier to evaluate whereas symptoms such as hallucinations are difficult to elicit or objectify and are rarely present continuously so that assessing transient change is not easy. Improvement in mania has also been reported (15). How far improvement is due to a nonspecific sedative effect remains to be evaluated.

Apo has a long history of use in the treatment of alcoholism (66). It is reported to exert an anti-craving effect in alcoholics. We found that both placebo and Apo eliminated subjective craving. This points to

TABLE 2. Oral apomorphine administration to chronic alcoholics

Group	Treatment	N	Duration (hrs)	Total Accumulated Dose (G)
A	Apomorphine po every 1-2 hrs	20	101.4±4.8 (71-155)	3.09±0.58[a] (0.67-11.2)
B	Apomorphine po every 1-2 hrs	20	12 hrs daily for 4-5 days	0.94±0.11[b] (0.36-2.37)

[a]Thirteen patients received a total of more than 2.0 G and three more than 5.0 G. [b]Nine patients received a total of more than 1.0 G. None of the patients developed schizophrenic-like symptoms. Schlatter, E.K.E. and Lal, S. (unpublished data).

the difficulty in evaluating the anti-craving effect of a drug in the absence of objective criteria for craving.

Apo-induced penile erections were first reported by Schlatter (65) and noted in subsequent reports (31, 66). This effect is abolished by pimozide and unaffected by methysergide whereas early morning erections are unaffected by either drug (41). The potential use of Apo in evaluating disorders of sexual potency requires exploration.

In our study with oral Apo (66) none of the 22 subjects in whom the blood urea nitrogen (BUN) was monitored developed azotaemia. The BUN was 14.0±1.5 (mg %) before Apo treatment and 14.1±0.9 after (P= NS). This contrasts with the observation of Cotzias et al. (19, 20) where 3 of 7 patients receiving oral Apo, 600-1400 mg/day, for an unspecified period of time, developed azotaemia which lasted 7-10 days after stopping the drug. NPA also induced azotaemia but only in doses much above the therapeutic dose (20).

APOMORPHINE AND ENDOCRINE STUDIES

Apo stimulates growth hormone (GH) and decreases prolactin (PRL) secretion in man (35, 36). Similar endocrine changes follow other directly or indirectly acting DA agonists. These observations point to an inverse DA regulation modulating GH and PRL secretion. In acromegalics, Apo induces a paradoxical decrease in the elevated GH values (12). In patients with PRL secreting tumours, Apo, L-dopa and bromocriptine lower the elevated PRL levels (55).

The presence of a stimulatory DA mechanism in the regulation of GH secretion in man (32) points to a postsynaptic locus of action of Apo. Several variables affect the Apo-induced GH response in normal subjects (Table 3). The response is reproducible (64) and is independent of stress effect (7, 39). The selectivity, reliability and rapidity of action of Apo compared with L-dopa (39) have led to the use of this Apo-induced endocrine response to evaluate DA function in a variety of psychiatric and neurological disorders and to investigate the effect of various psychoactive agents on central DA function in man (33, 34, 47). One limitation of this approach is that conclusions may not be applicable to brain regions outside the hypothalamic-pituitary axis (HPA).

Effect of Psychoactive Drugs on Apo-Induced GH Secretion

In keeping with the fact that neuroleptics block DA receptors chlorpromazine, pimozide and haloperidol antagonize the GH response to Apo (Table 4). Clozapine does not induce Parkinsonism. Further, behavioural,

TABLE 3. GH response to apomorphine in normal subjects

Variable	Effect	Reference
Gender	Diminished response in women	(23, 47)
Estrogen administration	Enhances response in pre and post-menopausal women	(23, 47)
Age	Decreased response with age	(53)
Obesity	Decreased response	(78)
Glucose loading	Decreased response	(23)
	No effect	(60)

TABLE 4. Effect of drugs on apomorphine-induced GH secretion

Drug	Class	Effect	Reference
Chlorpromazine	Neuroleptic	Antagonizes	(36)
Pimozide	Neuroleptic	Antagonizes	(41)
Haloperidol	Neuroleptic	Antagonizes	(64)
Clozapine	Neuroleptic	Antagonizes	(58)
Benztropine	Anticholinergic	No effect	(39)
Choline	Acetylcholine precursor	Enhances	(48)
Methysergide	Serotonin antagonist	No effect	(41)
Cyproheptadine	Serotonin antagonist	No effect	(64)
L-Tryptophan	Serotonin precursor	Little or no effect	(50)
Lithium	Anti-manic agent	No effect	(42)
Naloxone	Opiate antagonist	No effect	(43)
Levallorphan	Opiate antagonist	No effect	(43)
Baclofen	GABA-ergic agent	No effect	(59)
Sodium Valproate	GABA-ergic agent	No effect	(59)

biochemical and endocrinological indices of DA receptor blockade in animals following clozapine have been reported by Bürki et al. (8) to be either absent or only weakly present. These observations have led to the suggestion that the antischizophrenic effect of clozapine may not be mediated by DA receptor blockade (8). However, in man clozapine, like other neuroleptics, antagonizes Apo-induced GH secretion but unlike other neuroleptics has little or no effect on PRL secretion (34, 58). The weak effect of clozapine in elevating PRL concentrations cannot be explained on the basis of the potent anticholinergic effects of this drug (44, 58). These findings point to a differential effect of clozapine on functionally different DA systems in man. It is possible that there are differences in DA receptors that modulate PRL secretion and extrapyramidal function on the one hand and DA receptors that modulate GH secretion and anti-psychotic effects of tranquillizers on the other. The capacity of a drug to stimulate PRL secretion has been proposed as a screening test to detect potential antischizophrenic drugs. In light of findings with clozapine, inhibition of Apo-induced GH secretion may be a better indicator.

The failure of lithium, naloxone, levallorphan, baclofen or sodium valproate to modify the GH response to Apo suggests that the anti-manic effects of lithium and the putative antischizophrenic effects of narcotic antagonists or GABA-ergic agents are not mediated by DA receptor blockade or by modulating postsynaptic effects of DA. Preliminary observations that baclofen antagonizes the GH response to L-dopa (59) is in keeping with the view that baclofen inhibits the release of DA.

Anticholinergic agents potentiate DA mechanisms in the striatum. The failure of benztropine to enhance Apo-induced GH secretion point to different neurotransmitter interactions in the HPA. Whereas choline antagonizes basal ganglia DA function in man, choline enhances Apo-induced GH secretion (48). Whether the latter is mediated by increasing acetylcholine synthesis or by a muscarinic agonistic effect of choline itself is unclear.

Serotonin (5HT) modulates striatal DA function in animals. In man, the putative 5HT antagonists, methysergide and cyproheptadine, have no effect on Apo-induced GH secretion. Also, the 5HT precursor, L-tryptophan, in a dose sufficient to increase plasma free tryptophan levels almost 20-fold, and hence by inference brain tryptophan (88) and 5HT synthesis, has little or no effect on the GH response to Apo (50). These findings suggest that 5HT mechanisms have no major modulatory effect on DA function in man, at least in the HPA. It should be pointed out that the failure of some drugs to modify the GH response to Apo may be related to inadequate doses of experimental drug or to too large a dose of Apo.

Apo-Induced GH Secretion in Psychiatric and Neurological Disorders

Changes in Apo-induced GH secretion have been observed in certain extrapyramidal disorders (Table 5). The decrease in PD is in keeping with hypothalamic involvement in this disorder. In HC both a decrease and an increase have been observed. ST may be associated with a variety of extranuchal neurological symptoms (3) though the site and extent of the lesion are unknown (30). The normal GH response to Apo suggests that the lesion in ST, unlike other extrapyramidal disorders, does not extend to involve HPA DA function.

Chronic neuroleptic therapy induces DA receptor supersensitivity in animals (73, 76). Such a change in receptor function has been implicated in the pathophysiology of TD. In chronic schizophrenics withdrawn from chronic neuroleptic therapy (9.8±1.3 years) for two to fifteen weeks, the GH response to Apo was significantly lower than in controls (24). The GH

TABLE 5. GH response to apomorphine in psychiatric and neurological disorders

Diagnosis	GH Response	Reference
Unipolar depression	No change	(27, 54)
Bipolar depression	No change	(54)
Reactive depression	No change	(54)
Mania	Trend for decrease	(27)
Acute schizophrenia	Increase	(61)
Chronic schizophrenia	Decrease	(24)
" " "	No change	(74)
" " "	Bimodal response (mean unchanged)	(64)
Tardive dyskinesia	Decrease	(24)
" " "	No change	(74)
Huntington's chorea	Increase	(57)
" " "	Decrease	(52)
Parkinson's disease	Decrease	(6)
Dystonia musculorum deformans	No change	(6)
Spasmodic torticollis	No change	(45)
Hepatic dysfunction with or without encephalopathy	Decrease	(33)

response in patients with TD was significantly less than in patients without TD. The PRL response to Apo was similar in controls and patients withdrawn from neuroleptics. These data suggest that DA receptor sensitivity does not increase as a result of prior neuroleptic therapy, at least in the HPA. The diminished GH response, though not explicable on the basis of a persistent neuroleptic blockade of DA receptors, was considered a sequel to neuroleptic treatment rather than a consequence of the schizophrenic psychosis (24). The DA hypothesis of schizophrenia implicates an enhancement of DA mechanisms in brain. The findings of Ettigi et al. (24) and other investigators (64, 74), suggest that if there is supersensitivity in DA receptors in chronic schizophrenia, this does not extend to the tuberoinfundibular system. In contrast to chronic schizophrenia, Pandey et al. (61) found an enhanced GH response to Apo in acute schizophrenia. Confirmation of this finding is awaited.

There is evidence that DA neurotransmission is impaired in hepatic encephalopathy (56). The turnover of DA as assessed by the probenecid technique is unchanged (38), so that it is possible that DA receptor function is altered in hepatic coma. In patients with advanced hepatic dysfunction the GH response to Apo is decreased but this decrease is related to inadequate circulating levels of testosterone rather than to the presence or absence of coma (33). These observations suggest that adequate levels of testosterone are necessary for DA function at least in the HPA but that the occurrence of hepatic encephalopathy is independent of DA neurotransmission.

Apo-Induced GH Secretion and Sleep Deprivation

Sleep deprivation (SD) exerts an antidepressant effect in patients with an endogenous depression. In animals, rapid eye movement SD enhances the behavioural response to Apo (83). In contrast to animal studies and at variance with the DA model of manic-depressive illness, DA receptor function, as assessed by the GH response to Apo, is decreased in normal subjects following 24 hours total SD (49). Whether SD induces a similar effect in patients with an affective psychosis is unknown.

REFERENCES

1. Andermann, F., Carpenter, S., Gloor, P., Andermann, E., Wolfe, L.S., Lal, S., and Richardson, C. (1977): Can. J. Neurol. Sci., 4: 226.
2. Ashton, C., Anlezark, G., and Meldrum, B. (1976): Europ. J. Pharmacol., 39: 399-401.
3. Baxter, D.W., and Lal, S. (1979): Adv. Neurol., 24: 373-377.
4. Braham, J., and Sarova-Pinhas, I. (1973): Lancet, i: 432-433.
5. Braham, J., Sarova-Pinhas, I., and Goldhammer, Y. (1970): Brit. Med. J., 2: 768.
6. Brown, W.A., Van Woert, H., and Ambani, L.M. (1973): J. Clin. Endocr. Metab., 37: 463-465.
7. Brown, W.A., Krieger, D.T., and Van Woert, M.H. (1974): J. Clin. Endocr. Metab., 38: 1127-1130.
8. Bürki, H.R., Eichenberger, E., Sayers, A.C., and White, T.G. (1975): Pharmacopsychiatry, 8: 115-121.
9. Carroll, B.J., Curtis, G.C., and Koknen, E. (1977): Am. J. Psychiat., 134: 785-789.
10. Castaigne, P., Laplane, D., and Dordain, G. (1971): Res. Commun. Chem. Pathol. Pharmacol., 2: 154-158.

11. Cervantes, P., Lal, S., Smith, F., and Guyda, H. (1977): Acta Psychiat. Scand., 55: 214-219.
12. Chiodini, P.G., Liuzzi, A., Botalia, G., Cremascoli, G., and Silvestrini, F. (1974): J. Clin. Endocr. Metab., 38: 200-206.
13. Colpaert, F.C., Van Bever, W.F.M., and Leysen, J.E.M.F. (1976): Int. Rev. Neurobiol., 19: 225-268.
14. Corsini, G.U., Del Zompo, M., Cianchetti, C., Mangoni, A., and Gessa, G.L. (1976): Psychopharmacology, 47: 169-173.
15. Corsini, G.U., Del Zompo, M., Manconi, S., Cianchetti, C., Mangoni, A., and Gessa, G.L. (1977): Adv. Biochem. Pharmacol., 16: 645-648.
16. Corsini, G.U., Onali, P.L., Masala, C., Cianchetti, C., Mangoni, A., and Gessa, G.L. (1978): Arch. Neurol., 35: 27-30.
17. Corsini, G.U., Del Zompo, M., Gessa, G.L., and Mangoni, A. (1979): Lancet, i: 954-956.
18. Cotzias, G.C., Papavasiliou, P.S., Fehling, C., Kaufman, B., and Mena, I. (1970): New Engl. J. Med., 282: 31-33.
19. Cotzias, G.C., Lawrence, W.H., Papavasiliou, P.S., Düby, S.E., Ginos, J.Z., and Mena, I. (1972): Trans. Amer. Neurol. Assoc., 97: 156-159.
20. Cotzias, G.C., Papavasiliou, P.S., Tolosa, E.S., Mendez, J.S., and Bell-Midura, M. (1976): New Engl. J. Med., 294: 567-572.
21. Di Chiara, G., and Gessa, G.L. (1978): Adv. Pharmacol. Chemother., 15: 87-159.
22. Düby, S.E., Cotzias, G.C., Papavasiliou, P.S., and Lawrence, W.H. (1972): Arch. Neurol., 27: 474-480.
23. Ettigi, P., Lal, S., Martin, J.B., and Friesen, H.G. (1975): J. Clin. Endocr. Metab., 40: 1094-1098.
24. Ettigi, P., Nair, N.P.V., Lal, S., Cervantes, P., and Guyda, H. (1976): J. Neurol. Neurosurg. Psychiat., 39: 870-876.
25. Feinberg, M., and Carroll, B.J. (1979): Arch. Gen. Psychiat., 36: 979-985.
26. Feldman, F., Susselman, S., and Barrera, S.E. (1945): Am. J. Psychiat., 102: 403-405.
27. Garver, D.L., Pandey, G.N., Hengeveld, C., and Davis, J.M. (1977): Psychopharmacol. Bull., 13: 61-63.
28. Gessa, R., Tagliamonte, A., and Gessa, G.L. (1972): Lancet, ii: 981-982.
29. Granacher, J.P., and Baldessarini, R.J. (1975): Arch. Gen. Psychiat., 32: 375-380.
30. Lal, S. (1979): Canad. J. Neurol. Sci., 6: 427-435.
31. Lal, S., and de la Vega, C.E. (1975): J. Neurol. Neurosurg. Psychiat., 38: 722-726.
32. Lal, S., and Martin, J.B. (1980): In: Handbook of Biological Psychiatry, Vol. 3, edited by H.M. Van Praag, M.H. Lader, O.J. Rafaelsen, and E.J. Sachar, pp. 101-167, Marcel Dekker Inc., New York.
33. Lal, S., and Nair, N.P.V. (1979): In: Neuroendocrine Correlates in Neurology and Psychiatry, edited by E.E. Müller and A. Agnoli, pp. 179-194, Elsevier-North Holland Biomedical Press, Amsterdam.
34. Lal, S., and Nair, N.P.V. (1980): In: Neuroactive Drugs in Endo- crinology, edited by E.E. Müller, pp. 223-241, Elsevier-North Holland Biomedical Press, Amsterdam.
35. Lal, S., de la Vega, C.E., Sourkes, T.L., and Friesen, H.G. (1972): Lancet, ii: 661.

36. Lal, S., de la Vega, C.E., Sourkes, T.L., and Friesen, H.G. (1973):
    J. Clin. Endocr. Metab., 37: 719-724.
37. Lal, S., de la Vega, C.E., Garelis, E., and Sourkes, T.L. (1973):
    Psychiat. Neurol. Neurochirurg., 76: 113-117.
38. Lal, S., Aronoff, A., Garelis, E., Sourkes, T.L., Young, S.N., and
    de la Vega, C.E. (1974): Clin. Neurol. Neurosurg., 77: 142-154.
39. Lal, S., Martin, J.B., de la Vega, C.E., and Friesen, H.G. (1975):
    Clin. Endocrinol., 4: 277-285.
40. Lal, S., Allen, J., Etienne, P., Sourkes, T.L., and Humphreys, P.
    (1976): Clin. Neurol. Neurosurg., 79: 66-69.
41. Lal, S., Guyda, H., and Bikadoroff, S. (1977): J. Clin. Endocr.
    Metab., 44: 766-770.
42. Lal, S., Nair, N.P.V., and Guyda, H. (1978): Acta Psychiat., Scand.,
    57: 91-96.
43. Lal, S., Nair, N.P.V., Cervantes, P., Pulman, J., and Guyda, H.
    (1979): Acta Psychiat., Scand., 59: 173-179.
44. Lal, S., Mendis, T., Cervantes, P., Guyda, H., and de Rivera, J.L.
    (1979): Neuropsychobiology, 5: 327-331.
45. Lal, S., Hoyte, K., Kiely, M.E., Sourkes, T.L., Baxter, D.W.,
    Missala, K., and Andermann, F. (1979): Adv. Neurol., 24: 335-351.
46. Lal, S., Cervantes, P., and Nair, N.P.V. (1980): Psychiat. J.
    Univ. Ottawa, 5: 160-161.
47. Lal, S., Nair, N.P.V., Cervantes, P., and Guyda, H. (1980):
    Proceedingf of XI International Congress of the International
    Society of Psychoneuroendocrinology (in press), Elsevier-North
    Holland Biomedical Press, Amsterdam.
48. Lal, S., Etienne, P., Thavundayil, J., Nair, N.P.V., Collier, B.,
    Rastogi, R., Guyda, H., and Schwartz, G. (in press): J. Neural
    Trans.
49. Lal, S., Thavundayil, J., Nair, N.P.V., Etienne, P., Rastogi, R.,
    Schwartz, G., Pulman, J., and Guyda, H. (in press): J. Neural
    Trans.
50. Lal, S., Young, S.N., Cervantes, P., and Guyda, H. (1980): (in
    press), Pharmacopsychiatry.
51. Le, T., Seeman, P., Tourtellotte, W.W., Farley, I.J., and
    Hornykeiwicz, O. (1978): Nature, 274: 897-900.
52. Levy, C.H., Carlson, H.E., Sowers, J.R., Goodlett, R.E.,
    Tourtellotte, W.W., and Hershman, J.M. (1979): Life Sci., 24:
    743-750.
53. Maany, I., Frazer, A., and Mendels, J. (1975): J. Clin. Endocr.
    Metab., 40: 162-163.
54. Maany, I., Mendels, J., Frazer, A., Brunswick, D. (1979): Neuro-
    psychobiology, 5: 282-289.
55. Martin, J.B., Lal, S., Tolis, G., and Friesen, H.G. (1974): J.
    Clin. Endocr. Metab., 39: 180-182.
56. Morgan, M.Y., Jakobovits, A.W., James, I.M., and Sherlock, S.
    (1980): Gastroenterology, 78: 663-670.
57. Müller, E.E., Parati, E.A., Cocchi, D., Zanardi, P., and Caraceni,
    T. (1979): Adv. Neurol., 23: 319-334.
58. Nair, N.P.V., Lal, S., Cervantes, P., Yassa, R., and Guyda, H.
    (1979): Neuropsychobiology, 5: 136-142.
59. Nair, N.P.V., Lal, S., and Guyda, H. (1980): Pharmacol. Biochem.
    Behav. (in press).
60. Nilsson, K.O. (1975): Acta Endocrinol., 80: 230-236.

61. Pandey, G.N., Garver, D.L., Hengeveld, C., Erickson, S., Gosenfeld, L., and Davis, J. (1977): Am. J. Psychiat., 134: 518-522.
62. Quesney, L.F., Andermann, F., Lal, S., and Prelevic, S. (1980): Neurology (in press).
63. Reader, T.A., Champlain, J., and Jasper, H. (1976): Brain Res., 111: 95-108.
64. Rotrosen, J., Angrist, B., Gershon, S., Paquin, J., Branchey, L., Oleshansky, M., Halpern, F., and Sachar, E.J. (1979): Brit. J. Psychiat., 135: 444-456.
65. Schlatter, E.K.E. (1966): Quebec Psychopharmacology Association Meeting, 8 February, Montreal.
66. Schlatter, E.K.E., and Lal, S. (1972): Quart. J. Stud. Alc., 33: 430-436.
67. Schwab, R.S., Amador, L.V., and Lettvin, J.Y. (1951): Trans. Amer. Neurol. Assoc., 76: 251-253.
68. Smith, R.C., Tamminga, C.A., Haraszti, J., Pandey, G.N., and Davis, J.M. (1977): Am. J. Psychiat., 134: 763-768.
69. Sourkes, T.L., and Lal, S. (1975): Adv. Neurochem., 1: 247-299.
70. Strian, F., Micheler, E., and Benkert, O. (1972): Pharmacopsychiatry, 5: 198-205.
71. Struppler, A., and von Uexküll, T. (1953): Zeitschr. Klin. Med., 152: 46-57.
72. Symes, A.L., Lal, S., and Sourkes, T.L. (1976): Arch. Int. Pharmacodyn. Ther., 223: 260-264.
73. Symes, A.L., Lal, S., Young, S.N., Tsang, D., and Sourkes, T.L. (1977): Europ. J. Pharmacol., 43: 173-179.
74. Tamminga, C.A., Smith, R.C., Frohman, L.A., and Davis, J.M. (1977): Arch. Gen. Psychiat., 34: 1199-1203.
75. Tamminga, C.A., Schaffer, M.H., Smith, R.C., and Davis, J.M. (1978): Science, 200: 567-568.
76. Tarsy, D., and Baldessarini, R.J. (1977): Nature, 245: 262.
77. Tesarová, O. (1972): Pharmacopsychiatry, 5: 13-19.
78. Tolis, G., Lal, S., and Pinter, E. (1975): Symposium of the International Society of Psychoendocrinology, Visegrad, Publishing House of the Hungarian Academy of Sciences, pp. 335-339.
79. Tolosa, E.S. (1974): J. Amer. Med. Assoc., 229: 1579-1580.
80. Tolosa, E.S., and Sparber, S.B. (1974): Life Sci., 18: 1371-1380.
81. Tolosa, E.S. (1978): Arch. Neurol., 35: 459-462.
82. Tsang, D., and Lal, S. (1977): Canad. J. Physiol. Pharmacol., 55: 1263-1269.
83. Tufik, S., Lindsey, C.J., and Carlini, E.A. (1978): Pharmacology, 16: 98-105.
84. Van Tyle, W.K., Burkman, A.M. (1971): J. Pharm. Sci., 60: 1736-1738.
85. Van Woert, M.H., and Sethy, V.H. (1975): Neurology, 25: 135-140.
86. Vernier, V.G., and Unna, K.R. (1951): J. Pharm. Exp. Ther., 103: 365.
87. Von Uexküll, T. (1953): Verhandl. Deutsch Gesellsch. Inn. Med. Kong., 59: 104-107.
88. Young, S.N., Lal, S., Feldmuller, F., Sourkes, T.L., Ford, R.M., Kiely, M., and Martin, J.B. (1976): J. Neurol. Neurosurg. Psychiat., 39: 61-65.

Apomorphine and Other Dopaminomimetics,
Vol. 2: Clinical Pharmacology, edited by
G. U. Corsini and G. L. Gessa, Raven Press,
New York © 1981.

Behavioural Effects of Apomorphine in Man: Dopamine Receptor Implications

G. U. Corsini, M. P. Piccardi, A. Bocchetta, F. Bernardi, and M. Del Zompo

Institute of Clinical Pharmacology, University of Cagliari, 09100 Cagliari, Italy

Apomorphine has been used clinically for almost a century mainly to induce vomiting and, for this purpose is still used,although less frequently, today. Since 1967 when Ernst described its specific dopaminomimetic properties (24),the experimental use of apomorphine has greatly increased. Unlike dopamine (DA),when parenterally administered, apomorphine can easily cross the blood brain barrier and thus exert central effects. In rats, the behavioural effects of apomorphine have been shown to be dose-related : high doses (over 100 µg/kg subcutaneously) induce stereotipies and hypermotility that are reported to be due to the stimulation of DA receptors in the caudate nucleus and nucleus accumbens (24).These receptors are fundamental in controlling posture and motility and are considered as "classic" post-synaptic DA receptors. On the other hand, low doses of apomorphine (less than 50 µg/kg) induce inhibitory behaviour such as sedation (20) that seems to be due to the stimulation of a different type of DA receptors, defined "autoreceptors" or "pre-synaptic" or "self-inhibitory" receptors (6,32,21).

Behavioural effects in man.

Because of its strong emetic and hypotensive action, apomorphine is administered only in low doses to man, in whom it induces typical effects that can be chronologically divided into three distinct phases (Table 1).Vegetative changes such as hyper-salivation, bradicardia,

rhinorrhea, sweating, lacrimation, palpebral ptosis, pallor, arterial
hypotension and, when the dose is high enough, nausea and vomiting occur
5 to 10 minutes after its administration. 10 to 20 minutes after, subjects show yawning,sedation, and sometimes sound sleep (25,10).During
this phase (phase of the vigilance changes),repeated yawning is almost
constantly present and sedation which is partially a consequence of the
first phase,also shows typical features of psycho-motor inhibition.Sleep
appears more frequently in young subjects and is variable in onset and
duration (10).Sleep is rarely deep but more often limited to stages 1
and 2 and lacks completely of REM phases (8).However,spontaneous awake-
ning is pleasant and the subject refers a state of wellbeing. If the subject is not asleep,within 20 minutes after apomorphine administration,he
feels sad and miserable, displaying light headed feeling and tiredness.
This is the third phase of psychic changes that lasts 45-60 mins.(11).

TABLE 1

APOMORPHINE-INDUCED BEHAVIOURAL EFFECTS
IN MAN

1st Phase: Vegetative changes (5 to 10 mins)	Hypersalivation, Bradicardia, Rhinorrhea, Sweating, Lacrimation, Palpebral ptosis, Pallor, Hypo-tension, Nausea, Vomiting.
2nd Phase: Vigilance changes (10 to 20 mins)	Yawning, Sedation, Sleepiness, Sleep.
3rd Phase: Psychic changes (up to 50 mins)	Light headed feeling, Sadness, Tiredness.

It is obviously difficult to compare the above described symptomatology
obtained in humans with the effects observed in animals.However, the
possibility that apomorphine in man, at the dose until now used, may
produce signs of motor activation, can be easily ruled out. On the contrary, apomorphine-induced effects in man might be more related to the
kind of animal behaviour elicited by low doses of the drug. In fact the
prevailing sign in treated subjects is represented by sedation and by a
general reduction in motor performances. Whether this effect, similarly
to rats, is due to DA receptor stimulation, may be difficult to prove,
however, the following evidence may clarify this problem.

Pretreatment with DA receptor blockers.

When a subject, before receiving apomorphine, is treated with a specific DA receptor blocker like haloperidol (15-20 µg/kg intramuscularly 30 mins before) (Tab.2), the above described apomorphine-induced symptomatology does not appear at all (10).Haloperidol pretreatment prevents all the behavioural picture usually occurring after apomorphine administration. This result further confirms that, in man, apomorphine-induced effects are mediated through a DA receptor stimulation.

On the other hand, pretreatment with sulpiride, (2mg/kg intramuscularly 30 mins. before apomorphine), which is considered to be a rather specific blocker of the second type of DA receptors, prevents almost all apomorphine-induced effects (9,10,11,12). The subject under such treatment is wide awake and shows a normal behaviour but yawns repeatedly for several minutes (Tab.2).Yawning, the only behaviour unaffected by sulpiride, but prevented by haloperidol, may be therefore mediated by the activation of DA receptors of the "classic" type.

Pretreatment with domperidone (100 µg/kg intramuscularly 60 mins. before) (Tab.2), a dopamine receptor blocker that does not enter into the brain, prevents only the first phase of apomorphine-induced changes (13). Subjects under this treatment no longer suffer from hypotension, pallor,nausea, vomiting and sedation, occasionally show sleepiness and sleep episodes and frequently complain of malaise and deep sadness.This evidence indicates that the phase of the vegetative changes and partially sedation are mediated by the stimulation of DA receptors located in peripheral tissues or in brain areas outside the blood brain barrier. These receptors may be those present in area postrema however, we cannot exclude that those DA receptors present in other organs such as kidney, pituitary and stomach may also be involved.

TABLE 2

APOMORPHINE (10 µg/kg i.m.) INDUCED BEHAVIOURAL EFFECTS IN MAN			
Pretreatment with:	Haloperidol (20 µg/kg i.m.)	Sulpiride (2 mg/kg i.m.)	Domperidone (100 µg/kg i.m.)
Vegetative changes	O	O	O
Sedation	O	O	O
Sleep	O	O	X
Yawning	O	X	X
Psychic changes	O	O	X

O Absence
X Presence

DA receptors have been identified in dog area postrema (41) and their stimulation by apomorphine is responsible for the complex phenomena related to emesis. This area (chemoreceptor trigger zone), highly permeable to drugs, is connected to the dorsal vagal nucleus whose activation may induce an overall hyperactivity of the parasympathetic nervous system (5). Pallor, hypersalivation, bradicardia, rhinorrhea, sweating and lacrimation, which are commonly vomiting-related phenomena, might be the result of parasympathetic nervous system activation via stimulation of the chemoreceptor trigger zone (CTZ) by apomorphine. However, a direct effect of the drug on gastric motility has been described (48). It has been shown that DA receptors are present in gastric tissue and their stimulation by apomorphine decreases gastric motility, resulting in marked relaxation (48). Opposite effects are elicited by DA receptor blockers which increase gastric motility thus accelerating its emptying (30,40,48), an effect commonly provoked by radiologists during X-ray examinations. Unlike other dopaminomimetic drugs, apomorphine-induced hypotension is not a centrally mediated phenomenon in man, as suggested above and demonstrated by recent evidence in dogs (4). Arterial hypotension which is usually limited to a decrement of about 20 mm Hg, when subemetic doses of apomorphine are administered, might be a consequence of parasympathetic activation. However, this effect might also be due to stimulation of DA receptors which have been identified in dog renal artery (29). In fact, possible implications of these receptors in controlling arterial pressure have also been suggested in man (1).

More difficult to evaluate and quantitate, at least in man,is the apomorphine-induced sedative effect. In fact, the lack of appropriate rating scales to define this phenomenon, and the difficulty to differentiate it from sleepiness make our findings on apomorphine-induced sedation and its prevention by domperidone, uncertain and inconclusive.However, it is evident that, in man, apomorphine induces a decrease of attention, reactivity, and motor performances that is not merely correlated to sleep. When a subject treated with apomorphine is kept under stimulation by talking to him or by compelling him to perform different tasks, he displays difficulty in paying attention, in reacting properly and in speaking fluently. On the contrary, domperidone pretreated subjects, who may show sleep episodes after apomorphine if they are not stimulated, show quite normal reactivity, speech and attention, thus suggesting that this sedative effect in man seems to be a peripherally mediated phenomenon. This conclusion however, is in contrast to that observed in rodents in which apomorphine-induced hypomotility, commonly called "sedation" is not antagonized by domperidone (Corsini - unpublished results). It is possible that a better definition of "sedation", used too generally for different behaviours both in man and animals, will help to clarify this problem.

Apomorphine-induced sleep in man was first described in 1900 by Douglas (22). However, this effect is not frequently observed in adult subjects and is dependent on the environmental conditions (10). On the

contrary, young subjects or patients during acute manic episodes or subjects under barbiturate treatment always show sound sleep after apomorphine administration (16).

Which DA receptors are responsible for sleep induction is a difficult
question to answer but one might speculate that the "self-inhibitory"
ones, by decreasing dopaminergic activity, reduce this neuronal system
known to be involved in behavioural arousal (31). Actually, since the
physiologic role of dopaminergic pathways in the control of sleep induction needs to be further elucidated both in animal and in man, all hypotheses to this regard are a matter of speculation. Another sleep-related
phenomenon that is frequently induced by apomorphine is yawning. This
behaviour, which therefore seems to be under the control of the dopaminergic activity, is also elicited by drugs that increase cholinergic
stimulation (47). However, it is noteworthy that yawning is repeatedly
induced in rats, along with stretching and penile erection, by intracere-
bral administration of ACTH and β·MSH, thus indicating a peptidergic
neuromodulation of this behaviour (26). As described above, and as reported by different authors (2,45,26), apomorphine induces, in man, subjective feelings of malaise and deep sadness. These psychological modifications are not related to apomorphine-induced nausea and vomiting. In
fact, domperidone pretreated subjects who do not complain of nausea or
vomiting, frequently show these psychological symptoms which are often
so marked as to be suggestive of mental depression. Indeed, a depressive
state, similar to "melancolia gravis" has been reported in several subjects chronically treated with apomorphine (45), however, a subsequent
study performed under blind conditions did not confirm this finding
(33). Whether or not apomorphine has a depressant effect, needs to be
properly evaluated, and the following data on the actions of apomorphine
in different pathological conditions may better elucidate this problem,
in which possible implications of DA receptors are of great importance.

Effects in some pathological conditions.

Apomorphine has been reported to improve or worsen different psychiatric and neurological conditions which are summarized in Tab.3. The
drug is of therapeutic value in some mental disturbances such as schizophrenia (43),mania (11), or schizoaffective disorders (19), and in some
hyperkinetic syndromes such as acute dystonia (28),tardive dyskinesias
(7) or Huntington's chorea (46,12). Many early clinical observations, as
well as those of the past decade are discussed elsewhere in this volume
(e.g see Neumeyer, Lal).

Apomorphine has been used extensively in the treatment of agitated,
hospitalized mental patients. Bleuler reported the usefulness of the
drug in the treatment of schizophrenia (3) and other authors described
its effectiveness in some types of delusional states (23).

In 1977 we reported that the drug, at relatively low doses, markedly reduced the entire psychotic picture in some unmedicated, active, schizophrenic and manic patients, and this effect, although short lasting, was not related to the drug-induced sedation (11). Subsequently, in a double blind study, Tamminga et al. reported its effectiveness in chronic medicated schizophrenics (43) and recently these authors described the antipsychotic properties of N-n-propylnorapomorphine, a more potent analogue of apomorphine (44).

Actually, in this volume, we refer the data obtained by re-evaluation of diagnosis, social and therapeutic outcome of those psychotic patients who showed a marked improvement from apomorphine. These data are consistent with the fact that mostly schizoaffective patients of the manic type show to be sensitive to apomorphine-induced antipsychotic action (19).

Different neurological conditions associated with muscle spasms or movement disorders were reported very early on to be improved by apomorphine (27,37). More recently however, different authors have documented the beneficial effect of apomorphine on abnormal involuntary movements in choreic patients, and have claimed that this action was independent from its sedative properties (46,12).More attention has been paid to the effect of apomorphine in Parkinson's Disease,described for the first time in 1951 (38) and subsequently re-evaluated in more extensive studies by Cotzias et al. (14,15).Apomorphine improved rigidity and akinesia but revealed to be highly effective against tremor,a property not shared by L-DOPA or other dopaminomimetic drugs.These studies however, showed that upon chronic administration of the drug,tolerance to this effect and renal failure developed, thus limitating its clinical applications. All these effects, except that on Parkinson's Disease, are unexpected for a dopaminomimetic drug and may be interpreted as being due to the stimulation of the self-inhibitory DA receptors. According to this hypothesis,the action of the drug in epilepsy may also be considered.

TABLE 3

EFFECTS OF APOMORPHINE IN SOME PATHOLOGICAL CONDITIONS	
Improvement of Schizophrenia	(Corsini,1976 – Tamminga,1977)
" of G. de la Tourette	(Tolosa,1974 – Marsden,1975)
" of Tardive Dyskinesia	(Feinberg,1975)
" of Acute Dystonia	(Gessa,1972 – Corsini,1977)
" of Huntington's Chorea	(Tolosa,1974 – Corsini,1977)
" of Parkinson's Disease	(Schwab,1951 – Cotzias,1972)
Worsening of Epilepsy	(Del Zompo,1980)

In fact, apomorphine has been shown to worsen EEG patterns of epileptic patients (18), an effect which is usually induced by neuroleptic medication (35,42). On the contrary,in line with the classical hypothesis is the effect of apomorphine in Parkinson's disease (38,14);in this illness however, DA receptors present a supersensitivity (39) so that the apomorphine response under this condition may be altered and considered absolutely peculiar.

Pretreatment with DA receptor blockers.

When apomorphine is administered to patients affected by schizophrenia or by mania, a marked improvement in mental status can often be observed during the third phase (11,43).The amelioration regards formal thought disorders, hallucinations, delusions and inappropriate and bizzarre behaviour in schizophrenic patients,whilst in manic patients euphoria and psycho-motor excitement are notably improved.If apomorphine is administered to patients pretreated with haloperidol or sulpiride, it fails to induce mental changes (Tab.4).On the contrary,domperidone pretreatment does not antagonize the antipsychotic effect of apomorphine but it prevents the vegetative modifications induced by the drug.These findings suggest that central DA receptors of the self-inhibitory type may be responsible for such effects in mental patients.

A similar interpretation may be extended to the results obtained from patients affected by Huntington's chorea.Apomorphine during the third phase, induces a dose dependent decrease of abnormal involuntary movements (46,12).Pretreatment with haloperidol or sulpiride prevents this effect. On the contrary, pretreatment with domperidone, although affecting the first phase, does not alter the therapeutic action of apomorphine(12,17)(Tab.4).These results suggest that the apomorphine-induced improvement of choreic movements is due to a central action of the drug and that it is possibly due to stimulation of self-inhibitory DA receptors.

TABLE 4

IMPROVEMENT OF SOME PATHOLOGICAL
CONDITIONS BY APOMORPHINE

Pretreatment with:	Haloperidol (20 µg/kg i.m.)	Sulpiride (2 mg/kg i.m.)	Domperidone (100 µg/kg i.m.)
Schizophrenia	O	O	X
Huntington's D.	O	O	X
Parkinson's D.	O	X	X

O Absence
X Presence

On the contrary, similar considerations cannot be applied to apomorphine-induced improvement of the neurological disturbances in patients
affected by Parkinson's disease. In fact, apomorphine at relatively low
doses is known to improve, within 5 or 10 minutes after administration,
rigidity, akynesia and tremor (14,9). Pretreatment with haloperidol antagonizes this improvement. Pretreatment with sulpiride antagonizes all
the typical effects of apomorphine but does not antagonize the improvement of the neurological symptomatology(9). This suggests that such improvement is due, not to stimulation of self-inhibitory DA receptors,
but of "classic" post-synaptic ones (not blocked by sulpiride). As expected, pretreatment of these patients with domperidone did not alter
the therapeutic action of apomorphine whilst it did however modify many
of its side effects(1st phase of the vegetative changes) (13)(Tab.4).
This result underlines the usefulness of combining a peripheral DA receptor inhibitor with dopaminomimetic drugs in order to prevent most of the
side effects of the latter.

It is evident from all these data that further investigations are
needed in order to ascertain, confirm and define the antipsychotic action of apomorphine. The difficulty in performing double blind studies
with this drug, arises from the fact that apomorphine elicits multiple
side effects. To circumvent this problem, it may be necessary to use an
"active" placebo as a control treatment, that might simulate most of the
behavioural changes usually elicited by apomorphine. Among these changes
sedation is the most disturbing effect that may give rise to false positive evaluations especially in agitated patients, such as manics, whose
decrease in motor activity, induced by apomorphine, notably improves the
entire pathological feature, but does not necessarily imply that the
drug exerts an antipsychotic effect. This is the reason why a better evaluation of the antipsychotic effect of apomorphine has been performed on
subjects showing marked formal thought disorders with multiple delusions and hallucinations. In fact, in these patients, despite the sedation induced by apomorphine, a complete disappearance of their symptoms,
along with a conceptual and intellectual re-organization was easily evaluated. All these problems may account for the discrepancy actually present in the literature concerning the type of patients improved by apomorphine administration. As reported above, we found that patients with
schizoaffective disorders of manic type, rather than pure schizophrenics, were positively affected by apomorphine (19). This finding may
suggest that the drug acts primarily as an antimanic agent, a property
which may be connected to its depressant activity as shown in normal subjects (phase of psychic changes).The antipsychotic action of apomorphine
might be seen in light of the "dopaminergic hypothesis" of schizophrenia
and mania. Apomorphine, by stimulating self-inhibitory DA receptors, decreases brain dopaminergic activity, resulting in the same final effect
as that induced by neuroleptic drugs.

A similar mechanism of action may explain the apomorphine-induced improvement of abnormal involuntary movements in Huntington's disease. It

is known that neuroleptic medication notably improves choreic movements.
On the contrary, L-DOPA treatment worsens these symptoms in Huntingtonian patients or may induce abnormal movements in non choreic subjects.
This evidence indicates that the dopaminergic system has a key role in
the regulation of abnormal movements. Differently, the action of apomorphine in Parkinson's disease cannot be considered the result of a decrease of dopaminergic activity, since we would expect a worsening of the
symptoms, but, according to classic views, it is a consequence of dopaminergic activation due to a direct stimulation of post-synaptic DA receptors which are not only unimpaired by the disease, but are even hyper-
sensitive to the neurotransmitter (39).

CONCLUSION

Behavioural changes induced by apomorphine administration in man are,
in comparison to those elicited in rodents, more complex and various. In
fact, in rodents, the only observable behaviour is the hypo or the hypermotility and stereotipies in relation to dosages; in man, on the contrary, as shown in the present article, vegetative, motor and psychic
modifications occur after apomorphine administration. This more complex
feature provides useful indications, as this drug may act at various sites on different tissues.

However, all the data presented indicate that this drug acts with the
same mechanism at different sites, that is a stimulation of DA receptors which are known to be located in various organs other than brain.
The exact location and function of these DA receptors which can be activated by apomorphine is still matter for investigation, however, at least in brain, the data presented above suggest the possibility that apomorphine may act primarily on the "self-inhibitory" DA receptors. The
only exception is represented by Parkinson's Disease, in which a biochemical modification of DA receptors possibly modify their sensitivity
to apomorphine. The concept of "self-inhibitory" DA receptors is still
rather obscure: their existence is now strongly suggested by much experimental evidence but their anatomical and biochemical identification is
unclear. These receptors might be identified with "autoreceptors" present on the dopaminergic cell soma or with "presynaptic" receptors located, as shown in peripheral neurons, at the presynaptic level either on
noradrenergic or dopaminergic nerve terminals. Further, these receptors
may be identified with the "D_2" receptors which are sensitive to nanomo-
lar concentrations of apomorphine and are blocked specifically by substituted benzamides such as sulpiride or metoclopramide. However the "D_2"
receptor concept is based on only biochemical evidence which until now
did not undergo behavioural correlations.

Although the clinical usefulness of apomorphine is limited by a short
lasting action and by other limiting effects such as the induction of

tolerance, this drug proved to be a valuable tool in studying the dopaminergic system in man under physiological and pathological conditions. In fact, the use of apomorphine provided evidence for the presence of a different kind of DA receptor in human CNS and has suggested that a selective stimulation of such receptors may be of therapeutic value in some neurological and psychiatric diseases.

On this rational basis, different dopaminomimetic compounds have been practically used and found to be of therapeutic value in the same pathological conditions as those improved by apomorphine. This volume deals with these clinical trials and shows the advantages and limitations of such therapeutic approach.New dopaminomimetics with a high specificity for one or another type of DA receptor, as described in the first volume dealing with the pharmacology of apomorphine, should reveal to be of important therapeutic value.

REFERENCES

1). Agnati,L.F.,Bernardi,P.,Benfenati,F.,Adani,C.,Capelli,M.,Cocchi, V.,Zini,I.,Fresia,P.: This volume

2). Angrist,B.,Thompson,H.,Shopsin,B.,Gershon,S.(1975): Psychopharmacologia,44: 273-280.

3). Bleuler,E.(1911):Dementia praecox or the group of schizophrenias, translated by J.Zinkin and N.D.C.Lewis, pp.486,Int.Univ.Press,N.Y. 1950.

4). Bogaert,M.G.,Buylaert,W.A.,Willems,J.L.(1978):Br.J.Pharmacol.,63: 481-484.

5). Borison,H.L.(1974):Life Sci.,14: 1807-1817.

6). Carlsson,A.(1975):In:Pre- and Post-synaptic receptors, edited by E.Usdin and W.E.Bunney Jr, pp.49-65.Marcel Dekker,New York.

7). Carroll,B.J.,Curtis,G.L.,Kohmen,E.(1977): Am.J.Psychiat.,134: 785-789.

8). Cianchetti,C.,Masala,C.,Corsini,G.U.,Mangoni,A.,Gessa,G.L.(1979): Life Sci.,23: 403-408.

9). Corsini,G.U.,Del Zompo,M.,Cianchetti,C.,Mangoni,A.,Gessa,G.L. (1976): Psychopharmacologia, 47: 169-173.

10). Corsini,G.U.,Del Zompo,M.,Manconi,S.,Piccardi,M.P.,Onali,P.L., Mangoni,A.,Gessa;G.L.(1977): Life Sci.,20: 1613-1618.

11). Corsini,G.U.,Del Zompo,M.,Manconi,S.,Cianchetti,C.,Mangoni,A, Gessa,G.L.(1977):In: Advances in Biochemical Psychopharmacology, edited by E.Costa and G.L.Gessa,16:pp.645-648.Raven Press,New York

12). Corsini,G.U.,Onali,P.L.,Masala,C.,Cianchetti,C.,Mangoni,A.,Gessa, G.L.(1978): Arch.Neurol.,35: 27-30.

13). Corsini,G.U.,Del Zompo,M.,Gessa,G.L.,Mangoni,A.(1979): Lancet, 8123: 954-956.

14). Cotzias,G.C.,Papavasiliou,P.,Fehling,C.,Kaufman,B.,Mena,I.(1970): New Engl.J.Med., 282: 31-33.

15). Cotzias,G.C.,Papavasiliou,P.S.,Tolosa,E.S.,Mendez,J.S.,Bell-Midura M.(1976): New Engl.J.Med., 294: 567-572.

16). Del Zompo,M.,Piccardi,M.P.,Tocco,F.,Scano,M.L.,Corsini,G.U.(1979): Riv.Farm.Ter., 10: 61-72.

17). Del Zompo,M.,Burrai,C.,Tocco,F.,Piccardi,M.P.,Corsini,G.U.(1980): Pharmacology, (in publication).

18). Del Zompo,M.,Tocco,F.,Marrosu,F.,Passino,N.,Corsini,G.U.(1980): Arch.Neurol., (submitted for publication).

19). Del Zompo,M.,Pitzalis,G.F.,Burrai,C.,Tocco,F.,Corsini,G.U.:This volume.

20). Di Chiara,G.,Porceddu,M.L.,Fratta,W.,Gessa,G.L.(1977): Nature,277: 93-96.

21). Di Chiara,G.,Corsini,G.U.,Mereu,G.P.,Gessa,G.L.,Tissari,A.(1978): In: Advances in Biochemical Psychopharmacology, edited by P.J.Roberts et al.,19:pp.275-292,Raven Press,New York.

22). Douglas,C.J.(1900): Merck's Arch.,2: 212-213.

23). Douglas,C.J.(1908): Alien.Neurol.St.Louis.,29: 191-192.

24). Ernst,A.M.(1967): Psychopharmacology, 10: 316-323.

25). Feldman,F.,Susselman,S.S.,Barrera,S.E.(1945): Am.J.Psychiat.,102 : 403.

26). Ferrari,W.,Gessa,G.L.,Vargiu,L.(1963): Annals N.Y.Acad.Sci.,104: 330-343.

27). Gee,S.(1869): Tr.Clin.Soc.Lond., 2: 166-169.

28). Gessa,R.,Tagliamonte,A.,Gessa,G.L.(1972): Lancet,ii: 981-982.

29). Goldberg,L.I.,Volkman,P.H.,Kohli,J.D.,Kotake,A.N.(1977): In:Advances in Biochemical Psychopharmacology, edited by E.Costa and G.L.

Gessa,16:pp.251-256.Raven Press,New York.

30). Jacoby,H.I.,Brodie,D.A.(1967): Gastroenterology,52: 676-684.

31). Jones,B.E.,Bobillier,P.,Pin,C.,Jouvet,M.(1973): Brain Res., 58: 157-177.

32). Kebabian,J.W.,Calne,D.B.(1979): Nature,277: 93-96.

33). Lal,S.,De La Vega,C.E.(1975): J.Neurol Neurosurg.Psychiat., 38: 722-726.

34). Lal,S.:This volume.

35). Lyberi,G.,Last,S.L.(1956): Electroenceph.Clin.Neurophysiol., 8: 711-712.

36). Neumeyer,J.L.,Lal,S.,Baldessarini,R.J.: This volume.

37). Pierce,F.M.(1870): Brit.Med.J., 1:204.

38). Schwab,R.S.,Amador,L.V.,Lettvin,J.Y.(1951): Trans.Amer.Neurol.Ass. 76: 251-253.

39). Seeman,P.,Lee,T.,Rasput,A.,Farley,I.J.,Hornykiewicz,O.(1978): Nature, 273: 59-61.

40). Stadaas,J.O.,Aune,S. (1972): Scand.J.Gastroenterol., 7: 17-21.

41). Stefanini,E.,Clement-Cormier,Y.: This volume.

42). Stewart,L.F.(1957): Electroenceph.Clin.Neurophysiol., 9: 427-440.

43). Tamminga,C.A.,Schaffer,M.H.,Smith,R.C.,Davis,J.M.(1978): Science, 200,4341: 567-568.

44). Tamminga,C.A.,Defraites,E.G.,Gotts,M.A.,Chase,T.N.: This volume.

45). Tesarova,O.(1972): Pharmacopsychiatry.,5: 13-19.

46). Tolosa,E.S.,Sparber,S.B.(1974): Life Sci., 15: 1371-1380.

47). Urba-Holmgren,R.,Gonzales,R.M.,Holmgren,B.(1977): Nature, 267: 261-262.

48). Van Nueten,J.M.,Ennis,C.,Helsen,L.,Laduron,P.M.,Janssen,P.A.J. (1978): Life Sci., 23: 453-458.

Apomorphine and Other Dopaminomimetics,
Vol. 2: Clinical Pharmacology, edited by
G. U. Corsini and G. L. Gessa, Raven Press,
New York © 1981.

Dopamine Agonists in Reflex Epilepsy

Brian Meldrum and Gill Anlezark

Department of Neurology, Institute of Psychiatry, London SE5 8AF, United Kingdom

The most widely used classifications of epilepsy depend on EEG findings and the clinical pattern of the seizures, and not on the structural or biochemical basis of the disorder. However, seizure phenomena that are induced by specific stimuli or depend on a reflex mechanism can be differentiated from non-reflex epilepsy in terms of various physiological and pharmacological features. Forms of reflex epilepsy are readily modified by agents acting on monoaminergic transmission (13,23). This chapter is concerned with the effects of dopamine agonists.

The principal forms of reflex epilepsy are listed in Table 1. The specificity of the triggering stimulus is uncertain in the gerbil. Otherwise the genetic syndromes are characertised by a highly specific, monomodal stimulus. However, there is clear experimental evidence in mice and baboons that the full expression of the epileptic response is dependent on somatosensory inputs (from the vibrissae and somatic musculature in the mouse, from perioribital skin and muscles in the baboon).

TABLE 1. Principal forms of reflex epilepsy

	In Animals Species	Stimulus	In Man Epilepsy	Stimulus
Genetic				
	DBA/2 mice	sound	photosensitive	visual
	Gerbils Meriones ung.	?stress, novelty	"photoconvulsive"	pattern or flash
	Domestic hen Gallus dom.	flash		
	Baboon Papio papio	flash		
Acquired				
	Focal motor Rat (cobalt) Monkey (alumina)	somatic	focal motor myoclonus (action, posthypoxic, hyperosmolar)	somatosensory afferent movement (initiation) sensory (skin)

A role for muscle afferents in initiating and arresting cortical focal discharges has been demonstrated neurophysiologically in the monkey with chronic alumina oxide lesions.

In man the triggering or arrest of focal motor seizures by peripheral sensory stimulation or by active or passive limb movement was described by Jackson and Gowers in the nineteenth century, and is sometimes categorised as "movement epilepsy" (8,27). Similar triggering by sensory inputs or by the initiation of movement is familiar in several types of myoclonus (21). A role for somatic afferents in human photosensitive epilepsy has not been rigorously established.

AUDIOGENIC SEIZURES IN MICE

DBA/2 mice, 18-28 days of age, show a fixed sequence of seizure phenomena in response to a loud sound (wild running; clonic jerks, tonic extension; respiratory arrest). We have previously described prevention of the later stages of this response by dopamine agonists (see Table 2). The most potent agent is (-)N-n-propyl norapomorphine (26). We have recently evaluated a related tri-hydroxy aporphine, (-)2,10,11-trihydroxy-N-propylnoraporphine, (-)TNPA, (synthesised and supplied by Professor J. Neumeyer, see this volume). When administered intraperitoneally in the mouse this compound has a prolonged sedative action. In terms of ED_{50} for the clonic phase of the seizure response, it is equipotent with apomorphine (tested 30 minutes after drug administration).

TABLE 2. Dopamine agonists and audiogenic seizures in DBA/2 mice

Drug	Interval (minutes)	Clonic ED_{50} mg/kg	Reference
Apomorphine	20	0.7	(3)
(-)N-n-propylnor apomorphine	30	0.075	(6)
(-)TNPA	30	0.72	-
Ergocornine	45	1.1	(5)
Bromocryptine	60	5.0	(5)
LSD 25	30	9.3	(5)
Ergometrine	30	9.7	(2)

HANDLING SEIZURES IN GERBILS

Seizures precipitated by handling, "stress" or novelty in susceptible strains of Meriones unguiculatus are susceptible to many extraneous influences making evaluation of drug effects aleatory. A protective effect of apomorphine, 1 mg/kg was originally reported (10). In a more recent study protection was found only after apomorphine, 16 mg/kg (31).

PHOTOSENSITIVE EPILEPSY IN THE BABOON

Dopamine agonists protect against the paroxysmal EEG and myoclonic responses to photic stimulation in Papio papio (Table 3). In this model of epilepsy seizure responses are potently modified by drugs acting on serotoninergic transmission (24). The relatively greater potency of LSD 25 and ergometrine in the baboon compared with the mouse are thus probably attributable to effects on serotoninergic rather than dopaminergic transmission.

(-)TNPA, 0.02 mg/kg, produced a mild sedative effect but did not modify myoclonic responses to photic stimulation. However, complete protection was seen for 3-7 hours after (-)TNPA, 0.5 and 2.5 mg/kg, given intravenously. These doses were also followed by pupil dilatation, yawning, slowing of EEG background rhythms, and at the highest dose, by excess salivation and piloerection.

TABLE 3. Abolition of myoclonic responses to photic-stimulation in the baboon, Papio papio

Drug	Minimal dose mg/kg	Duration of protection (minutes)	Reference
Apomorphine	0.5	30-45	(23)
(-)NPA	0.2	180	(6)
(-)TNPA	0.5	180-300	-
Ergocornine	1.0	30-60	(4)
Ergometrine	1.0	150	(4)
LSD 25	0.1	45-60	(4)
Bromocryptine	>4	-	(4)

FOCAL MOTOR SEIZURES IN THE RAT

Focal spikes induced in the motor cortex of the rat by the chronic implantation of a cobalt-gelatine pellet are inhibited by apomorphine, 0.5-2 mg/kg, intraperitoneally, or by lisuride, 0.1-0.5 mg/kg, i.p.(12). Bromocryptine, 10 or 20 mg/kg, is protective (after latent periods of 3-4 hours or 1-2 hours, respectively). Bilateral focal injections of dopamine, 25 µg in 2 µl, or apomorphine, 60 µg in the striatum also block the EEG spike activity.

OTHER ANIMAL MODELS OF EPILEPSY

The myoclonic jumping behaviour induced in guinea pigs by the injection of high doses of L-5-hydroxytryptophan is stimulus-sensitive and can be blocked by dopamine agonists, such as apomorphine, 0.5 mg/kg, L-dopa, 400 mg/kg (+ carbidopa); or lergotrile mesylate, 50 mg/kg (34,35).

Protection is not seen following dopamine agonists when seizures are induced by convulsant drugs, in rodents or baboons. Indeed, pentylenetetrazol seizures in rats are exacerbated by apomorphine (33). In baboons pretreated with a subconvulsant dose of allylglycine, the administration of apomorphine, 1 mg/kg, or ergocornine, 1 mg/kg, leads to the occurrence of generalised seizures (4,23).

In electroshock seizures in rodents dopamine agonists produce effects that vary according to the species employed and the experimental methodology (20).

Flash-evoked after discharges in the rat cortex, which, like pentylenetetrazol seizures have been proposed as a model for absence seizures or petit mal, are not modified by apomorphine, 0.2-7.5 mg/kg (15).

Apomorphine, 10 mg/kg, given daily before amygdaloid stimulation, does not influence the development of kindled seizure responses in the rat (7).

PHOTOSENSITIVE EPILEPSY IN MAN

A definite protective effect of low doses of apomorphine has recently been observed in patients with photosensitive primary cortical reticular epilepsy (29). Brief stroboscopic stimulation was used to induce a photoconvulsive response on the EEG at intervals of 1.5-3 minutes. These responses were no longer seen 15 minutes after apomorphine, 1.2-1.5 mg subcutaneously. They remained absent for approximately 45 minutes. Only a third of the patients experienced nausea or vomiting and this was an earlier and much less sustained effect than blockade of the photoconvulsive response.

REFLEX MYOCLONUS IN MAN

Stimulus-sensitive myoclonus may occur in patients with or without other signs of epilepsy. Its pathological basis includes post-anoxic brain damage (Lance-Adams syndrome), various degenerative disorders, and metabolic/osmotic stresses such as uraemia and disorders of sodium balance. The reflex trigger may be either spontaneous movement ("action" or "intention" myoclonus) or external stimulation ("sensory myoclonus"). Electrophysiologically two forms can be distinguished:- cortical reflex myoclonus and reticular reflex myoclonus (21).

Lhermitte and colleagues (17) described a powerful therapeutic effect of chronic L-dopa (up to 2.5 g daily, orally) or of L-dopa acutely plus an inhibitor of peripheral dopa-decarboxylase, in a case of post-anoxic myoclonus. Subsequently an equivocal effect of apomorphine, 0.5 mg, s.c., in action myocolous has been reported (33). However, there is a clear need for further studies of reflex myocolous that take into account the varying aetiological groups and physiological mechanisms.

OTHER TYPES OF EPILEPSY IN MAN

A preliminary study of the effects of low doses of apomorphine in patients with various types of seizures, including primary generalised (absences) and partial seizures with elementary and complex symptomatology (focal motor and temporal lobe seizures) has failed to show any protective action in these patients (11).

DOPAMINE ANTAGONISTS IN EPILEPTIC SYNDROMES

In the principal animal models discussed (DBA/2 mice, photosensitive baboons, cobalt foci in rats) the protective effects of apomorphine can be antagonised by appropriate doses of phenothiazines or other dopamine antagonists (5,12,23). Administration of the dopamine antagonists alone enhances the incidence of spontaneous cortical EEG spike discharges (e.g. haloperidol, 0.6-1.2 mg/kg in the baboon; pimozide, 1 mg/kg i.p., in the rat) (12,23). The incidence of photically-induced spike and wave discharges in the baboon EEG is greatly enhanced by haloperidol, although the incidence of myoclonic responses is little changed (23).

In other animal models of epilepsy enhancement, depression or no change in seizure threshold is reported depending on dose and model. High doses of chlorpromazine are protective in several models (e.g. chlorpromazine has an ED_{50} of 4.4 mg/kg against pentylenetetrazol, and of 64 mg/kg against maximal electroshock seizures in the mouse)(16). Effects of high doses of neuroleptics do not provide any precise information about the role of dopamine in these forms of epilepsy. However, they are in strong contrast with drugs blocking GABA-ergic transmission which invariably induce generalised seizures (22). Indeed it appears likely that at the cellular level dopamine agonists depend on the integrity of other inhibitory systems in order for their protective effect to be manifest. Thus when inhibitory processes are impaired by pentylenetetrazol or allyglycine apomorphine becomes proconvulsant (23,32).

ANATOMICAL SITE OF ACTION OF DOPAMINE AGONISTS

An action of apomorphine and other dopamine agonists on the nigro-striatal, meso-limbic or meso-cortical dopaminergic systems could provide a unified explanation for the effects seen in all types of reflex epilepsy. However, an action at the retinal level has to be considered in the case of photosensitive epilepsy. Thus changes in the metabolic activity in the superior colliculus of the rat following apomorphine (as shown by the ^{14}C-deoxyglucose technique) are dependent on an intact retina (19). The same technique (18) also demonstrates changes in metabolic activity following systemic apomorphine in regions not receiving a dopaminergic input (e.g. the cerebellum). Thus indirect means of modulating seizure threshold may be involved.

However, the following observations support a primary action on the nigro-striatal and meso-cortical dopaminergic systems:-

1) Direct intrastriatal injections of DA agonists block focal cortical spikes in the rat (12). Upward diffusion of the agonists into the cortex was not excluded by the technique employed.

2) Lesions of the caudate exacerbate audiogenic seizures in the rat (14).

3) Electrical stimulation of the caudate at low frequency can diminish focal cortical spiking due to cobalt in the cat (29).

4) Imbalance between dopaminergic and cholinergic activity employed within the striatum can produce epileptiform phenomena (9).

5) Activity within the meso-cortical dopamine system is apparently reduced by rhythmic visual stimulation (30). Thus dopamine agonists could be restoring an intracortical inhibitory tone that may be deficient during sensory stimulation.

6) Electrophysiological studies indicate that striatal units play an important role in integrating sensory inputs (visual and proprioceptive) with ongoing movements (1). They also show that an interaction between afferent activity and motor output is crucial to the development of later stages of reflexly evoked epileptic phenomena (25).

CONCLUSION

Dopamine agonists block the reflex induction of a variety of seizure phenomena. This finding has yet to find an application in therapy. Newer dopamine agonists or a combination of apomorphine with an antagonist that blocks nausea and autonomic effects (such as domperidone) might be useful in some forms of myoclonus and photosensitive epilepsy. The finding suggests new experimental approaches to understanding the interaction between sensory inputs and motor output in the basal ganglia and cortex.

ACKNOWLEDGEMENT

We thank The Wellcome Trust and the Medical Research Council for financial support.

REFERENCES

1. Anderson,R.J., Aldridge,J.W., and Murphy,J.T.(1979): Brain Res., 173:489-501.
2. Anlezark,G.M., Horton,R.W., and Meldrum,B.S.(1978): Biochem. Pharmacol., 27:2821-2828.
3. Anlezark,G.M., and Meldrum,B.S.(1975): Brit.J.Pharmacol., 53:419-421.
4. Anlezark,G.M., and Meldrum,B.S.(1978): Psychopharmacol., 57:57-62.
5. Anlezark,G., Pycock,C., and Meldrum,B.S.(1976): Eur.J.Pharmacol., 37:295-302.
6. Ashton,C., Anlezark,G., and Meldrum,B.S.(1976): Eur.J.Pharmacol., 39:399-401.
7. Callaghan,D.A., and Schwark,W.S.(1979): Neuropharmacol., 18:541-545.
8. Chauvel,P., Louvel,J., and Lamarche,M.(1978): Electroenceph.clin. Neurophysiol., 45:309-318.
9. Cools,A.R., Hendriks,G., and Korten,J. (1975): J.Neural Transmission, 36:91-105.
10. Cox,B., and Lomax,P.(1976): Pharmacol.Biochem.Behav., 4:263-267.
11. Del Zompo,M., Marrosu,F., Tocco,F., Passinu,N., and Corsini,G.U. (1981): Arch.Neurol. (submitted).
12. Farjo,I.B., and McQueen,J.K.(1979): Brit.J.Pharmacol., 67:353-360.
13. Horton,R., Anlezark,G., and Medlrum,B.(1980): J.Pharmacol.exp. Therap., 214:437-440.
14. Kesner,R.P.(1966): Exp.Neurol., 15:192-205.
15. King,G.A., and Burnham,W.M.(1980): Psychopharmacol., 69:281-285.
16. Krall,R.L., Penry,J.K., White,B.G., Kupferberg,H.J., and Swinyard, E.A.(1978): Epilepsia, 19:409-428.
17. Lhermitte,F., Marteau,R., and Degos,C.F.(1972): Rev.Neurol., 126: 107-114.
18. McCulloch,J., Savaki,H.E., McCulloch,M.C., and Sokoloff,L.(1979): Nature, 282:303-305.
19. McCulloch,J., Savaki,H.E., McCulloch,M.C., and Sokoloff,L.(1980): Science, 207:313-315.
20. McKenzie,G.M., and Soroko,F.E. (1972): J.Pharm.Pharmacol., 24: 686-701.
21. Marsden,C.D.(1980): Research and clinical forums, 2:31-45.
22. Meldrum,B.S.(1979): In: GABA-Neurotransmitters, edited by P.Krogsgaard-Larsen, J.Scheel-Krüger, and H.Kofod, pp.390-405. Munksgaard, Copenhagen.
23. Meldrum,B.S., Anlezark,G., and Trimble,M.(1975): Eur.J.Pharmacol., 32:203-215.
24. Meldrum,B.S., Anlezark,G.M., Ashton,C.G., Horton,R.W., and Sawaya, M.C.B.(1977): In: Epilepsy: Post-traumatic Epilepsy, Pharmacological Prophylaxis of Epilepsy, edited by J.Majkowski, Polish Chapter of ILEA, Warsaw, pp.139-153.
25. Menini,C.H.(1976): J.Physiol.(Paris): 71:5-44.
26. Menon,M.K., Clark,W.G., and Neumeyer,J.L.(1979): Eur.J.Pharmacol., 52:1-9.

27. Murphy,J.T., Kwan,H.C., McKay,W.A., and Wong,Y.C.(1980): Can.J. Neurol.Sci., 7:79-85.
28. Mutani,R., and Fariello,R.(1969): Brain Res., 14:749-753.
29. Quesney,L.F., Andermann,F., Lal,S., and Prelevik,S.(1980): Neurology (Minneap.), in press.
30. Reader,T.A., Champlain,J., and Jasper,H.(1976): Brain Res., 111: 95-108.
31. Schonfeld,A.R., and Glick,S.D.(1980): Neuropharmacology, 19:1009-1016.
32. Soroko,F.E., and McKenzie,G.M.(1970): Pharmacologist, 12:253.
33. Van Woert,M.H., and Sethy,V.H.(1975): Neurology, 25:135-140.
34. Volkman,P.H., Lorens,S.A., Kindel,G.H., and Ginos,J.Z.(1978): Neuropharmacol., 17:947-955.
35. Weiner,W.J., Carvey,P.M., Nausieda,P.A., and Klawans,H.L.(1979): Neurology, 29:1622-1625.

Apomorphine and Other Dopaminomimetics,
Vol. 2: Clinical Pharmacology, edited by
G. U. Corsini and G. L. Gessa, Raven Press,
New York © 1981.

Dopaminergic and Nondopaminergic Elements in Schizophrenia

B. Angrist and J. Rotrosen

Psychiatry Service, Veterans Administration Medical Center, New York, New York 10010; Department of Psychiatry, New York University School of Medicine, New York, New York 10016

The purpose of this paper is to acquaint the reader with an evolving concept regarding the etiopathogenesis of schizophrenia and to provide some data in its support.

The extensive literature suggesting both the importance of dopaminergic over-activity in schizophrenic disorders and the limitations of the dopamine hypothesis have been reviewed by Meltzer and Stahl (1976). More recently a refined view of this formulation has emerged in which a role for dopamine is related to positive, productive schizophrenic symptomatology only (Johnstone et al 1978, Crow 1980). Thus Johnstone et al (1978A) reported that the therapeutic effect of ∝ Flupenthixol was limited to positive schizophrenic symptoms, and Meltzer (1979) in a more recent review of the dopamine hypothesis, suggested that dopaminergic mechanisms may be relevant only to the "phase of acute psychosis which is present in some but not all forms of schizophrenia".

In their 1976 review Meltzer and Stahl suggested that dopaminergic over-activity in schizophrenia was "probably due to some other basic defect". The same year saw the beginning of a line of investigation suggesting that in some schizophrenic patients "the underlying process--- is a brain disease which produces multiple deficits" (Owens and Johnstone 1980).

In 1976 Johnstone et al reported ventricular dilatation in some chronic schizophrenic patients and a correlated impairment of performance on tests of cognitive function. The same group, following this line of investigation has subsequently demonstrated: (1) not only a correlation between increased ventricular size in schizophrenic patients and intellectual impairment but also a relationship between impaired cognition and negative schizophrenic symptoms "affectual flattening, retardation, poverty of speech" (Johnstone et al 1978B), (2) that negative but not positive schizophrenic symptoms predicted a poor social outcome one year after an acute episode of schizophrenic illness (Johnstone et al 1979), (3) that negative schizophrenic symptoms correlated highly significantly with poor cognitive test performance, defective ward behavior, and neurological signs in a large group of chronically institutionalized schizophrenic patients (Owens and Johnstone 1980).

Weinberger et al (1980 confirmed that some chronic schizophrenic patients showed enlarged cerebral ventricles and demonstrated that these patients showed a poorer response to neuroleptic treatment than a matched group of schizophrenic patients without ventricular enlargement. Donnelly et al (1980) subsequently demonstrated associated cognitive defects in a sample of these patients.

Recently Crow (1980) has synthesized these findings in a formulation which states:

"It seems that two syndromes can be distinguished in those diseases currently described as schizophrenic and that each may be associated with a specific pathological process. The first (the type I syndrome, equivalent to 'acute schizophrenia' and characterized by the positive symptoms - delusions, hallucinations, and thought disorder) is in some way associated with a change in dopaminergic transmission; the second process (the type II syndrome, equivalent to the 'defect state', and characterised by the negative symptoms - affective flattening and poverty of speech) is unrelated to dopaminergic transmission but may be associated with intellectual impairment and, perhaps, structural changes in the brain. Type I symptoms are reversible; type II symptoms, which are more difficult to define, may indicate a component of irreversibility. The former predict a potential response to neuroleptics; the latter are more closely associated with a poor long-term outcome. Episodes of type I symptoms may be followed by development of the type II syndrome, and both may be present together. Type II symptoms, however, define a group of illnesses of graver prognosis."

This formulation suggests that positive (dopaminergic) schizophrenic symptoms would be expected to increase after amphetamine and to decrease after neuroleptics, while negative (presumably brain disease related) symptoms should be less consistently changed by either intervention.

We have recently studied correlations between psychopathology change after an acute dose of amphetamine and after chronic neuroleptic treatment (Angrist et al 1980). By reanalysing these data we assessed the effect of both amphetamine and neuroleptics on positive vs negative schizophrenic symptoms and determined whether the anticipated differential effects on positive symptoms indeed occurred.

The methods used are detailed in the previous study (Angrist et al 1980). Briefly, 21 schizophrenic patients who consented to participate remained neuroleptic-free for 6-15 days or more (mean 9.9 ± 0.7 days) before receiving amphetamine. All met the research diagnostic criteria (RCD) of Spitzer et al (1978) for schizophrenia; 10 were acute or sub-acute, and 11 were chronic or subchronic.

Subjects received 0.5mg/kg of d-amphetamine orally. Unstructured clinical interviews were done before and every hour after drug was given. The BPRS was administered before and 3 h after amphetamine aministration.

After rating amphetamine-induced changes in psychopathology, subjects were treated with neuroleptics. Treatment duration ranged from as little as 7 days (in rapid responders who could be discharged) to 5-6 weeks of high dose treatment. All but one subject were able to be discharged at the end of the study. Psychopathology was rated with the BRPS weekly and at termination.

In this data analysis, changes in psychopathology after amphetamine and after neuroleptics were compared with baseline levels via paired t-tests. Comparisons of change were made for:

1. Total psychopathology.

2. Positive schizophrenic symptomatology consisting of factors 3,4, and 5 of the BPRS. These factors are No. 3 thought disturbance (conceptual disorganization, grandiosity, hallucinatory behavior, and unusual thought content); No. 4 activation (tension, mannerisms and postering, and excitement); No. 5 hostile suspiciousness (hostility, suspiciousness, and uncooperativeness).

3. Negative schizophrenic symptomatology consisted of the withdrawal-retardation factor (emotional withdrawal, motor retardation, and blunted affect; Guy 1976).

In addition, for reasons that will be discussed below, separate analyses were done for changes in the emotional withdrawal vs. the motor retardation and blunted affect items of this factor.

Our findings with respect to changes in psychopathology, for total BPRS scores and for both positive and negative schizophrenic symptoms (as defined above) are shown in Table 1. A further subdivision in the negative symptoms (emotional withdrawal vs. motor retardation and blunted affect) is also indicated.

Table 1. The effects of acute amphetamine and chronic neuroleptic treatment on two different types of schizophrenic psychopathology

	Baseline	Post-amphetamine	Postneuro-leptic treatment
Total BPRS	36.5 ± 2.05	42.8 ± 2.6 $P < 0.01$	29.8 ± 1.5 $P < 0.01$
Positive symptoms	21.3 ± 1.7	26.6 ± 2.3 $P < 0.001$	15.4 ± 1.05 $P < 0.001$
Negative symptoms	8.09 ± 0.42	8.85 ± 0.43 $P < 0.05$	7.66 ± 0.55 NS
Emotional withdrawal	3.47 ± 0.28	4.38 ± 0.33 $P < 0.001$	2.85 ± 0.26 $P < 0.02$
Motor retardation and blunted affect	4.66 ± 0.36	4.47 ± 0.37 NS	4.85 ± 0.40 NS

P refers to change from baseline (Paired t-test, two tailed)

Total psychopathology scores were signicicantly increased by amphetamine and diminished by neuroleptic treatment Most of this change could indeed be accounted for by changes in positive schizophrenic symptoms.

The lack of significant effect of neuroleptic treatment on negative
schizophrenic symptoms was also consistent with Crow's formulation. The
finding that negative symptoms were increased by amphetamine at a level
just reaching significance however, was not.

We suspected that methadologic problems in scoring the "emotional
withdrawal" item of the negative symptom cluster accounted for the effect
of amphetamine on this factor. The "cue" for this item is "Rate only the
degree to which the patient gives the impression of failing to be in
emotional contact with other people in the interview situation". It
should be noted however that two types of pathologic emotionality are
scored as positive via this cue. Impaired capacity for a quantitatively
adequate emotional response (classical schizophrenic emotional blunting
and deterioration) would indeed be scored positively but so also would
brisk but incongruant emotionality (pervasive anger, for example in response to persecutory delusions or degrading auditory hallucinations,
regardless of the interviewer's demeanor). Both types of emotional pathology produce defects in emtional contact during the interview;
incongruant emotionality, however, might be expected to be related more
to positive than negative symptoms according to this clinical interpretation.

Separating the Withdrawal-Retardation Factor into its components,
emotional withdrawal 'vs' motor retardation and blunted affect', supports
the interpretation that the increase in negative symptoms seen after
amphetamine was largely due to our scoring incongruent emotionality as
'emotional withdrawal'. Motor retardation and blunted affect were not
significantly changed by administration of either amphetamine or neuroleptics. Emotional withdrawal, however, indeed showed a pattern of drug
response similar to that of positive schizophrenic symptoms. Mean scores
for this item were highly significantly increased by amphetamine ($P < 0.001$)
as well as being significantly diminished by neuroleptics. ($P < 0.02$) If the
methololologic problems involved in scoring the "Emotional Withdrawal" item
of the BPRS are taken into account (see Guy 1976, p162, for further
discussion of these problems), We believe that these results rather
strongly support the formulation proposed by Crow. Not only is the "Type
1 syndrome improved by neuroleptics, but it is also intensified by amphetamine. The 'Type II syndrome, however, is relatively uninfluenced by
either of these manipulations of dopaminergic systems.

We believe that Crow's formulation constitutes an importmant refine-
ment of the 'Dopamine Hypothesis' of schizophrenia. It takes into
account both the probable role of dopaminergic mechansims in the pathogenesis of productive schizophrenic symptoms and the limitations of this
concept in explaining all clinical aspects of schizophrenic illness. It
is certainly consistent with the very common clinical experience
represented by the patient whose florid (and presumably dopaminergicly
mediated) psychopathology is effectively reduced by neuroleptics, but
who remains incapacitated to some degree by a residual schizophrenic
defect state - the presumed sequallae of the "brain disease" postulated
by Owens and Johnstone. This concept is also consistent with very fundamental data on the course of schizophrenia prior to neuroleptics recently presented by Winokour (1980). When the severity of individual
schizophrenic symptoms was followed over time it was found that positive
symptoms tended to decline while negative symptoms either remained
stable or worsened.

Further research in this area might specifically address the relationships between positive and negative symptoms' predominance and ventricular enlargement on CAT scan in young schizophrenics with minimal neuroleptic treatment histories. In addition, the elevated activity of adenylate kinase in cerebrospinal fluid (CSF) from some schizophrenic patients (Alm et al 1979) lends support for the "brain disease" concept. Adenylate kinase is an intracellular enzyme normally undetectable in CSF; however in some neurologic disorders, elevated CSF adenylate kinase has been reported as a nonspecific marker of compromised cellular integrity (Firthz et al 1977). A positive correlation between elevated adenylate kinase activity in CSF, negative symptoms, and neuroanatomical pathology would lend support to the type I, type II concept.

The formulation presented here is consistent with viral and autoimmune hypotheses of schizophrenia (See Torrey and Peterson 1976 and Matthysse and Matthysse 1978 for reviews). In this context it is interesting to note that one of the subepidemics in the pandemic of encephalitus lethargica (a presumably viral encephalitus with a known propensity for attacking dopaminergic systems) took a hyperkinetic form in which a violent agitation rather than somnolence was the presenting sign (Economo 1931). The sequallae of this disease included not only Parkinsonism, but also both emotional deterioration strikingly reminiscent of that seen in chronic schizophrenia and frank psychoses. Economo spoke of a "psychic torpor" in which patients "remain unoccupied for hours without suffering boredom". The American Psychiatric Association's Diagnostic and Statistical Manual (DSM II 1968) specifically noted that in some survivors of this disease, "the outstanding feature is apparent indifference to persons and events ordinarily of emotional significance, such as the death of a family member". By analogy the most characteristic course of schizophrenia with its episodes of psychosis and progressive decline of function could be seen as representing episodes of cellular inflammation and irritability followed by cell drop out and progressive deficit.

Finally, Crow's formulation might influence treatment approaches. Negative symptomatology might be an important index of poor prognosis. More important, the use of neuroleptics might be reserved specifically for the treatment or prevention of positive schizophrenic symptoms.

References

1. Alm, P.O., Frithz, G., and Ronquist, G. (1979): ACTA Psychiatrica Scand., 59:517-524.
2. American Psychiatric Association Committee on Nomenclature and Statistics (1968): Diagnostic and Statistical Manual of Mental Disorders, 2nd Edition (DMS II). Published by the American Psychiatric Association, 1700 W. 18th St., N.W., Washington, D.C. 20009 USA, section 292.2 p 27.
3. Angrist, B., Rotrosen, J., Gershon, S. (1980): Psychopharmacology, 67:31-38.
4. Crow, T.J. (1980): Brit. Med. J., 280:66-68.
5. Donnelly, E.F., Weinberger, D.R. and Waldman, I.N. (1980): J. Nerv. Ment. Dis., 168:305-308.
6. Economo, C. (1931): Encephalitus Lethargica its sequellae and treatment. Translated K.O. Newman. Oxford U. Press, London: Humphrey Milford pp 125,126,131,132,135,136.

7. Frithz, G., Ericsson, P. and Ronquist, G. (1977): Uppsala J. Med. Sci. 82:11-14.
8. Guy, W. (1976): E.C.D.E.U. assessment manual for psychopathology, Washington, D.C.: U.S. Department of Health, Education and Welfare, pp 160,162,167.
9. Johnstone, E.C., Crow, T.J., Frith, C.D., Husband, J., Kreel, L. (1976): Lancet, 2:924-926.
10. Johnstone, E.C., Crow, T.J., Frith, C.D., Carney, M.W.P., Price, J.S. (1978a): Lancet, 1:848-851.
11. Johnstone, E.C., Crow, T.J., Frith, C.D., Stevens, M., Kreel, L., Husband, J. (1978b): Acta Psychiat Scand, 57:304-324.
12. Johnstone, E.C., Frith, C.D., Gold, A. and Stevens, M. (1979): Brit J Psychiat, 134:28-33.
13. Matthysse, S. and Matthysse, A.G. (1978): In Psychopharmacology a Generation of Progress edited by M.A. Lipton, A. Di Mascio and K. Killam, Raven Press, New York pp 1125-1129.
14. Meltzer, H.Y., Stahl, S.M. (1976): Schizophr Bull, 2:19-76.
15. Meltzer, H.Y. (1979): In Disorders of the Schizophrenic Syndrome edited by L. Bellak Basic Books New York p 113.
16. Owens, D.G. and Johnstone, E.C. (1980): Brit. J. Psychiat., 136:384-395.
17. Spitzer, R.L., Endicott, J., Robins, E. (1978): Arch. Gen. Psychiat., 35:733-782.
18. Torrey, E.F. and Peterson, M.R. (1976): Schizophrenia Bull, 2:136-146.
19. Weinberger, D.R., Bigelow, L.B., Kleinman, J.E., Klein, S.T., Rosenblatt, J.E. and Wyatt, R.J. (1980): Arch. Gen. Psychiat., 37:11-13.
20. Winokour, G. (1980): Presented at a symposium "Schizophrenia as a Brain Diasease", October 6 & 7, Iowa City, Iowa USA.

Acknowledgements

These studies were supported in part by a grant from the Schizophrenia Research Program of the Scottish Rite Foundation and by USPHS Grants MH00137 and MH29587 from the NIMH.

Apomorphine and Other Dopaminomimetics,
Vol. 2: Clinical Pharmacology, edited by
G. U. Corsini and G. L. Gessa, Raven Press,
New York © 1981.

Phenylethylamine, Dopamine, and Norepinephrine in Schizophrenia

Richard J. Wyatt, *Egidio A. Moja, Farouk Karoum, David M. Stoff,
Steven G. Potkin, and Joel E. Kleinman

*Adult Psychiatry Branch, Division of Special Mental Health Research, Intramural Research Program,
National Institute of Mental Health, Saint Elizabeths Hospital, Washington, D.C. 20032; *Institute of
Neurology, University of Cagliari, 09100 Cagliari, Italy*

Amphetamine produces many of its behavioral, biochemical, and pharmacological actions by altering catecholaminergic--most often dopaminergic--systems. Amphetamine is of considerable interest to neuropsychiatrists (17) because in addition to a number of clinically beneficial properties, amphetamine can produce a paranoid psychosis, which closely mimics paranoid schizophrenia. Because amphetamine is not normally found in humans, interest (13,18) has focused on the endogenously produced amphetamine-like compound phenylethylamine (PEA). Phenylethylamine is not only the chemical backbone of amphetamine (amphetamine is α-methyl-phenylethylamine) but produces many behavioral changes in animals that are similar to those produced by amphetamine. Further, since PEA is present in humans it might well be involved in normal physiological process as an endogenous stimulant as well as in pathological processes such as schizophrenia.

We have been particularly interested in the possibility that elevated PEA might be related to the cause of paranoid schizophrenia in some persons. This concept was first put forth by Fischer and colleagues in 1968 (5). They found increased PEA concentrations in the urines of a small number of schizophrenic patients (Table 1). Although Fischer in a subsequent study (6) confirmed his original finding of elevated PEA, two other groups (14,16) using more refined techniques, but very few patients, did not find PEA elevations. We examined the 24-hour urinary PEA excretion in populations both from Washington, D.C. (12) and from Bombay, India (8). In both populations, paranoid schizophrenic patients had higher PEA excretion rates than nonparanoid schizophrenic patients and controls.

In an examination of subjects living in Sardinia, we were able to collect afternoon four-hour urines. Urine was collected in plastic bottles containing 1 ml of 10% EDTA. It was frozen at -15°C within two hours after collection, and shipped to our laboratory in Washington, D.C. There it was analyzed for PEA and phenylacetic acid (the major metabolite of PEA). The values expressed in Table 2 are per mg creatinine. (Twenty-four-hour collections were not obtainable and, unfortunately, in our experience there has been too much variability in a four-hour urine collection to adequately reflect a 24-hour collection.) All subjects were interviewed by a psychiatrist using a semistructured interview (12), either in their hometown or as a patient in the Ospedale di is Mirionis in Cagliari. Subjects were diagnosed schizophrenic, but no attempt was made to subgroup the patients.

Table 1. Mean Urinary Phenylethylamine in Chronic Schizophrenic and Control Patients (N)

Study	Controls	All Schizophrenics	
Fischer et al., 1968 (5)	35.5 ug/l (N=11) (range 22-44)	N.R.* (N=7) (25-800 ug/liter)	
Fischer et al., 1972 (6)	336 ug/24 hr (N=17) (105-775)	1484 ug/24 hr (N=4) (960-2700)	
Schweitzer et. al., 1975 (14)	10.3 ug/24 hr (N=18) (0-78.5)	.9 ug/24 hr (N=3) (0-2.6)	
Suzuki and Yagi, 1977 (16)	15.9 ug/24 hr (N=9) (9.4-26.6)	9.3 ug/24 hr (N=5) (4.9-12.6)	
		P	NP
Potkin et al., (1979) (12)	8.5 ug/24 hr (N=32)	18.8 ug/24 hr (N=16)	7.36 ug/24 hr (N=15)
Jeste et al., 1980 (8)	4.1 ug/24 hr (N=19)	8.3 ug/24 hr (N=39)	5.0 ug/24 hr (N=11)

*N.R. = Not Reported

P=Paranoid; NP= Nonparanoid

Table 2. Four-Hour Urine Collection (expressed as Mean + S.D., ug/mg creatinine) Phenylethylamine (PEA) and Phenylacetic acid in normal controls and Schizophrenic Patients from Sardinia

	Controls	Patients
PEA (N-15)	5.62 ± 1.8	6.55 ± 3.6
Phenylacetic acid (N=14)	39.1 ± 7.1	76.7 ± 12.1*

*Two-tailed t-test, $p < .02$

All patients had been hospitalized one to four times during psychotic episodes, but all had less than six months of total lifetime hospitalization (mean age of males=33, females=32). The controls were hospital personnel (mean age of males=38, females=26). As a group the schizophrenic patients had a nonsignificant trend toward elevated urinary PEA, and almost a doubling (two-tailed t-test t=2.7; p< .02) in phenylacetic acid.

Our interest in PEA stems from the finding of decreased monoamine oxidase (MAO) activity in the peripheral platelets, lymphocytes, and muscle of schizophrenic patients (19), as well as the finding of altered catecholamine metabolism in the autopsied brains of schizophrenic patients. The decreased MAO activity (platelet, lymphocyte, and muscle) found in schizophrenic patients is type B, for which the perferred substrate is PEA. While it is unclear to what degree the enzyme activity is lowered by factors secondary to being schizophrenic, like neuroleptics, a number of studies suggest that the paranoid or hallucinating schizophrenic patients have the greatest decrease. Whether or not the decreased MAO activity found in these paranoid schizophrenic patients is sufficient to cause a corresponding increase in urinary PEA is unknown.

Another finding of related interest is the elevated norepinephrine concentrations found in the nucleus accumbens of some paranoid schizophrenic patients at autopsy. Increased norepinephrine in the nucleus accumbens was first found by Farley et al. (4) and has been subsequently confirmed by several groups (1,3), including our own (Table 3) (9). Lake et al. (10) have also found elevated norepinephrine in the CSF of paranoid schizophrenic patients.

Table 3. Mean (+S.D.) Catecholamines and Metabolites in Human (N) Nucleus Accumbens (ng/mg protein)

	CPS	CUS	Others	Normals
NE	*2.54+1.62 (N=10)	0.99+0.69 (N=8)	0.56+0.35 (N=8)	0.82+0.60 (N=12)
MHPG	**1.61+0.77 (N=10)	1.14+0.50 (N=9)	1.14+0.46 (N=8)	0.71+0.4 (N=13)
DA	65.1+18.4 (N=10)	52.2+14.7 (N=9)	66.7+22.3 (N=8)	59.8+34.5 (N=13)
HVA	104.5+31.9 (N=10)	109.8+16.9 (N=7)	93.4+20.6 (N=7)	90.5+17.5 (N=13)
DOPAC	6.89+2.11 (N=10)	8.87+3.80 (N=8)	9.51+5.37 (N=7)	10.37+6.00 (N=14)

*One-way ANOVA: Df(3,34); F=7.51; p<0.001; p<0.01 relative to CUS, Other psychiatric patients and Normals with Neuman-Keul.
**One-way ANOVA: Df(3,36); F=5.34; p<0.005; p<0.01 relative to normals with Neuman-Keul.
CPS=Chronic Paranoid Schizophrenic; CUS=Chronic Undifferentiated Schizophrenic. NE=Norepinephrine; DA=Dopamine; HVA=Homovanillic Acid

We have recently raised the question whether there might be a connection between the elevated urinary PEA concentrations and norepinephrine in the nucleus accumbens of paranoid schizophrenic patients. Elevated PEA in the urine probably reflects elevated PEA in blood. Since PEA readily crosses the blood-brain barrier, it follows that PEA may be elevated in the brain as well.

In one study (11), Rhesus monkeys adapted to chronic primate chairs were given single PEA doses (75 mg/kg intramuscularly). Cerebrospinal fluid norepinephrine and dopamine were measured serially before and after PEA administration. While dopamine was increased slightly (about 25%) between three and six hours after PEA administration, norepinephrine was found to be markedly increased--by as much as nearly 400% in the first three hours, and remained elevated over a nine-hour time period.

To determine not only if acute PEA administration increased norepinephrine in the CSF, but also whether chronic PEA increased norepinephrine in the brain itself, PEA (100 mg/kg) was administered to rats intragastrically twice daily for 10 days (Fig. 1). The rats were sacrificed two hours after the last dose. Of the various brain areas analyzed, norepinephrine concentrations were selectively and significantly increased in only the hypothalamus (36% above controls) and the nucleus accumbens (96% above controls). Norepinephrine's major metabolite, 3-methoxy-4-hydroxyphenylglycol (MHPG) was also increased in the hypothalamus (47% above controls), but remained normal in the nucleus acumbens. In contrast, dopamine was not changed, but 3-4-dihydroxyphenylacetic acid (DOPAC) was slightly increased. These biochemical findings of increased norepinephrine concentrations in the nucleus accumbens after administration of PEA are consistent with findings that application of PEA to the nucleus accumbens potentiates PEA stereotypy (2) and hyperactivity (7).

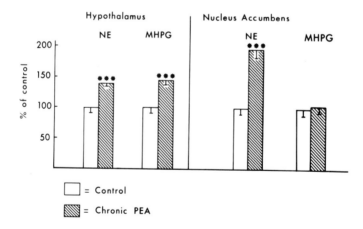

FIG. 1. Concentration of norepinephrine (NE) and 3-methoxy-4-hydroxyphenyl-glycol (MHPG) in hypothalamus and nucleus accumbens in rats given 100 mg/kg PEA twice daily for 10 days.

In order to understand how brain catecholamines might be changed by PEA, Stoff and Gale (15) studied the effects of PEA on striatal tyrosine hydroxylase. Phenylethylamine (600 mg/kg) was given intragastrically to rats twice daily for 14 days. The Vmax for striatal tyrosine hydroxylase increased 20%, an effect lasting for at least 10 days after the last PEA dose. This effect was not blocked by concurrent administration of haloperidol.

In summary, we studied PEA because of its close similarity to amphetamine. Phenylethylamine may be elevated in some paranoid schizophrenic patients, perhaps in association with decreased MAO activity. Unlike amphetamine, PEA appears to work by altering norepinephrine metabolism, and not by altering dopamine metabolism.

REFERENCES

1.   Bird, E. D., Spokes, E. G., and Iversen, L. L. (1979): Science, 204:93-94.

2.   Borison, R. L., Havdala, H. S., and Diamond, B. I. (1977): Life Sci., 21:117-122.

3.   Carlsson, A. (1979): In: Catecholamines: Basic and Clinical Frontiers, edited by E. Usdin, I. J. Kopin, and J. D. Barchas, pp. 4-19. Pergamon Press, New York.

4.   Farley, I. J., Price, K. S., McCullough, E., Deck, J. H., Hordynski, W., and Hornykiewitz, O. (1978): Science, 200:456-457.

5.   Fischer, E., Heller, D., and Miro, A. A. (1968): Arzneimittel-Forsch, 18:1486-1489.

6.   Fischer, E., Spatz, H., Saavedra, J. M., Reggini, H., Miro, A. H., and Heller, V. (1972): Biol. Psychiatry, 5:139-142.

7.   Jackson, D. M., Andén, N. E., and Dahlstrom, A. A. (1975): Psychopharmacologica (Berl.), 45:139-149.

8.   Jeste, D. V., Doongaji, D. R., Sheth, A. S., Apte, J. S., Potkin, S. G., Karoum, F., Panjwani, D., Datta, M., Thatte, R., and Wyatt, R. J.: Brit. J. Psychiatry, submitted.

9.   Kleinman, J. E., Bridge, T. P., Karoum, F., Speciale, S., Staub, R., Zalcman, S., Gillin, J. C., and Wyatt, R. J. (1979): In: Catecholamines: Basic and Clinical Frontiers. edited by E. Usdin, I. J., Kopin, and J. D. Barchas, pp. 1845-1848. Pergamon Press, New York.

10. Lake, C. R., Sternberg, D. E., van Kammen, D. P., Ballenger, J. C., Ziegler, M. G., Post, R. M., Kopin, I. J., and Bunney, W. E. (1980): Science, 207:331-333.

11. Perlow, M. J., Chiueh, C. C., Lake, C. R., and Wyatt, R. J. (1980): Brain Res., 186:469-473.

12. Potkin, S. G., Karoum, F., Chuang, L-W., Cannon-Spoor, H. E., Phillips, I., and Wyatt, R. J. (1979): Science, 206:470-471.

13. Sandler, M., and Reynolds, G. P. (1976): Lancet, 1:70-71.

14. Schweitzer, J. W., Freedhoff, A. J., and Schwartz, R. (1975):   Biol. Psychiatry, 10:277-285.

15. Stoff, D. M., and Gale, K. (1980): Neuroscience Abstracts, November 1980.

16. Suzuki, S., and Yagi, L. (1977): Clin. Chim. Acta, 78:401-410.

17. Woodrow, K. M., Reifman, A., and Wyatt, R. J. (1978): In: Neuropharmacology and Behavior, edited by B. Haber, and M. Aprison, pp. 1-18. Plenum Press, New York.

18. Wyatt, R. J. (1978): In: Nature of Schizophrenia, edited by L. Wynne, R. Cromwell, R., and Matthysse, pp. 116-125. John Wiley and Sons, New York.

19. Wyatt, R. J., Potkin, S. G., and Murphy, D. L. (1979): Am. J. Psychiatry, 136:377-385.

*Apomorphine and Other Dopaminomimetics,
Vol. 2: Clinical Pharmacology*, edited by
G. U. Corsini and G. L. Gessa, Raven Press,
New York © 1981.

Effects of Apomorphine on Schizophrenia

John M. Davis, *Carol Tamminga, **Martin H. Schaeffer,
and †Robert C. Smith

*Department of Psychiatry, University of Chicago, Department of Psychiatry, University of Illinois, and
Illinois State Psychiatric Institute, Chicago, Illinois 60601; *Department of Psychiatry, University of
Maryland, Baltimore, Maryland 21228; **Department of Psychiatry, University of Chicago, Chicago,
Illinois 60601; †Texas Research Institute for Mental Sciences, Houston, Texas 77025*

As all effective antipsychotic drugs inhibit dopamine neurotransmission, it would follow that new drugs could be developed that inhibit dopamine transmission in a manner different from existing drugs as well as the conventional "me too" method of drug screening. Among the physiologic regulators of dopaminergic neurotransmission are presynaptic dopamine receptors, sometimes called autoreceptors, which reside on the presynaptic dopaminergic cell and regulate dopamine-neurotransmission via synthesis and release. The classical dopamine presynaptic stimulus is apomorphine, which at a certain dose range appears to stimulate presynaptic dopamine receptors and reduce dopamine neurotransmission. Based on the early pharmacologic work characterizing these presynaptic dopamine receptors (1,3,6,7),- our group administered apomorphine s.c. to schizophrenics in roughly the same mg per kg dose as used in animals as a presynaptic agonist. Much higher doses of apomorphine would be expected to stimulate postsynaptic receptors for one would hypothesize worsening of the psychosis.

The vomiting produced by apomorphine clouds the issue of its antipsychotic effect in man. In addition, we were particularly interested, for theoretical reasons, in the use of apomorphine along with conventional neuroleptic drugs. Since apomorphine stimulates both pre-and postsynaptic receptors, it might be expected that at a certain dose the predominant stimulation would be presynaptic and at a much higher dose the predominant stimulation might be postsynaptic. However, even at low doses, there might be some postsynaptic effect which may cloud its presynaptic action. Based on the assumption that apomorphine might have a greater affinity for presynaptic receptors and that conventional neuroleptics, such as chlorpromazine or thioridazine, might have a greater affinity for postsynaptic receptors, we felt that the two drugs might have an additive or synergistic effect to reduce dopamine transmission and consequently to reduce schizophrenic symptomatology. Since blockade of postsynaptic receptors results in a feedback-induced increase in dopamine synthesis, this increase may partly work in some broad sense in the opposite direction from the antidopamine pharmacologic effect intended. Stimulation of presynaptic receptors might counteract or overcome this feedback augmentation of dopaminergic synthesis. Thus, apomorphine, by stimulating presynaptic receptors, may result in a decrease in dopamine synthesis and/or release and also might contradict any feedback effects consequent to dopamine blockage by the chlorpromazine-type receptor blocker. Empirical evidence is needed to substantiate the various assumptions of this rationale. It seems reasonable to try the combination of drugs in man to see if an antipsychotic effect would be observed.

All our studies were double blind. Low dose apomorphine produced a modest decrease in psychotic symptoms in two schizophrenics when given alone (4). Another patient showed a very slight increase in psychosis. Of particular interest is one unusually florid schizophrenic who had continuous hallucinations. This patient took part in a dose-ranging study receiving doses from 1 to 6 mg.s.c. for morphine or placebo on 12 different days in addition to the standard dose of butaperazine (40mg/day). Generally, apomorphine resulted in a reduction of psychosis in comparison to placebo injections when all drug days were compared to all placebo days. Since the intensity of her schizophrenic illness fluctuated somewhat from day to day, perhaps a more sensitive test compared the patients' response to apomorphine with the closest placebo day. In 7 of 9 comparisons, psychosis was decreased following apomorphine to a greater extent than following placebo. Moreover, the symptoms benefited by apomorphine where those which characterized the schizophrenic illness-hallucinations and delusions, thought disorder and paranoid ideation.

These initial observations were verified in double-blind, random assignment studies of 18 severely-disturbed chronic schizophrenic patients (5). These patients received a constant low dose (subtherapeutic) of neuroleptics over several weeks. Each patient still manifested florid schizophrenic symptoms despite the low dose neuroleptic, so there was considerable potential for improvement. Each patient received two injections, one apomorphine (3 mg), one placebo. The order of injection was determined by randomization. No nausea or vomiting occured because of the antivomiting effect of the neuroleptic

The effect on schizophrenia appeared roughly 20 minutes after the injection and lasted from 40 to 60 minutes. Psychotic symptoms were evaluated using a modification of the New Haven Schizophrenia Scale, an instrument which evaluates florid schizophrenic symptoms, such as hallucinations, delusion etc. Apomorphine substantially decreased these schizophrenic symptoms in 9 patients and had little effect in the other 9. The magnitude of the reduction was such that when considering all 18 patients together, the intensity of schizophrenia was slightly reduced below baseline evaluation (1.67$\pm$ .9) with placebo but a decrease substantially of 6.22$\pm$ .4 with apomorphine (p<.02). At the time we were doing these studies, Corsini and his collaborators (2) were performing a clinical trial of apomorphine in schizophrenia and observing here that apomorphine had an antipsychotic effect, a finding presented at a previous symposium in Sardinia in 1976. Since neither investigator could have been aware of the other investigator's work at the time these initial studies were done, the findings of both groups independently replicate the other's work.

It is possible to screen a presynaptic agonist which may have an antidopamine effect by the use of animal models and/or by biochemical pharmacologic technique in order to find a long-acting orally administered presynaptic agonist to which tolerance does not develop. The empirical demonstration by both Corsini and his coworkers (2) and by our group (4,5) that an acute dose of apomorphine does benefit schizophrenic symptoms in man plus the theoretical rationale provide some justification that such a screening process might in fact yield a new antipsychotic drug acting through this mechanism of action. It is particularly important to look for antipsychotics with a novel mechanism of action since there is always a possibility that producing an antidopamine effect in a different way from receptor blockade may have a lesser risk of tardive dyskinesia. Such a drug could be used alone or in addition to conventional dopamine receptor blocking drugs.

REFERENCES

1. Carlsson, A. (1975): In: Presynaptic and Postsynaptic Receptors, edited by E. Usdin and W. E. Bunney, p.49, New York.

2. Corsini, G. U., Del Zompo, M., Momoni, S., Cianchetti, C., Mangoni, A., Gessa, G. L. (1977): Advances in Biochemical Psychopharmacology, 16:645-648.

3. Kehr, W., Carlsson, A., Lindquist, M., Magnusson, T., Atack, C. (1972): J. Pharm. Pharmacol. 24:744.

4.   Smith,R.C.,Tamminga,C.,Davis,J.M. (1977): J.Neurol.Trans-
      mission. 40:171-176.

5.   Tamminga,C.,Schaeffer,M.H.,Smith R.C.,Davis ,J.M. (1978):
      Science 200:567-566.

6.   Walters,J.R.,Bunney,B.S.,Roth,R.H. (1974): Adv.Neurol. 9:136

7.   Walters,J.R.,Roth,R.H. (1975): In: Antipsychotic drugs,
      Pharmacodynamics and Pharmacokinetics, p.147, Pergamon
      Press, New York.

Apomorphine and Other Dopaminomimetics,
Vol. 2: Clinical Pharmacology, edited by
G. U. Corsini and G. L. Gessa, Raven Press,
New York © 1981.

Apomorphine and *N-n*-Propylnorapomorphine in the Treatment of Schizophrenia

C. A. Tamminga, E. G. DeFraites, M. D. Gotts, and T. N. Chase

Maryland Psychiatric Research Center, University of Maryland, Department of Psychiatry, Baltimore, Maryland 21228 and the Experimental Therapeutics Branch, National Institute of Neurological and Communicative Disorders and Stroke, National Institutes of Health, Bethesda, Maryland 20205

The treatment of psychotic illness with neuroleptic drugs, although successful in large numbers of schizophrenic patients continues to be beset with serious difficulties. Not only are particular persons unresponsive to neuroleptic administration, but serious adverse effects not infrequently complicate chronic use. New compounds and therapeutic strategies to treat the psychotic symptoms of schizophrenia thus continue to be sought.

The antipsychotic effect of neuroleptic drugs is generally attributed to their ability to block postsynaptic dopamine receptors, thus diminishing dopamine-mediated synaptic transmission (2,12). Recent data suggests that multiple types of dopamine receptors exist, distinguished by location (1), receptor binding properties (5,15), and pharmacologic response (6); these receptor subtypes appear to mediate different neural responses. A body of evidence supports the hypothesis that stimulation of the purported dopamine autoreceptor, located on the dopamine neuron itself, may diminish dopamine-mediated neural transmission, an action similar to neuroleptic drugs (7,12). Selective dopamine autoreceptor agonist treatment would then be predicted to have antipsychotic efficacy in schizophrenic patients with active psychotic symptoms. This hypothesis was originally tested in schizophrenic patients using apomorphine in the dose ranges thought to activate the dopamine autoreceptor (13). Subsequent experiments tested potent ergot dopamine agonists,e.g. bromocriptine and CF 25-397 (14). More recently, 10,11-dihydroxy-N-n-propylnorapomorphine (NPA) has been evaluated in a preliminary trial in patients with active schizophrenic psychosis.

METHODS AND RESULTS

Apomorphine. Patients (n=18) diagnosed as having chronic schizophrenic illness by the Research Diagnostic Criteria (RDC) received a 3 mg dose of apomorphine administered subcutaneously in a placebo-controlled, double-blind, random crossover design. All patients remained on their chronic neuroleptic therapy but sustained a 40-50% reduction in their accustomed dosage 1-2 weeks before the apomorphine test. A significant decrease in psychotic symptoms was observed 20 and 40 min following apomorphine administration, compared with placebo (6.0$\pm$ 1.5 vs.1.4$\pm$ 1.4, mean $\pm$ SEM, respectively, Psychosis Change Scale). The significant mean change could be accounted for by half of the patients (n=9) who responded with a clinically apparent diminuition in psychotic symptoms; the other 9 patients failed to respond. No diagnostic subtype significantly distinguished the responder from the nonresponder group (Fig.1).

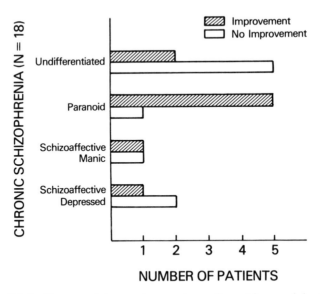

FIG.1. RDC diagnostic categories for the schizophrenic subjects (n=18) who received 3 mg apomorphine subcutaneously. Some individuals improved following apomorphine (hatched bar) while others showed no change from placebo administration (open bar).

Ergot Dopamine Agonists. Ergot family dopamine agonists, including bromocriptine and CF 25-397, were tested in schizophrenic patients using a double-blind, placebo-controlled, crossover design with a subchronic administration schedule. Piribedil, a nonergot mild dopamine agonist was similarly tested. None of these agents, after 7 days of oral treatment, significantly altered psychotic symptoms (Table 1).

Table 1. Psychosis Score

Medication	N	Drug	Placebo	Significance
Bromocriptine	6	23+4	20+8	NS
CF 25-397	8	23+4	23+4	NS
Piribedil	6	22+2	23+2	NS

N-n-propylnorapomorphine. NPA is a dopamine agonist chemically related to apomorphine; because of the previously demonstrated antipsychotic properties of apomorphine the therapeutic potential of NPA was explored in schizophrenic subjects. Data from acute dose studies are available. Four patients with an RDC diagnosis of schizophrenia, free from all neuroleptic drugs for 4-6 weeks, received single oral doses of NPA beginning at 5 mg and increasing to 40 mg/dose; 24-48 hrs separated each single dose administration. Psychosis was evaluated immediately prior to and at 2 and 4 hrs following each oral dose. Placebo doses were randomly inserted into the rising dose sequence to maintain the double-blind, placebo-controlled design. After receiving NPA each patient showed improvement at one of the dose levels between 10 and 40 mg (Fig.2). Overall, the patient group evidenced a mean 23% diminuition in symptoms (Table 2). While there was some decrease in anxiety and in manic-like behaviours, the predominant change occurred in psychotic symptoms.

COMMENTS

NPA (fig.3) is a structural analogue of apomorphine several times more potent as a dopamine agonist(8). It induces stereotypies and stimulates locomotor behaviour with 10 times the potency of apomorphine (8,11). Like apomorphine, NPA is thought to exert its dopamine agonist action through direct stimulation of dopamine receptors; both stimulate adenylate

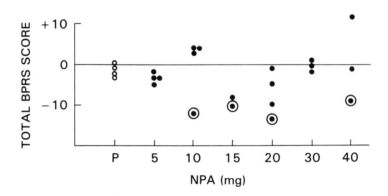

FIG.2. Change in BPRS score for each of the 4 patients during the 4 hrs following oral NPA administration at the dose indicated. Circled dots represent the NPA dose level at which the maximal decrease in BPRS score occurred in each patient.

Table 2.

PEAK DOSE RESPONSE
(Mean ± SEM)

	NPA	Placebo
BPRS: Total Score	−11 ± 1.1	−1 ± 1.6
BPRS: Percent Decrease	23%	2%
BPRS: Psychosis Subscale	−4.3 ± 1.1	−.55 ± 2.1
BPRS: Anxiety Subscale	−2.0 ± 1.1	−.18 ± .28

cyclase activity with similar potency (9). Presumably, NPA
has parallel dose-specific potential as apomorphine for stimulating either postsynaptic dopamine receptors or dopamine
autoreceptors. However, NPA does exert actions which are
different from either apomorphine or dopamine when directly
applied to specific brain areas. When dopamine, apomorphine
or NPA are directly applied to the striatum or nucleus accumbens rather than administered peripherally, differences in
potency as well as varying effects on locomotor and stereotypic behaviours became apparent. Such observations suggest
that pharmacologically distinct types of dopamine receptors
may exist in different terminal areas (10).

Early clinical trials with NPA evaluated its usefulness
as an antiparkinsonian drug (4). Its efficacy upon oral administration and lack of significant nephrotoxic properties,
compared to apomorphine, recommended its clinical application at that time. Its use in Parkinson's disease has not been
further developed despite the fact that those first clinical
experiments demonstrated antiparkinsonian efficacy and possible usefulness in some L-dopa-resistant parkinsonian patients.

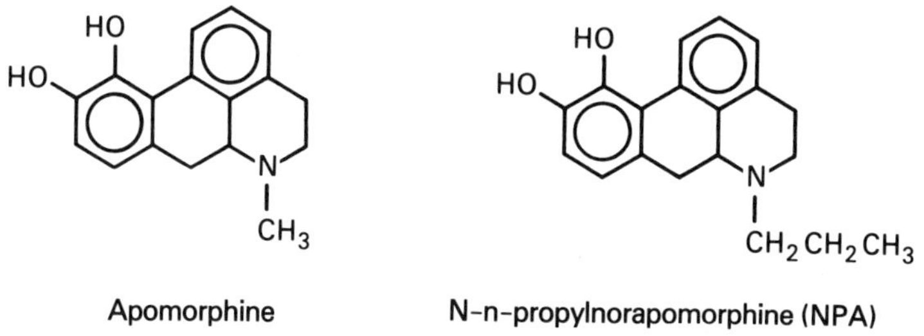

Apomorphine   N-n-propylnorapomorphine (NPA)

FIG.3. Chemical structure of apomorphine and NPA.

The theory of dopamine autoreceptor stimulation therapy
in hyperdopaminergic syndromes has matured; the use of NPA
in these studies is suggested by previous clinical investigations which have reported apomorphine to have antipsychotic
activity. The data reported here are consistent with the

hypothesis that NPA has antipsychotic potential when given acutely. Testing beyond this limited sample is necessary to verify these results. Moreover, if NPA is demonstrated to have antipsychotic potential, conditions for its therapeutic application need to be determined: optimal dose, potential combination treatment, and tolerance effects.

If further clinical study shows NPA has antipsychotic efficacy upon acute administration the question of tolerance upon chronic administration will need to be considered. Repeated administration of NPA and apomorphine result in tolerance to a wide range of drug effects, including behavioural, biochemical and neurophysiological actions. Furthermore, in the Cotzias study of NPA in parkinsonism, patients treated with the compound gradually developed tachyphylaxis to its therapeutic effect (4). Antiparkinsonian activity was preserved by gradual dose increases or by concomitant treatment with suboptimal doses of other agents. The tolerance to NPA effect was explained then by postulating a gradual accumulation of the 0-methylated apomorphine metabolite, apocodeine, which has antidopaminergic properties, progressively antagonizing the direct dopamine agonist effect on NPA (16). Whereas drug tolerance is commonly related to changes in receptor sensitivity, this hypothesis of metabolic interference was put forth to explain why apomorphine, distinct from other direct acting dopamine agonists, induces tolerance acutely. Even if tolerance develops upon repeated administration in drug naive subjects, the data of Ungerstedt (this volume), suggest that the effect of apomorphine in chronic neuroleptic-treated animals differs remarkably from its effects in drug-naive subjects. Since most, if not all, schizophrenic patients are chronically neuroleptic-treated individuals, the production of tolerance may differ in this population from non-drug treated persons.

REFERENCES

1. Carlsson,A.(1975): In: Basal Ganglia, edited by M.O.Yahr, pp.181-189. Raven Press, New York.
2. Carlsson,A. and Linquist,M.(1963): Acta Pharmacol.Toxicol 20: 140-146.
3. Costall,B.,Naylor,R.J.,Cannon,J.G. and Lee,T.(1977): J Pharm.Pharmacol., 29: 337-342.
4. Cotzias,G.C.,Papavasilious,P.S.,Tolosa,E.S.,Mendez,J.S., and Bell-Midara,M.(1976): New Engl.J.Med.,294: 567-572.

5. Creese,I., and Snyder,S.H.(1980): In: <u>Catecholamines:</u> <u>Basic and Clinical Frontiers.</u>, edited by E.Usdin,I.Kopin and J.Barchas. Peramon Press, New York.

6. Kebabian,J.W.,and Calne,D.B.(1979): <u>Nature</u> 277: 93-96.

7. Kehr,W.,Carlsson,A.,and Lindquist,M.(1972): <u>J.Pharm.</u> <u>Pharmacol</u>,24: 744-747.

8. Menon,M.K.,Clark,W.G., and Neumeyer,J.L.(1978): <u>Europ.J.</u> <u>Pharmacol.</u>,52: 1-9.

9. Miller,R.J.,Kelly,P.H., and Neumeyer,J.L.(1976): <u>Europ.</u> <u>J.Pharmacol.</u>,35: 77-83.

10. Neumeyer,J.L.,and Dafeldecker,W.P.(1977): <u>J.Med.Chem.</u>, 20: 190-196.

11. Neumeyer,J.L.,Reinhard,J.F.,Dafeldecker,W.P.,Guarino,J., Kosersky,D.S.,Fuxe,K.,and Agnati,L.(1976): <u>J.Med.Chem.</u>, 20: 190-196.

12. Snyder,S.H.,Banerjee,S.P.,Yamamura,H.I.,and Greenberg,D. (1974): <u>Science</u>, 184: 1243-1250.

13. Tamminga,C.A.,Schaffer,M.H.,Smith,R.C., and Davis,J.M. (1978): <u>Science</u>,200: 567-568.

14. Tamminga,C.A. and Schaffer,M.H.(1979): <u>Psychopharmacology</u> 66: 239-242.

15. Titeler,M.,Tedesco,J.L.,and Seeman,P.(1978): <u>Life Sci.</u>, 23: 587-592.

16. Tolosa,E.S.,Cotzias,G.C.,Burckhardt,P.G.,Tang,L.C., and Dahl,K.E.(1977): <u>Exper.Neurol.</u>,55:56-66.

17. Walters,J.R.,and Roth,R.H.(1974): <u>J.Pharmacol.Exp.Ther.</u>, 191: 82-91.

Apomorphine and Other Dopaminomimetics,
Vol. 2: Clinical Pharmacology, edited by
G. U. Corsini and G. L. Gessa, Raven Press,
New York © 1981.

Experiences with Dopamine Agonists in Depression and Schizophrenia

Leo E. Hollister

Departments of Medicine, Psychiatry, and Pharmacology, Stanford University School of Medicine and Veterans Administration Medical Center, Palo Alto, California 94304

The introduction of levodopa as a treatment for Parkinson's disease in 1967 opened a new approach to treatment of nervous system diseases: replenishment of deficient neurotransmitters by loading with their precursors. One of the major hypotheses in 1967 was that endogenous depression was due to decreased aminergic neurotransmission, primarily that of norepinephrine or serotonin. Administration of amounts of levodopa comparable to doses used in Parkinson's disease might be a way to remedy the postulated norepinephrine deficiency of some depressions. At that time (1968) we were unaware of a defect in this logic, namely while levodopa increases dopamine concentrations in brain rather substantially, even large amounts do not much change norepinephrine concentrations. Also, we were not aware that similar studies were being conducted at the National Institute of Mental Health.

Study #1. Levodopa in Depressed Patients

We sought to identify mainly patients considered to have depression of the endogenous type, primarily those who also showed psychomotor retardation. None of the patients were currently on any other antidepressant drug. The dose of levodopa for the initial trials started with 150 mg/day orally with rapid increments to 1500 mg/day at the end of two weeks and 3 g/day during the third week of treatment. We expected eventually to use as much as 10 g/day to get optimal results.

For reasons that are obvious, this study was terminated after five depressed patients were treated. Their data are summarized in Table 1. Two patients had relatively mild illnesses (De and Fra); one (De) showed minimal improvement, while the other (Fra) showed marked worsening after having received 6 g/day of levodopa orally. Of the remaining three patients, each of whom had moderate degrees of depression, one was unchanged and the other two became worse, all on 3 g/day of levodopa orally. Thus, four of the five patients were judged to have done worse than expected from conventional antidepressant drugs. Side effects or exacerbated symptoms included the following: nausea and vomiting, apathy, insomnia, excitement, tremor, mannerisms, unusual thought content and disorganized thinking. No specific laboratory abnormalities were associated with the drug.

TABLE 1. Summary data on five depressed patients treated with levodopa

Pt	Age	Sex	Diagnosis	Duration Treatment	Max.Dose	BPRS Pre-Score	BPRS Post-Score	Global
De	51	M	Retarded	3 wks	3000 mg	13.5	7.0	Min
Fre	42	M	Retarded	3 wks	3000 mg	32.5	30.5	Un
Ha	50	M	Retarded	3 wks	3000 mg	22.5	30.0	Worse
Ba	56	F	Agitated	18 days	3000 mg	47.0	56.0	Worse
Fra	42	F	Anxious	7 days	6000 mg	10.0	43.0	Worse

Meanwhile, the National Institute of Mental Health group had reported substantial improvement in some patients treated with either large doses of levodopa alone or smaller doses in combination with a peripheral decarboxylase inhibitor (1,2). We interpreted our experience as indicating that levodopa would not become an effective treatment for depression, nor did we feel that further exploration of higher doses would be useful.

Because of the psychotic-like symptoms shown by these depressed patients during treatment with levodopa, as well as reports of such symptoms in patients with Parkinson's disease treated with this drug, we decided to try the drug in schizophrenics (3). By the time that we were able to start this study, a report on five schizophrenic patients treated with doses of 1 to 2 g/day of levodopa orally indicated that four had become worse, even though three were also receiving doses of antipsychotic drugs (4).

Study #2. Levodopa in Schizophrenics

We chose three patients clearly diagnosed as schizophrenic. Two patients were still psychotic while the other was in partial remission. Results on these three patients (we stopped the study after their treatment was complete) are summarized in Table 2. Two patients (Co and De) became clearly more psychotic, one on a daily dose of 3 g of levodopa, the other on a daily dose of 9 g. It was of some interest that the latter patient had been receiving a substantial amount of antipsychotic drugs, yet levodopa administration was still able to aggravate the psychosis.

Thus, our findings substantiated the fact that levodopa in the doses usually given for treating Parkinson's disease made schizophrenics worse, even when they presumably had postsynaptic dopamine receptors blocked by substantial doses of antipsychotic drugs.

TABLE 2. Summary data on three schizophrenics treated with levodopa

Pt	Age	Sex	Diagnosis	Duration treatment	Max.dose	Other drugs	Outcome
Co	27	M	Paranoid	2 wks	3000 mg	None	Hostile Uncooperative Agitated Maximum security ward
Ke	49	M	Undiff.	3 wks	3000 mg	Reserpine 1 mg/day	No change
De	28	M	Undiff.	3 wks	9600 mg	Thioridazine 800 mg/day Trifluoperazine 40 mg/day Chlorpromazine 1200 mg/day	Bizarre behavior Incoherant Inappropriate laughter Increase in psychosis

A few years later, we were intrigued by two reports that low doses of levodopa had a beneficial effect in schizophrenics. In both cases, levodopa was added to already existing doses of antipsychotic drugs. Twenty-five of 84 schizophrenics so treated showed moderate or marked improvement and only five became worse (5). Another group confirmed this phenomenon in a controlled cross-over trial involving 18 outpatients with simple schizophrenia (6). These controversial reports led us to speculate that levodopa in low doses selectively stimulated presynaptic inhibitory dopamine receptors, reducing the impulse flow and release of dopamine from nerve terminals.

Study #3. Low Dose Levodopa in Schizophrenia

Three schizophrenic patients were selected for study in the psychiatric clinical research center of the hospital. All had been relatively resistant to treatment with antipsychotic drugs. Their treatment with these drugs was not altered during the experimental protocol. Levodopa was started in a daily dose of 100 mg with similar increments daily until a level of 500 mg/day was reached. At this point plasma growth hormone concentration was measured just before and 45 minutes after a dose of levodopa. If no growth hormone response was observed, doses were to be increased by further increments until a rise occurred. Then the dose would be reduced to a level which showed no evidence of postsynaptic activity as determined by the growth hormone concentrations.

The data are summarized in Table 3. Only in patient #2 was growth hormone increased, but we decided to continue his small dose rather than reduce it further. One might have expected this patient to have become worse, due to evidence of postsynaptic receptor stimulation, but he did not. On the other hand, two patients who showed no growth hormone response from 500 mg/day of levodopa, clearly became worse even though covered by substantial doses of antipsychotic drugs.

TABLE 3. Summary data on three schizophrenics treated with low-dose levodopa

Pt	Age	Sex	Diagnosis	Duration Treatment	Max.dose	Other drugs	Outcome
#1	41	M	Undiff.	10 days	500 mg	Fluphenazine 40 mg/day	Loose associations, more delusional auditory hallucinations, excited
#2	24	M	Undiff.	6 wks	500 mg	Fluphenazine 20 mg/day Flu.decanoate 50 mg IV q 2 wks	No change
#3	40	M	Paranoid	10 days	500 mg	Thiothixene 40 mg/day Chlorpromazine 600 mg/day Flu.decanoate 25 mg IV q wk	More paranoid, excited

Despite this discouraging result with small doses of levodopa, the idea of stimulating selectively presynaptic autoreceptors still seemed tenable. Evidence that apomorphine might have such a selective effect was considerably more compelling than for levodopa (7–11). Further, one group had reported benefit in schizophrenics treated with apomorphine, a report later confirmed by another group (12,13).

Study #4. High-Dose Apomorphine

Rather than use the low doses previously reported, we reasoned that if patients were concurrently being treated with antipsychotic drugs, one might be able to use much higher doses of apomorphine, and still retain a selective action. To measure whether or not postsynaptic receptors were being stimulated by apomorphine, we decided to monitor by observing for clinical signs of nausea or vomiting, as well as by the response of serum concentrations of human growth hormone and prolactin to doses of apomorphine. We expected that nausea and vomiting, increased growth hormone or decreased prolactin levels would provide clues to postsynaptic receptor activity that would allow us to test the highest possible doses with selective presynaptic action.

We first did an open study on two patients. Apomorphine was prepared freshly in ethanolic solution for oral administration; we assumed the oral:parenteral ratio to be about 100:1. Results are summarized in Table 4. One can see that during treatment with apomorphine, postsynaptic activity, as judged by the measures used, was not evident; but that patients became clearly more agitated and more psychotic.

TABLE 4. High-dose oral apomorphine study in schizophrenics maintained on antipsychotic drugs

Date	Daily dose (qid)	Anti-Psychotic Treatment	Total BPRS Score	Agitation	Δ serum HGH	Δ serum prolactin
W.H.						
10/31/77	7.5	Fluphena-zine 20 mg	50	0	0	−11
11/1	15.0		40	3	+3	−13
11/2	30.0		39	4	0	−15
11/3	60.0		58	4	+3	−15
11/4	120.0		50	4	0	− 8
11/5	0					
11/9			65			
11/16	0		74	4	+15	
11/18	30.0					
11/23	11.25		80	4	+2	
11/30			69	4		
W.M.						
11/14/77	7.5	CPZ 606 Thiothix-ene 40 mg	55	0	0	− 8
11/15	15.0		31	3	+1	0
11/16	30.0		47	4	0	− 2
11/17	60.0		66	3	0	− 1
11/18	120.0		58	4	0	− 4
11/19	15.0					
11/25			73	4	0	
11/30			Agitated; refused to continue			

Thus, once again, evidence suggested that even under the protection of antipsychotic drugs, a dopamine agonist could aggravate schizophrenia, despite little evidence of postsynaptic dopaminergic action on receptors mediating non-psychiatric effects.

Study #5. Low-dose Apomorphine

Having failed with the original hypothesis, we decided to replicate the reports of amelioration of schizophrenia by low doses of apomorphine. Our first study was a non-blind trial with five schizophrenic patients treated with four-times daily oral doses of apomorphine or placebo/no treatment. After a baseline period of about two weeks during which only the current antipsychotic drug treatment was given, patients were started on doses of 2.5 mg of apomorphine orally four times daily; some doses being raised to as much as 7.5 mg four times daily. Treatment lasted over a three-week period followed by a period of placebo treatment.

Results from this open study are summarized in Table 5. All BPRS ratings done during placebo or no-treatment periods were compared with ratings done during the treatment period. The initial results looked to be somewhat favorable although not clinically impressive.

This phase of the study was followed by a blind controlled trial that involved 11 patients, very carefully selected to meet the current Research Diagnostic Critiera for schizophrenia. Three of these patients were among the five previously treated in the open study. During the first week of the nine-week study, all patients were placed on placebo After that, the four remaining two-week periods were randomly allocated to treatment with placebo or apomorphine. The dose of apomorphine was kept constant at 5 mg four times daily orally. The placebo was a quinine solution that mimicked the bitter taste of apomorphine in solution.

Results are summarized in Table 5. No evidence of a therapeutic effect of apomorphine was found. One patient, also on thiothixene 30 mg/day, had a marked exacerbation of psychosis after 8 days on apomorphine and was dropped from the study. Thus, with oral doses of apomorphine given to patients already receiving neuroleptics, it was impossible to show any augmentation of the antipsychotic action by apomorphine. Even were apomorphine to have an ameliorating effect in schizophrenia, it would not add to present drug treatment.

TABLE 5. Low-dose oral apomorphine in schizophrenia-open and blind studies

Open study	Placebo	Apomorphine	Max. qid Dose (mg)	Concurrent antipsychotics
Br	44	35	7.5	Trifluoperazine, 10 mg/day
Pl	61	50	7.5	Haloperidol, 120 mg/day
Mo	49	45	2.5	Fluphenazine decanoate, 37.5 mg IM q week
We	49	48	5.0	Haloperidol, 20 mg/day
Tr	58	53	5.0	Haloperidol, 40 mg/day
Blind study				
Br	40	42	5.0	Trifluoperazine, 10 mg/day
We	45	40	5.0	Haloperidol, 20 mg/day
Mo	43	49	5.0	Fluphenazine decanoate, 37.5 mg IM weekly
Bo	42	43	5.0	Trifluoperazine, 20 mg/day
Ha	60	53	5.0	Fluphenazine, 20 mg/day
Bol	51	52	5.0	Thiothixene, 60 mg/day
Wa	38	41	5.0	
Fi	43	47	5.0	
Do	40	46	5.0	
Dob	32	34	5.0	Trifluoperazine, 10 mg/day

DISCUSSION

This series of studies dating from 1968 indicates primarily that dopamine agonists can aggravate schizophrenia even in patients being treated with effective doses of neuroleptics. Further, such aggravation can occur without any evidence that the agonist is working postsynaptically to produce either clinical or neuroendocrine effects mediated through dopamine. Thus, one may conclude that dopamine receptors pertinent to schizophrenia may not be as readily blocked with antipsychotic drugs as is desirable.

The idea of selective presynaptic receptor blockade as another approach to treating schizophrenia is of great interest. Our studies failed to confirm the previous reports, but differences in doses, routes of administration and concurrent treatment keep the question open. What may be the case is that even if an ameliorative action is to be had, it will not augment the therapeutic effects of existing antipsychotic drugs.

SUMMARY

Levodopa aggravated psychotic-like behavior and thinking in patients with depression. It was not a practical treatment for this disorder. It also aggravated psychotic-like symptoms in schizophrenics, both at high and at low dose, even in the presence of effective doses of antipsychotic drugs. Apomorphine in high doses given orally aggravated the psychotic symptoms of schizophrenics, even though they continued treatment with previously effective doses of neuroleptics. At low doses, apomorphine failed to augment the beneficial effects of antipsychotic drugs. Attempts to manage schizophrenia by selective blockade of presynaptic dopamine receptors may be difficult, and possibly of limited clinical utility.

Work reported in this chapter was funded by grant MH-03030 and the Research Services of the Veterans Administration. Collaborators in these various studies included Drs. Wendell Lipscomb, John Prusmack, Helena Calil, Shigeyuki Nakano, Kenneth L. Davis and Philip Berger.

REFERENCES

1. Braham, J. and Sarova-Pinhas, I. (1973) Apomorphine in dystonia musculorum deformans. Lancet 1:432-433.
2. Bunney, W.E., Janowsky, D.S., Goodwin, F.K., Davis, J.M., Brodie, H.K.H., Murphy, D.L. and Chase, T.W. (1969) Effect of l-dopa on depression. Lancet 1:885-886.
3. Celesia, G.G. and Barr, A.N. (1970) Psychosis and other psychiatric manifestations of levodopa therapy. Arch. Neurol. 23:193-200.
4. Corsini, G.U., Del Zompo, M., Manconi, S., Cianchetti, C., Mangoni, A. and Gessa, G.L. (1977) Sedative, hypnotic and antipsychotic effects of low doses of apomorphine in man. In: Advances in Biochemical Psychopharmacology, Vol. 16, E. Costa and G.L. Gessa, Eds. pp 645-648, Raven Press, New York.

5. Cotzias, G.C., Mena, I., Papavasiliou, P.S. and Mendez, J. (1974) Unexpected findings with apomorphine and their possible consequences. In: Advances in Neurology, Vol. 5, pp 295-299, Raven Press, New York.

6. Costall, B. and Naylor, R.J. (1973) On the mode of action of apomorphine. Europ. J. Pharmacol. 21:350-361.

7. Duby, S.E., Cotzias, G.C., Papavasiliou, P.S. and Lawrence, W.H. (1972) Injected apomorphine and orally administered levodopa in Parkinsonism. Arch. Neurol. 27:474-480.

8. Gerlach, J. and Luhdorf, K. (1975) The effect of 1-dopa on young patients with simple schizophrenia treated with neuroleptic drugs. Psychopharmacologia 44:105-110.

9. Goodwin, F.K., Brodie, H.K.H., Murphy, D.L. and Bunney, W.E. (1970) Administration of a peripheral decarboxylase inhibitor with 1-dopa to depressed patients. Lancet 1:908-911.

10. Inanaga, K., Nakazawa, Y., Inoue, K., Tachibana, H., Oshima, M., Kotorii, T., Tanaka, M. and Ogawa, N. (1975) Double-blind controlled study of 1-dopa therapy in schizophrenia. Folia Psychiatr. Neurol. Jpn 29:123-143.

11. Tamminga, C.A., Schaffer, M.H., Smith, R.C. and Davis, J.M. (1978) Schizophrenic symptoms improve with apomorphine. Science 200:567-568.

12. Tolosa, E.S. (1974) Paradoxical suppression of chorea by apomorphine. JAMA 229:1579-1580.

13. Yaryura-Tobias, J.A., Diamond, B. and Merlis, S. (1970) The action of 1-dopa on schizophrenic patients: A preliminary report. Curr. Ther. Res. 12:528-531.

Apomorphine and Other Dopaminomimetics,
Vol. 2: Clinical Pharmacology, edited by
G. U. Corsini and G. L. Gessa, Raven Press,
New York © 1981.

Antipsychotic Effect of Apomorphine: A Retrospective Study

M. Del Zompo, G. F. Pitzalis, F. Bernardi, A. Bocchetta,
and G. U. Corsini

Department of Clinical Pharmacology, University of Cagliari, 09100 Cagliari, Italy

Several lines of evidence suggest a relationship between some psychotic states and central dopaminergic hyperactivity (6,20,40,2). It has been suggested that the antipsychotic action of neuroleptics is a consequence of a decrease in central dopaminergic transmission (7,9,19). On the contrary, drugs that enhance dopaminergic activity appear to produce some schizophrenic symptoms in non-psychotic subjects and exacerbate existing schizophrenic symptoms (36). L-DOPA can induce psychoses that can be indistinguishable from schizophrenia in non schizophrenics, and can cause marked exacerbation of symptomatology when administered to schizophrenics (1). More attention has been directed towards amphetamine or amphetamine-like substances such as methylphenidate which also demonstrated to be powerful in inducing psychosis and in activating pre-existing schizophrenic symptomatology (4). However, L-DOPA, amphetamine and methylphenidate clearly affect both dopamine and noradrenaline, although many reports have suggested that these psychotomimetic actions are mediated through the dopaminergic system (39). This is the reason why, in an attempt to explore the hypothesized relationship between dopamine and schizophrenia, many authors examined the clinical effects of drugs that promised to be more specific dopaminergic agonists (2,12,43).

Angrist and Gershon found that oral administration of piribedil caused worsening of psychiatric status in 4 out of 7 schizophrenic patients and induced a paranoid state and a syndrome of auditory hallucinosis in 2 non schizophrenics. However, these effects were far less dramatic than those noted in other studies with amphetamine. On the contrary, acute intravenous piribedil and apomorphine did not show psychotogenic effects. A very high dose of apomorphine (24 mg) has been infused in 1 hour by these authors without observing any stimulant or euphoriant effects (2).

Particularly apomorphine, which is considered to be the most specific stimulant of DA receptors, failed to activate schizophrenic symptoms or to induce psychosis in non schizophrenics (15). There is only one case in literature suggesting its psychotogenic potential which has been reported by Strian (42),however, this patient was a parkinsonian patient, under L-DOPA treatment.

On the contrary, apomorphine has been usefully administered to mental patients for more than 80 years: at the beginning of the century, Douglas described its effectiveness as a sedative (23) and later on,in 1911, Bleuler reported its usefulness either alone or in combination with antimuscarinic agents in the management of various forms of psychosis, including schizophrenia (5). In fact, apomorphine not only does not activate psychotic symptoms but paradoxically seems to ameliorate schizophrenic status. In 1977 we described the effect of an acute administration of non emetic doses of apomorphine in different actively ill psychotic patients (12);we reported that a few minutes after intramuscularly administered apomorphine, some subjects showed a sudden and marked improvement of all the psychotic picture. This effect, even though short lasting and accompanied by other disturbing effects, was time related to the drug action; the patient then returned to his previous mental condition. Subsequently, the antipsychotic effect of apomorphine was further evaluated in a double blind study, however, due to the multiple side effects induced by the drug, even at lower doses, we were doubtful as to the complete blindness both of the psychiatrist and of the patient. Double blind studies however, have been performed by Tamminga et al.(43) and other investigators (38), using video tape techniques, and similar findings in chronic schizophrenics have been reported.

In order to clarify some aspects of this action of apomorphine, we re-evaluated a selected number of patients who had been treated with the drug during the first trial. Each of these patients, selected on the basis of a well documented response to the apomorphine administration (either positive or negative), as appeared from their clinical records, was re-interviewed and complete anamnestical data and the long term outcome were investigated under blind conditions. In the present study we also re-evaluated the diagnosis of these patients by applying the criteria of Spitzer et al.(41). Unlike previous findings, the data obtained are consistent with the fact that schizoaffective patients of manic type, rather than schizophrenics, are mostly affected by the antipsychotic effect of apomorphine.

Materials and Methods

Among the psychotic patients who had had apomorphine administration (apomorphine test) in the first trial in 1975, we selected those cases whose clinical records with anamnestical data and a complete description of the psychic changes induced by apomorphine administration (including Brief Psychiatric Scale scores before and after the treatment), were available. Only those patients who showed an improvement of more than 75% according to the BPRS scores (Responders) or no improvement (Non responders) were selected. The cases which met these criteria were 18, seventeen females and one male, aged from 18 to 47 years. 9 patients were evaluated as apomorphine "responders" and 9 as "non responders". All cases were rediagnosed according to the criteria of Spitzer et al.(41) under blind conditions and the anamnestical data at the time of apomorphine administration were re-evaluated. All these patients, and some relatives as well, were recontacted and interviewed at our Institute. Each patient was evaluated for psychiatric, occupational, marital and residential status according to the criteria of Tsuang et al.(45).

Results

The mean age at the time of apomorphine administration was 28.77 years for responders and 30.77 for non responders (Tab.1), being the difference between the two groups not statistically significant. Similarly, the mean age of these two groups of patients at the onset of the disease was not significantly different (Tab.1). These data indicate that the antipsychotic effect of apomorphine is not related to age of patients or onset of the disease.

TABLE 1

APOMORPHINE TEST (N° OF PATIENTS)	AGE AT ONSET OF DISEASE (YRS) (MEAN ± SD)	AGE AT TIME OF TEST (YRS) (MEAN ± SD)
RESPONDERS (9)	26.87 ± 6.7	28.77 ± 4.9
NON RESPONDERS (9)	25.00 ± 8.7	30.77 ± 5.5
t-test	ns	ns

Furthermore, if the number of psychotic episodes sustained by each patient before apomorphine administration is considered, no significant difference was observed between the two groups (2.5 versus 3.4) (Tab.2). On the contrary, the mean duration of these episodes is slightly longer for non responders (2.6 months) than for responders (1.5 months) (Tab.2).

TABLE 2

APOMORPHINE TEST (N° of PATIENTS)	N° OF EPISODES BEFORE TEST	DURATION OF EPISODES (mths)
	mean ± SD	mean ± SD
RESPONDERS (9)	2.5 ± 0.7	1.5 ± 0.4
NON RESPONDERS (9)	3.4 ± 0.9	2.6 ± 0.6
t-test	ns	ns

When we considered the side effects induced by apomorphine in our patients, we evaluated the variable appearance of nausea, vomiting, sweating, yawning, sedation and sleep in the two groups (Tab.3). However, short lasting sleep episodes which began 30-40 mins. after drug administration were described in 7 out of the 9 responders, and in only one of the non responders. This difference between the two groups suggests that apomorphine-induced sleep might be related to its antipsychotic action. It is noteworthy that long lasting episodes of sound sleep induced by apomorphine were observed in agitated manic patients, in young subjects or in patients under barbiturate treatment (21).

TABLE 3

SIDE EFFECTS INDUCED BY APOMORPHINE		
	RESPONDERS (N°pt/9)	NON RESPONDERS (N°pt/9)
Nausea	2	2
Vomiting	1	1
Sweating	2	1
Yawning	5	6
Sedation	4	3
Sleep	7	1

Unexpectedly, and partially in contrast with our previous findings (12), by re-evaluating the diagnoses of our patients under blind conditions with more selective criteria , we found quite evident difference of diagnoses between the two groups. The diagnostic criteria we used

revealed that 7 out of the 9 responders were classified as suffering
from schizoaffective disorders of the manic type. Two patients were
classified as schizophrenics (one paranoid and one disorganized)(Tab.4)

TABLE 4

	APOMORPHINE RESPONDERS		
PTS	EPISODE DIAGNOSIS	PTS	EPISODE DIAGNOSIS
1	Schizoaffective D. (manic type)	6	Schizoaffective D. (manic type)
2	Schizoaffective D. (manic type)	7	Schizoaffective D. (manic type)
3	Schizoaffective D. (manic type)	8	Schizophrenia (paranoid)
4	Schizoaffective D. (manic type)	9	Schizophrenia (disorganized)
5	Schizoaffective D. (manic type)		

ACCORDING TO SPITZER ET AL. - R.D.C., 1977

On the contrary, 8 out of the 9 non responders were judged as schizophrenics (five paranoids and three disorganized) and one was evaluated
as a schizoaffective patient of the depressed type (Tab.5). This evidence strongly suggests that mainly schizoaffective patients (manic type),
rather than schizophrenics, are sensitive to the antipsychotic effect
of apomorphine. The presence of a schizoaffective patient of depressed
type in the group of non responders suggests that apomorphine may act
mainly during manic episodes.

The long term outcome of the psychiatric symptoms and also the occupational status of our patients, proved to be in agreement with the diagnostic evaluation. In fact, most of the responders had a "good" occupational status (7 patients); on the contrary, 5 out of the 9 non responders had a "poor" occupational situation and only 3 patients of this
group were classified as having a "good" status (Fig.1).The psychiatric
conditions of 6 responders were judged as "good" while only one patient
in the group of non responders had this positive evaluation (fig.1).The
assessment also of the "residential" and "marital" status in our patients, revealed a difference, even though not marked, between the two
groups, further indicating a better social outcome for responders in
relation to non responders. Consistent with these data is the fact that
neuroleptic medication represented the prevailing treatment in both

TABLE 5

APOMORPHINE NON RESPONDERS

PTS	EPISODE DIAGNOSIS	PTS	EPISODE DIAGNOSIS
1	Schizoaffective (depressed type)	6	Schizophrenia (paranoid)
2	Schizophrenia (paranoid)	7	Schizophrenia (disorganized)
3	Schizophrenia (paranoid)	8	Schizophrenia (disorganized)
4	Schizophrenia (paranoid)	9	Schizophrenia (disorganized)
5	Schizophrenia (paranoid)		

ACCORDING TO SPITZER ET AL. - R.D.C., 1977

groups, but 7 out of the 9 responders were under lithium therapy, and in none of these patients was the lithium therapy withdrawn (Tab.6). On the contrary, none of the non responders was under lithium therapy, although in 2 of them, lithium was administered, but only for a short period.

DISCUSSION

Paradoxically, apomorphine, a specific stimulant of dopamine receptors, not only is devoid of psychotomimetic properties, but even exerts an antipsychotic action. Because of its short lasting effect, it is obviously difficult to define this action in terms of evaluating which symptoms are selectively improved and how much. Furthermore, this phenomenon cannot be easily accepted without some scepticism since we are not accustomed to observing such a sudden switch into normality by a psychotic patient and it may appear unreasonable that all symptoms of a chronic mental disease could cease in a few minutes. However, it is known that few milligrams of apomorphine make an incapacitated parkinsonian patient able to walk and move normally in a very short time, thus releasing him from the symptoms of such a chronic and progressive illness (35,18,11). It is quite amazing to observe this phenomenon for the first time and if it were not so clear it would give rise to some scepticism.

Figure 1

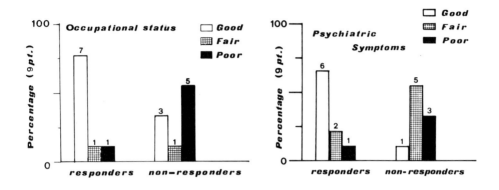

Further, the same low dosage of apomorphine abruptly reduces the abnormal involuntary movements of patients affected by Huntington's Chorea, a chronic and progressive disease (13), and this effect also is usually observed with surprise. Actually, a decrease of rigidity and tremor or a reduction of movements can be easily evaluated by means of different apparatus (13).On the contrary, different problems make the psychometric evaluation of apomorphine-induced psychic changes, difficult and complex. The short time of drug action does not allow the proper assessment of all symptoms in order to meet all the requirements of a fixed rating scale and often for some behavioural evaluations, a quite lengthy period of observation is necessary. Further, the presence of multiple side effects, besides interfering with the psychiatric interview, complicates considerably the possibility of carrying out a double blind study. For this reason, it may be necessary to use an "active" placebo as a control treatment that might simulate most of the behavioural changes usually elicited by apomorphine. Among these changes, sedation is the most interfering effect that may give rise to wrong evaluations, especially in agitated patients, such as manics, whose decrease in motor activity, induced by apomorphine, remarkably improves the entire pathological feature, but does not necessarily imply that the drug exerts an antipsychotic effect.

This is the main reason why a more appropriate evaluation of the antipsychotic effect of apomorphine was performed on those mental patients who showed marked formal thought disorders with multiple delusions

TABLE 6

APOMORPHINE TEST (N° of PATIENTS)	UNDER LITHIUM THERAPY AT PRESENT	WITHDRAWAL OF LITHIUM THERAPY
	N° of PTS	N° of PTS
RESPONDERS (9)	7	0
NON RESPONDERS (9)	0	2

and hallucinations. In fact, in these patients, despite the sedation induced by apomorphine, a complete disappearance of their symptoms, along with a conceptual and intellectual re-organization was easily evaluated. In order to prevent sedation and other disturbing effects as well, such as nausea and hypotension, we recently administered domperidone, a dopamine receptor blocker which does not enter into the brain (29),in combination with apomorphine (14,16). Domperidone pretreatment antagonizes most of the side effects induced by apomorphine (phase of the vegetative changes),but does not interfere with its antipsychotic action (17). All these problems may account for the discrepancy actually present in the literature concerning the kind of patients improved by apomorphine administration. As reported above, we found that patients with schizoaffective disorders of manic type, rather than pure schizophrenics, were positively affected by this drug. Further, our patients were not under neuroleptic treatment when apomorphine was administered. In fact, we observed that neuroleptic medication abolished almost completely all apomorphine-induced effects in these patients (12).On the contrary, the data reported by Tamminga and coworkers (43) indicate that apomorphine improves mostly chronic schizophrenics.Furthermore, these patients, when tested with apomorphine, were all under neuroleptic medication. Similar findings were subsequently obtained by these authors with N-n-propylnorapomorphine, a more potent analogue of apomorphine (44).

These conflicting data cannot be ascribed to the diagnostic criteria applied since, in both studies, the patients were classified according to the criteria of Spitzer et al.(41). One might speculate that two completely different phenomena induced by apomorphine were actually observed. The improvement of mental conditions described by Tamminga in chronic schizophrenics under neuroleptic medication might be similar to that observed after L-DOPA treatment.In fact, there have been several reports of positive therapeutic effects of L-DOPA on schizophrenic patients.

These reports, based on uncontrolled (46,31) and controlled (24,27,25) studies, deal with the positive therapeutic effects, especially in the areas of communication and rapport, when L-DOPA was added to neuroleptic treatment. On the contrary, our data are consistent with the hypothesis that apomorphine acts primarily as an antimanic agent. In fact, we further observed that one of our schizoaffective patients, who, during a manic episode, showed a marked improvement by apomorphine, in a subsequent episode, but of the depressive type, failed to have any beneficial effect from the drug The social, psychiatric, marital and residential status of the patients who showed a positive response from apomorphine administration, further strengthened the concept that these subjects were affected by schizoaffective disorders. In agreement with these results is the finding that most of these patients were under lithium therapy with a good outcome. This result may be of particular interest since apomorphine administration might provide a predictive indication for lithium therapy. Nevertheless, if one considers the difficulty of diagnosing schizoaffective patients during their first episodes, it is reasonable to suggest that apomorphine administration might represent a useful diagnostic tool.

However, there is much disagreement about the concept of the schizoaffective psychosis, which actually represents a nosological enigma. In fact, different authors suggested that schizoaffective psychosis is a heterogenous entity including different pathological states (34). Once, this entity was considered as a subtype of schizophrenia (28), but more recently, it has been listed, at least for the manic type, among affective disorders (32). Considering the fact that clinical, genetic, prognostic and therapeutic aspects of this psychosis have a definite relationship with the major affective disorders. It is conceivable therefore, that this effect of apomorphine, observed in our patients, might be primarily related to an antimanic action of the drug. Actually, the antimanic properties of apomorphine were described in our previous study (12), however, for the reasons presented above, it was extremely difficult to assess an antipsychotic action on pure manic patients, also because , as already described, these patients frequently show marked sleep episodes after apomorphine, thus limiting a proper psychiatric interview. Consistently, other dopaminergic agonists such as piribedil, were described as having antimanic activities at relatively low doses(33). These data provide some support for the concept that dopaminergic mechanisms are involved in manic illness.

In agreement with a current view on the mechanism of action of dopamine agonists administered at relatively low doses both in animals and humans (8,17,22), the antimanic effect of apomorphine might be due to a direct stimulation of the so called "self-inhibitory" dopamine receptors (autoreceptors or presynaptic dopamine receptors) whose activation decreases firing rate and dopamine turnover of the dopaminergic neurons themselves (8,22). Gessa et al.(26,37) reported evidence that chronic tricyclic administration in rats, is associated with an attenuated decrease in sedation and dopamine turnover following apomorphine challenge. These data are consistent with the concept that self-inhibitory dopamine receptors involved in the regulation of tyrosine hydroxylase and dopamine turnover may be desensitized during the course of chronic tricyclic antidepressant treatment.

These biochemical findings, recently confirmed by single unit studies (10) and by ^{3}H-apomorphine binding studies (30),suggest the importance of self-inhibitory dopamine receptors in regulating switch processes in affective illness.

REFERENCES

1. Angrist,B.M.,Sathananthan,G.,Gershon,S.(1973): Psychopharmacologia, 31:1-12.

2. Angrist,B.M.,Thompson,H.,Shopsin,B.,Gershon,S.(1975): Psychopharma-cologia, 44:273-280.

3. Baldessarini,R.J.(1977): New.Engl.J.Med., 297:988-995.

4. Bell,D.S.(1965): Brit.J.Psychiat., 111:701-707.

5. Bleuler,E.(1911): In: Dementia praecox or the group of schizo-phrenias, translated by J.Zinkin and D.C.Lewis,p.486,Int.Univ.Press New York,1950.

6. Bowers,M.B.(1974): Arch.Gen.Psychiat., 31:50-54.

7. Bunney,B.S.,Walters,J.R.,Roth,R.H. et al.(1973): J.Pharmacol.Exp. Ther., 185:560-571.

8. Carlsson,A.(1975): In: Receptor-mediated control of dopamine metabolism., edited by E.Usdin and W.E.Bunney Jr, pp.49-65, Marcel Dekker,New York.

9. Carlsson,A.(1978): Am.J.Psychiat., 135: 164-173.

10. Chiodo,L.A.,Antelman,S.M.(1980): Science, 210: 799-801.

11. Corsini,G.U.,Del Zompo,M.,Cianchetti,C.,Mangoni,A.,Gessa,G.L.(1976) :Psychopharmacologia, 47: 169-173.

12. Corsini,G.U.,Del Zompo,M.,Manconi,S.,Cianchetti,C.,Mangoni,A,Gessa, G.L.(1977): In: Advances in Biochemical Psychopharmacology, edited by E.Costa and G.L.Gessa, 16:pp.645-648,Raven Press,New York.

13. Corsini,G.U.,Onali,P.L.,Masala,C.,Cianchetti,C.,Mangoni,A.,Gessa, G.L.(1978): Arch.Neurol., 35:27-30.

14. Corsini,G.U.,Del Zompo,M.,Gessa,G.L.,Mangoni,A.(1979): Lancet, 8123:954-956.

15. Corsini,G.U.,Bernardi,F.,Marrosu,F.,Gessa,G.L.(1980): In: Neuro chemistry and Clinical Neurology, edited by L.Battistin and G. Hashim,A.Lajtha,pp.225-237,Alan Liss inc.,New York.

16. Corsini,G.U.,Burrai,C.,Toccafondi,F.,Del Zompo,M.,Gessa,G.L.(1981): Neurology,: submitted for publication.

17. Corsini,G.U.,Piccardi,M.P.,Bocchetta,A.,Bernardi,F.,Del Zompo,M. :This volume.

18. Cotzias,G.C.,Papavasiliou,P.S.,Fehling,C.,Kaufman,B.,Mena,I.(1970): New.Engl.J.Med., 282: 31-33.

19. Creese,I.,Burt,D.R.,Snyder,S.H.(1975): Life Sci., 17:993-1002.

20; Crow,T.J.,Deakin,J.F.W.,Johnston,E.C.et al.(1976): Lancet, ii: 563-566.

21. Del Zompo,M.,Piccardi,M.P.,Tocco,F.,Scano,M.L.,Corsini,G.U.(1979): Riv.Farm.Ter., 10: 61-72.

22. Di Chiara,G.,Corsini,G.U.,Mereu,G.P.,Tissari,A.,Gessa,G.L.(1978): In: Advances in Biochemical Psychopharmacology, edited by P.J. Roberts,G.N.Woodruff and L.L.Iversen,19:pp.275-293,Raven Press, New York.

23. Douglas,C.J.(1900): Merck's Arch.,2:212-213.

24. Fleming,P.,Makar,H.,Hunter,K.R.(1970): Lancet, ii: 1186.

25. Gerlach,J.,Luhdorf,K.(1975): Psychopharmacologia, 44:105-110.

26. Gessa,G.L.,Serra,G.,Argiolas,A.: This volume

27. Inanaga,K,Nakazawa,Y.,Inoue,K.,et al.(1975): Folia Psychiatr.Neurol Jpn., 29: 123-143.

28. Kolb,L.C.(1973): Modern Clinical Psychiatry, ed.8., W.B.Saunders & Co,Philadelphia.

29. Laduron,P.M.,Leysen,J.E.(1979): Biochem.Pharmacol., 2: 2161-2165.

30. Muller,P.,Seeman,P.(1979): Eur.J.Pharmacol., 55: 149-157.

31. Ogura,C.,Kishimoto,A.,Nakao,T.(1976): Curr.Ther.Res.,20:308-318.

32. Pope,H.G.Jr,Lipinski,J.F.,Cohen,B.M.,Axelrod,D.T.(1980): Am.J. Psychiat., 137: 921-927.

33. Post,R.M.,Gencer,R.H.,Carman,S.J.(1976): Lancet, 24:203-204.

34. Procci,W.R.(1976): Arch.Gen.Psychiat., 33: 1167-1178.

35. Schwab,R.S.,Amador,L.V.,Lettvin,J.Y.(1951): Trans.Amer.Neurol.Ass., 76: 251-253.

36. Segal,D.S.,Janowsky,D.S.(1978):In: Psychopharmacology: a generation of progress, edited by M.A.Lipton,A.Di Mascio,K.F. Killan,pp.1113-1123,Raven Press,New York.

37. Serra,G.,Argiolas,A.,Klimek,V.,Fadda,F.,Gessa,G.L.(1979): Life Sci. 25:415-424.

38. Smith,R.C.,Tamminga,C.A.,Davis,J.M.(1977): J.Neural Trans., 40: 171-176.

39. Snyder,S.H.(1972): Arch.Gen.Psychiat., 27:169-179.

40. Snyder,S.H.(1976): Am.J.Psychiat., 133:197-202.

41. Spitzer,R.L.,Endicott,J.,Robins,E.(1977): Research Diagnostic Criteria (RDC) for a selected group of functional disorders, 3rd Edit,New York State Psychiatric Institute,Biometrics research,N.Y.

42. Strian,F.,Micheler,E.,Benkert,O.(1972): Pharmacopsychiatry, 5: 198-205.

43. Tamminga,C.A.,Schaffer,M.H.,Smith,R.C.,Davis,J.M.(1978): Science, 200: 567-568.

44. Tamminga,C.A.,De Fraites,E.G.,Gotts,M.A.,Chase,T.N.:This volume.

45. Tsuang,M.P.,Woolson,R.F.,Fleming,J.A.(1979): Arch.Gen.Psychiat., 36: 1295-1301.

46. Yaryura-Tobias,J.A.,Diamond,B.,Merlis,S.(1970): Curr.Ther.Res., 12: 528-531.

*Apomorphine and Other Dopaminomimetics,
Vol. 2: Clinical Pharmacology,* edited by
G.U. Corsini and G.L. Gessa, Raven Press,
New York © 1981.

Dopamine Agonists in Affective Illness: Implications for Underlying Receptor Mechanisms

Robert M. Post, Neal R. Cutler, David C. Jimerson,
and William E. Bunney, Jr.

*Section on Psychobiology, Biological Psychiatry Branch, National Institute of Mental Health,
Bethesda, Maryland 20205*

Introduction

Pharmacological data as well as direct measurement of dopamine metabolites in cerebrospinal fluid of affectively ill patients provide some support for the concept that dopaminergic mechanisms are involved in manic-depressive illness. Randrup et al. (64), reviewing the literature on effects of neuroleptics in mania as well as in agitated and psychotic depression, suggested the involvement of dopamine in affective illness. These data and formulations are now supported by several clinical trials of dopamine agonists in affective illness (25,57,70), in addition to a rapidly growing literature regarding the possible alterations of presynaptic dopaminergic autoreceptors in the mechanism of action of antidepressant treatments including the tricyclic antidepressants, monoamine oxidase inhibitors, and electroconvulsive therapy (8,9,27,69). In approximately one half of the studies utilizing baseline cerebrospinal fluid levels of the dopamine metabolite homovanillic acid (HVA) or its accumulation following probenecid, values in depressed patients were significantly lower than those in normal and neurological controls (60). Although values in the manic phase generally were not higher than those in controls, they tended to be significantly elevated compared to the depressed phase of the illness. Moreover HVA accumulations following probenecid were significantly higher in manic patients treated with neuroleptics than in non-manic patients receiving similar doses of either pimozide or the more routine neuroleptics thioridazine and chlorpromazine (61). While not unambiguous, these data provide some indirect support for the idea that dopamine metabolism may be altered in affective illness.

Piribedil in Depression: Evidence for Receptor Effects

Gessa and associates (27,69) reported evidence that chronic tricyclic administration is associated with an attenuated decrease in HVA following apomorphine challenge. These findings are compatible with the notion that presynaptic dopamine autoreceptors involved in the regulation of tyrosine hydroxylase and dopamine turnover may be desensitized during the course of chronic tricyclic antidepressant treatment with the typical tricyclics as well as the atypical compounds such as iprindole. These investigators also noted similar findings following treatment with monoamine oxidase inhibitors and electroconvulsive treatment. These results are also consistent with the findings of Modigh and associates (44), as well as Green and associates (29) and Evans et al. (21), of increased responsivity to dopamine active agents following repeated electroconvulsive treatment in rats. Single unit studies of Chiodo and Antelman (8-10) have recently extended these biochemical findings. These investigators reported that following treatment with a variety of antidepressant modalities, including tricyclic antidepressants, monoamine oxidase inhibitors, and electroconvulsive shock, there was an attenuated inhibitory response of single dopamine neurons to a systemic challenge with low doses of apomorphine. Moreover, Chiodo and Antelman suggest that there is a progressive development of dopaminergic autoreceptor subsensitivity that evolves over time following initial treatments whether or not chronic treatment is maintained. They suggest that relatively acute treatment with tricyclic antidepressants or electroconvulsive therapy might in itself be sufficient to initiate biochemical changes that result in the later emergence of antidepressant effects.

We wish to reconsider the antidepressant effects of the dopamine agonist piribedil in light of these new postulated mechanisms involving desensitization of dopaminergic autoreceptors based on biochemical and electrophysiological data in the laboratory. We have treated 17 depressed patients with the putative dopamine agonist piribedil (ET-495). While a considerable body of evidence supports the notion that piribedil is a dopamine receptor agonist (13,14,16,23) some investigators have suggested that piribedil's activating effects on behavior are mediated through antagonism of dopaminergic inhibitory receptors (12) or by acting as an antagonist of the DA_1 (adenylate cyclase dependent) dopamine receptor (47). In addition to its effects on dopaminergic receptors, several investigators have reported that piribedil, particularly in high doses, can also affect noradrenergic metabolism (23, 24,33). Thus, much remains to be clarified regarding the specificity of piribedil's effects on dopaminergic receptors as well as precisely which class of dopamine receptors are involved in the mediation of piribedil's behavioral and biochemical effects in animals and man. It does appear, however, that piribedil shares many actions with those of other dopaminergic agonist compounds and, importantly, inhibits the firing of dopaminergic neurons when iontophoresed directly on presumed dopamine autoreceptors (77). These data, taken in conjunction with the findings that piribedil is of some utility in the treatment of parkinsonism (6,22,41,42,66,71) and decreases CSF accumulations of HVA in parkinsonian (7) and depressed patients (57), supports the notion that piribedil possesses dopaminergic agonist properties sufficient for some inferences to be drawn from clinical trials in affectively ill patients regarding dopaminergic mechanisms.

As illustrated in Fig. 1, 12 of 16 patients showed some improvement during treatment with moderate doses of piribedil (range 100 to 200 mg per day) for an average of approximately five weeks duration. Following double-blind placebo discontinuation of the drug, several patients showed mild relapses in depressive symptomatology while several

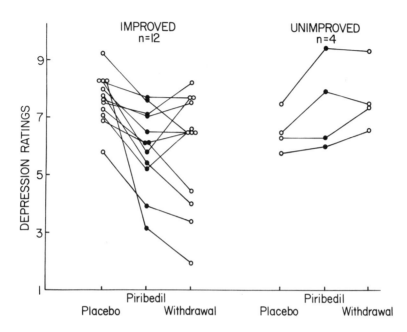

EFFECTS OF PIRIBEDIL ON DEPRESSED PATIENTS

other patients continued to show notable clinical improvement of sufficient magnitude that discharge planning could be begun and further
pharmacological intervention on an acute basis was no longer necessary.
As discussed in more detail elsewhere (57,58), several of these patients had previously been nonresponsive to more routine antidepressant
modalities prior to their double-blind clinical trial with piribedil.
Two patients illustrated in the figure showed little change or slight
worsening during piribedil administration, while two patients showed
exacerbation of symptomatology. One experienced prominent dysphoric
activation, increased anger and sexual interest during treatment with
piribedil, while the other showed worsening of agitated psychotic
depressive symptomatology. An additional patient, discussed in detail
elsewhere (26), during treatment with piribedil developed rapid cycling
manic episodes which persisted following the double-blind discontinuation of the drug and which partially responded to institution of the
dopamine receptor antagonist pimozide.

In light of the positive effects of indirect and direct dopamine
agonists on motor function in parkinsonian patients, we were interested
in whether improvement in our depressed patients was occurring initially or solely in the motor sphere rather than in other components of the
depressive syndrome. As illustrated in Fig. 2, in a patient with only
a mild to moderate response to piribedil as assessed by blind global
nurses' ratings in Fig. 1, most of the components of the depressive
syndrome appeared to respond positively to treatment with piribedil.
These data supported our clinical impression that in patients who im-

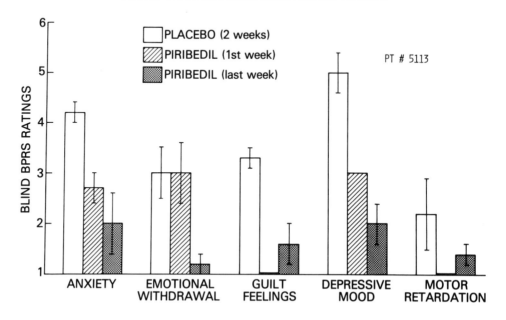

PIRIBEDIL-INDUCED IMPROVEMENT IN DIFFERENT SYMPTOM AREAS IN AN INDIVIDUAL DEPRESSED PATIENT

proved, change did not occur solely in the motor sphere, but also included depressive mood, anxiety, and other symptoms, as rated by nurses on the BPRS.

Our clinical data are consistent with those of several other investigators suggesting that dopaminergic agonists may be useful in the treatment of some patients with depressive symptomatology. Shopsin and Gershon (70) reported initial improvement in depression in seven patients treated with piribedil, although they noted relatively uniform dysphoric activation as the patients continued their clinical trial and the dose of piribedil was increased. Gerlach et al. (25) have found positive effects on depressive mood in a large series of patients treated with the ergot dopamine agonist bromocriptine. It is also of interest that van Praag and Korf (75) reported that L-DOPA improved depression in retarded patients with low HVA in cerebrospinal fluid. In this regard it is noteworthy that Van Scheyen (76) found that those with lower HVA in cisternal fluid responded best to an antidepressant trial with nomifensine. A similar inverse relationship between pre-treatment HVA accumulations following probenecid administration and degree of antidepressant response was noted in our patients with piribedil (57).

The doses of piribedil which were associated with improvement in the majority of depressed patients studied were sufficient to decrease HVA accumulations in cerebrospinal fluid (Fig. 3), as well as CSF prolactin (Fig. 4) (34). As illustrated in Fig. 5, an oral dose of 100

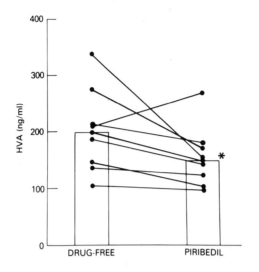

PIRIBEDIL-INDUCED DECREASE IN HVA ACCUMULATIONS IN CSF

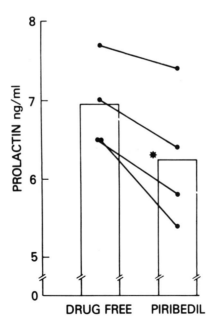

EFFECTS OF PIRIBEDIL ON PROLACTIN IN CSF

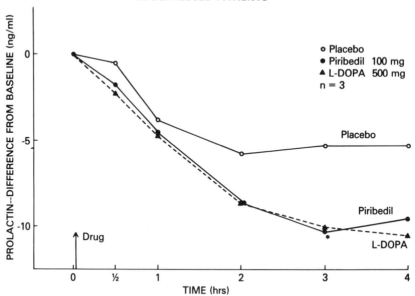

mg of piribedil produced serum prolactin decreases of equal magnitude
to 500 mg of L-DOPA. However, when nine depressed patients were administered apomorphine (0.75 mg subcutaneously) before and during chronic
piribedil administration, no significant effect of chronic piribedil
treatment on plasma prolactin was noted (35). These findings of the
lack of effect of chronic treatment with piribedil on basal plasma
prolactin or decreases following apomorphine are subject to several
possible interpretations. Although one might have expected chronic
dopaminergic agonist treatment to desensitize dopamine receptors and
lead to a decreased prolactin response to apomorphine, it is possible
that tolerance developed to this effect, similar to that demonstrated
for tolerance development to HVA increases in animals and patients
maintained on chronic neuroleptics (55). It is also possible that the
regulation of plasma prolactin which presumably occurs at the pituitary
level, does not reflect mechanisms occurring in the central nervous
system and particularly in the striatum. Considerable evidence supports the notion of a differential time course and/or effect of psychotropic agents on striatal versus pituitary dopaminergic function (53).
Further, the lack of effect of chronic piribedil treatment on apomorphine-induced prolactin suppression would be consistent with the formulations of Cools and van Rossum (12) and Offermeier and van Rooyen (47)
that piribedil and apomorphine are acting at different dopaminergic
receptor sites.
    Although there was no direct endocrine evidence of desensitization
of dopaminergic autoreceptors during chronic treatment with piribedil,

our clinical findings of improvement in depressed patients treated with this dopamine agonist are not inconsistent with the formulations of Serra et al. (69), Gessa et al. (27), and Chiodo and Antelman (8,9) suggesting that desensitization of autoreceptors initiated by a variety of antidepressant treatment modalities would indirectly lead to increased dopaminergic function. It is possible that chronic treatment with moderate doses of a direct acting dopamine agonist such as piribedil or bromocriptine could similarly desensitize presynaptic autoreceptors, especially since recent data suggest that these receptors have an increased sensitivity to agonists compared to postsynaptic receptors (28). It is also possible that piribedil and bromocriptine are effective in depression because of actions directly at postsynaptic receptors when administered at sufficiently high doses. Further basic and clinical investigation is required to separate these and other alternatives regarding the possible specific site or sites of action of these putative dopamine agonists in relation to their effects on affective symptomatology. To the extent that agents such as piribedil and bromocriptine are acting through dopaminergic mechanisms, these preliminary clinical trials do support the notion of involvement of dopaminergic mechanisms in at least some symptom components of affective illness.

Apomorphine: Endocrine and Diurnal Effects on Hypothermia

In an effort to assess dopaminergic receptor function in affectively ill patients compared to controls, apomorphine (0.75 mg subcutaneous) was administered to medication-free patients and normal volunteers so that hypothermic, behavioral, and endocrine responses could be compared. Cutler et al. (17) reported that in male subjects and in depressed post-menopausal females, significant decreases in apomorphine hypothermia were noted at 9:00 p.m., but not at 9:00 a.m. (Fig. 6). These data suggested differences in dopaminergic responsivity occurring diurnally, as assessed by hypothermic response to apomorphine. Other measures of behavioral response, as well as side-effects such as shivering and nausea, were not significantly different at the p.m. compared to a.m. time points.

In male depressed patients studied at 9:00 a.m., significantly greater apomorphine-induced decreases in prolactin (but not increases in growth hormone) were noted compared with male normal volunteer subjects (35). These data further support possible alterations in dopaminergic receptor function in affective illness and paradoxically suggest increases in dopamine receptor response in at least some phases of depressive illness as measured by this peripheral neuroendocrine indice. Again, it is possible that alterations in prolactin response are not correlated with dopaminergic receptor function in other areas of brain (Fig. 7), but these data raise the possibility that at least peripheral dopaminergic receptors might be hyper-responsive in male depressed patients compared to normal control subjects.

These findings are also of interest in relation to postulated dopamine receptor changes that could occur during the course of a prolonged depressive episode where postulated decreases in dopaminergic neurotransmitter function could lead to a secondary or compensatory increase in receptor sensitivity, leading to an increased vulnerability to a switch into mania, as postulated by bunney and associates (5). These findings of altered prolactin responsivity in depressed patients are consistent with those of Asnis et al. (1) and may be usefully

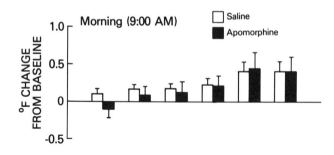

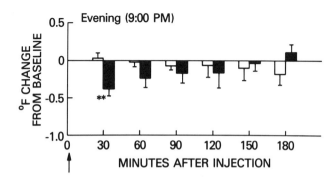

considered in light of our findings of the occurrence of state-dependent tardive dyskinesia.

State-Dependent Tardive Dyskinesia

We have recently reported the observations that depressed patients with rapidly cycling manic-depressive illness show marked exacerbation of tardive dyskinesia during depressive phases and notable remissions with the onset of each manic episode (18). Ratings of dyskinesia were performed on the involuntary movements rating scale during both depressed and manic episodes, as rated independently by nursing observers. As illustrated in Fig. 8, in a patient studied during a medication-free interval, there were marked increases in severity of rated dyskinesias occurring with each depressive period (shaded area), as characterized by increased severity of depression ratings and absence of mania ratings. Following each manic episode, dyskinesias disappeared or were attenuated.

These findings would appear inconsistent with conventional theories of tardive dyskinesia and affective illness. That is, dopaminergic receptor supersensitivity has been the postulated mechanism for tardive dyskinesia developing in the late phases of neuroleptic administration (11,50) and upon neuroleptic withdrawal (72). If dopaminergic excesses which have been postulated to occur during mania were interacting with hypothetically supersensitive dopamine receptors based on

⑦

INDICES OF BRAIN
DOPAMINERGIC RECEPTOR FUNCTION

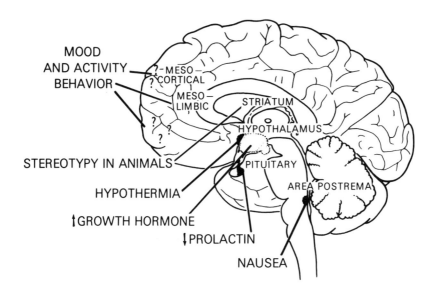

previous chronic neuroleptic administration, one might expect an exacerbation of tardive dyskinesia during the manic phase of the illness, which was opposite to that repeatedly observed in our case studies. Thus, these observations of state-dependent dyskinesia, if supported in larger patient populations, might suggest that theories of dopaminergic alterations in affective illness and/or tardive dyskinesia may require modification. As indicated above, it is possible that depressed patients during some phase of their illness may have increased dopamine receptor responsivity. It is possible that this could develop secondary to the postulated decreases in dopaminergic function, as reflected in many studies of low HVA in cerebrospinal fluid of depressed patients, or it is conceivable that such decreases in HVA are themselves secondary to a primary increase in receptor sensitivity. Whatever the ultimate mechanism, these findings of state-dependent tardive dyskinesia do appear to suggest the utility of exploring alternative neurotransmitter substances and neurotransmitter mechanisms underlying the occurrence of tardive dyskinesia and/or affective illness.

It would also appear, however, that these findings of marked exacerbation and remission of a neurological syndrome such as tardive dyskinesia occurring in close association with affective disturbances, adds further evidence for a biological dysfunction occurring during manic and depressive phases of the illness. We are cognizant of the fact that classical descriptions of oral-buccal-lingual dyskinesias were reported by Kraepelin (40) and de Fursac (20) in the pre-neuroleptic era, and that Tepper and Haas (74) have recently reviewed the literature on the occurrence of spontaneous dyskinesias in patients without a history of prior neuroleptic administration. Both of the

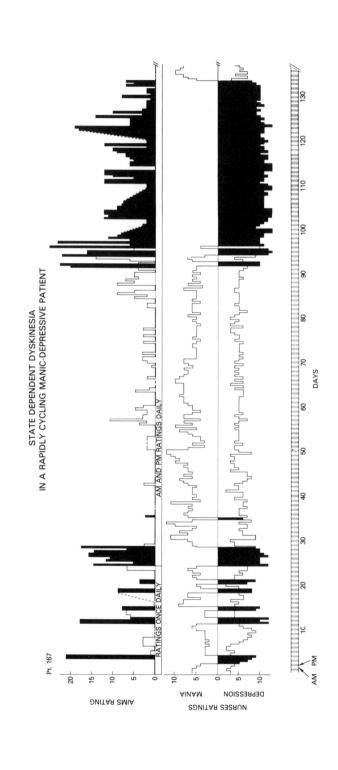

STATE DEPENDENT DYSKINESIA
IN A RAPIDLY CYCLING MANIC-DEPRESSIVE PATIENT

patients included in our study had received several thousand grams of chlorpromazine equivalents and thus were at high risk for the development of tardive dyskinesia. Nevertheless, even if the dyskinesias were not neuroleptic related and were of the "spontaneous" variety (74), their notable recurrence during depressive phases and essential disappearance during mania would still support the notion of a biochemical disturbance occurring differentially in mania and depression of sufficient magnitude to affect these oral-buccal-lingual dyskinesias.

Dopamine Agonist and Psychomotor Stimulant Behavioral Sensitizaton: Relationship to Affective Illness

A variety of data support the concept that repeated administration of psychomotor stimulants (36,37,56,68) and direct (43,46) and indirect (38) dopamine agonists may result in increases in some behavioral parameters rather than tolerance. In particular, a number of studies have documented increases in either locomotor or hyperactivity or in stereotypy following repeated, intermittent (54) administration of these substances.

These findings are of interest in relation to the suggestion that presynaptic receptor desensitization may also account for this progressive behavioral augmentation. Schwartz et al. (67) and Martres et al. (43) suggest on the basis of pharmacological data that the increasing severity of apomorphine-induced stereotypic climbing in mice might result from presynaptic receptor desensitization following repeated administration. Chiodo and Antelman (10) have also recently reported electrophysiological data based on recordings from dopaminergic neurons that psychomotor stimulants such as amphetamine not only result in a less prominent inhibitory response to apomorphine, but some dopaminergic neurons show a switch from inhibition to activation following this pretreatment. Muller et al. (45) also provide biochemical data consistent with such a formulation and note that decreases in ^{3}H-apomorphine binding occurred under conditions designed to maximally assess dopaminergic autoreceptor binding activity. Moreover, several other investigators have reported paradoxical increases in tritiated agonist or antagonist binding following acute (4,63) or chronic (32,38, 65,73,78) stimulant or dopamine agonist administration. The possibility thus remains that increases in postsynaptic receptor function, as well as a variety of other mechanisms, could be considered as candidates for the increase in behavioral responsivity noted following acute and chronic direct and indirect dopamine agonist treatment.

Preliminary data in man suggest there are alterations in several end-points in response to repeated dopamine agonist administration. Nine subjects received two doses of apomorphine (0.75 mg subcutaneously) 24 and 12 hours prior to a rechallenge at 9:00 p.m. In response to this third apomorphine injection subjects had significantly attenuated hypothermic responses as well as a significantly enhanced rebound hyperthermia compared to the first apomorphine injection 24 hours earlier (19). These data are consistent with the formulation of Costentin et al. (15), as well as Schwartz and associates (67), that hypothermic responses show only tolerance on repeated administration, but hyperthermia (like other dopaminergic end-points such as stereotypy) may be capable of showing sensitization upon repeated dopamine agonist challenge. It remains to be clarified the nature of the receptor mechanisms underlying this altered responsivity to repeated dopamine agonist administration in man.

We have suggested elsewhere that repeated psychomotor stimulant administration may be a useful model for some aspects of manic illness (51,52,59), particularly the tendency for patients to show an increased rapidity (62) of manic onsets and an increased vulnerability to affective recurrences as a function of number of prior episodes (18,30, 31,39). The model of behavioral sensitization may be useful in order to conceptualize, test, and rule out possible mechanisms which could underlie the apparent sensitization that many patients with recurrent affective illness experience. We raise the issue not only whether some of the treatments for depressive illness, such as the tricyclics and monoamine oxidase inhibitors which hypothetically desensitize presynaptic receptors among other neurotransmitter and receptor effects, may be increasing the vulnerability to switches into mania, but also whether endogenous dopaminergic alterations could also be occurring in a long-term fashion leading to an increased vulnerability to recurrences of further episodes. This conceptual framework also raises interesting questions regarding the mechanism of action of psychotropic drugs useful in the acute and prophylactic treatment of recurrent affective illness -- lithium carbonate and the recently studied drug carbamazepine (2,3,48,49) -- which we introduced in part because of its effects on a variety of sensitization models (59).

References

1. Asnis, G.M., Nathan, R.S., Halbreich, U., Halpern, F.S., Sachar, E.J. (1980): Am. J. Psychiatry 137:1117-1118.
2. Ballenger, J.C., Post, R.M. (1978): Communications in Psychopharmacology 2:159-175.
3. Ballenger, J.C., Post, R.M. (1980): Am. J. Psychiatry 137:782-790.
4. Baudry, M., Martres, M.P., Schwartz, J.C. (1977): Life Sci. 21: 1163-1170.
5. Bunney, W.E., Jr., Post, R.M., Andersen, A.E., Kopanda, R.T. (1977): Communications in Psychopharmacology 1:393-405.
6. Chase, T.N., Woods, A.C., Glaubiger, G.A. (1974): Arch. Neurol. 30:383-386.
7. Chase, T.N., Shoulson, I. (1975): In: Advances in Neurology, Vol. 9, edited by D.B. Calne, T.N. Chase, and A. Barbeau, pp. 383-392. Raven Press, New York.
8. Chiodo, L.A., Antelman, S.M. (1980): Science 210:799-801.
9. Chiodo, L.A., Antelman, S.M. (1980): Eur. J. Pharmacol. 66:255-256.
10. Chiodo, L.A., Antelman, S.M. (In press, 1980): Biol. Psychiatry.
11. Clow, A., Jenner, P., Theodorou, A., Marsden, C.D. (1979): Nature 278:59-61.
12. Cools, A.R., van Rossum, J.M. (1980): Life Sci. 27:1237-1253.
13. Corrodi, H., Farnebo, L.O., Fuxe, K., Hamberger, B., Ungerstedt, U. (1972): Eur. J. Pharmacol. 20:195-204.
14. Costall, B., Naylor, R.J. (1974): Naunyn-Schmiedeberg's Arch. Pharmacol. 285:71-81.
15. Costentin, J., Protais, P., Schwartz, J.C. (1975): Nature 257:405-407.
16. Creese, I., Burt, D.R., Snyder, S.H. (1975): Life Sci. 17:993-1002.

17. Cutler, N.R., Post, R.M., Bunney, W.E., Jr. (1979): Communications in Psychopharmacology 3:375-382.
18. Cutler, N.R., Post, R.M. (1980): Sci. Proc. Am. Psychiatr. Assoc. 133:71, Abstract #28.
19. Cutler, N.R., Post, R.M., Bunney, W.E., Jr. (1980): In: New Research Abstracts, 133rd Annual Meeting of the American Psychiatric Association, Abstract #NR44.
20. de Fursac, J.R. (1918): Manual of Psychiatry. Third Edition. Edited and translated by A.J. Rosanoff. John Wiley & Sons, New York.
21. Evans, J.P.M., Grahame-Smith, D.G., Green, A.R., Tordoff, A.F.C. (1976): Br. J. Pharmacol. 56:193-199.
22. Feigenson, J.S., Sweet, R.D., McDowell, F.H. (1976): Neurology 26:430-433.
23. Fuxe, K., Corrodi, H., Hokfelt, T., Lidbrink, P., Ungerstedt, U. (1973): J. Pharm. Pharmacol. 25:409-411.
24. Garattini, S., Barreggi, S., Marc, V., Calderini, G., Marsella, P.L. (1974): Eur. J. Pharmacol. 28:214-216.
25. Gerlach, J. (1980): Personal communication.
26. Gerner, R.H., Post, R.M., Bunney, W.E., Jr., (1976): Am. J. Psychiatry 133:1177-1180.
27. Gessa, G.L. (1980): Presented at the Symposium of Clinical Pharmacology of Apomorphine and Other Dopaminomimetics, Sardinia, Italy, September 28 - October 2, 1980.
28. Grace, A.A., Bunney, B.S. (1979): Eur. J. Pharmacol. 59:211-218.
29. Green, A.R., Heal, D.J., Grahame-Smith, D.G. (1977): Psychopharmacology 52:195-200.
30. Grof, P., Angst, J., Haines, T. (1974): In: Symposia Medica Hoest Vol. 8: Classification and Prediction of Outcome of Depression, edited by F.K. Schattauer, pp. 141-148. Schattauer Verlag, New York.
31. Grof, P., Zis, A.P., Goodwin, F.K., Wehr, T.A. (1978): Sci. Proc. Am. Psychiatr. Assoc. 131:179-180.
32. Howlett, D.R., Nahorski, S.R. (1979): Brain Res. 161:173-178.
33. Jenner, P., Marsden, C.D. (1975): Eur. J. Pharmacol. 33:211-261.
34. Jimerson, D.C., Post, R.M., Skyler, J., Bunney, W.E., Jr. (1976): J. Pharm. Pharmacol. 28:845-847.
35. Jimerson, D.C., Cutler, N.R., Post, R.M., Rey, A.C., Gold, P.W., Brown, G.M., Bunney, W.E., Jr. (1980): Presented at the Annual Meeting of the Society of Biological Psychiatry, Boston, September, 1980.
36. Kilbey, M.M., Ellinwood, E.H. (1977): In: Advances in Behavioral Biology, Volume 21: Cocaine and Other Stimulants, edited by E.H. Ellinwood and M.M. Kilbey, pp. 409-430. Plenum Press, New York.
37. Klawans, H.L., Margolin, D.I. (1975): Arch. Gen. Psychiatry 32:725-732.
38. Klawans, H.L., Hitri, A., Nausieda, P.A., Weiner, W.J. (1977): In: Animal Models in Psychiatry and Neurology, edited by I. Hanin and E. Usdin, pp. 351-364. Pergamon Press, New York.
39. Kraepelin, E. (1904): Lectures in Clinical Psychiatry. Translated and edited by T. Johnstone. Hafner Publishing Co., New York.
40. Kraepelin, E. (1907): Clinical Psychiatry, edited by A.R. Ross, abstracted and adapted from the 7th German edition of Kraepelin's Lehrbuch der Psychiatrie. McMillan and Company, Ltd. London.
41. Laubie, M., Schmitt, H., LeDourec, J.C. (1969): Eur. J. Pharmacol. 6:75-82.

42. Lieberman, A.N., Shopsin, B., LeBrun, Y., Boal, D., Zolfaghari, M. (1975): In: Advances in Neurology, Vol. 9, edited by D.B. Calne, T.N. Chase, A. Barbeau, pp. 399–407. Raven Press, New York.

43. Martres, M.P., Costentin, J., Baudry, M., Marcais, H., Protais, P., Schwartz, J.C. (1977): Brain Res. 136:319–337.

44. Modigh, K. (1975): J. Neural Trans. 36:19–32.

45. Muller, P., Seeman, P. (1979): Eur. J. Pharmacol. 55:149–157.

46. Nausieda, P.A., Weiner, W.J., Kanapa, D.L., Klawans, H.L. (1978): Ann. Neurol. 20:1183–1188.

47. Offermeier, J., van Rooyen, J.M. (1980): In: Abstracts of the 12th Collegium Neuro-Psychopharmacologicum, Gothenburg, Sweden, June, 1980, edited by C. Radouco-Thomas and J. Garcin, p. 284, Abstract #492. Plenum Press, New York.

48. Okuma, T., Inanaga, K., Otsuki, S. Sarai, K., Takahashi, R., Hazama, H., Mori, A., Watanabe, M. (1979): Psychopharmacology 66: 211–217.

49. Okuma, T. Kishimoto, A., Inoue, K., Matsumato, H., Ogura, A., Matsushita, T., Naklao, T., Ogura, C. (1973): Folia Psychiatr. Neurol. Jpn. 27:283–297.

50. Owen, F., Cross, A.J., Waddington, J.L., Poulter, M., Gamble, S.J., Crow, T.J. (1980): Life Sci. 26:55–59.

51. Post, R.M. (1975): Am. J. Psychiatry 132:225–231.

52. Post, R.M. (1977): In: Animal Models in Psychiatry and Neurology, edited by I. Hanin and E. Usdin, pp. 201–210. Pergamon Press, New York.

53. Post, R.M. (1978): In: Psychopharmacology: A Generation of Progress, edited by M.A. Lipton, A. Dimascio, and K.F. Killam, pp. 1323–1335. Raven Press, New York.

54. Post, R.M. (1980): Life Sci. 26:1275–1282.

55. Post, R.M., Goodwin, F.K. (1975): Science 190:488–489.

56. Post, R.M., Kopanda, R.T., Black, K.E. (1976): Biol. Psychiatry 11: 403–419.

57. Post, R.M., Gerner, R.H., Carman, J.S., Gillin, J.C., Jimerson, D.C., Goodwin, F.K., Bunney, W.E., Jr. (1978): Arch. Gen. Psychiatry 35:609–615.

58. Post, R.M., Gerner, R.H., Jimerson, D.C., Carman, J.S., Rey, A.C., Bunney, W.E., Jr. (1979): Psychologie Medicale 11:30–41.

59. Post, R.M., Ballenger, J.C. (In press, 1980): In: Handbook of Biological Psychiatry, Vol. II, edited by H.M. van Praag, M.H. Lade, O.J. Rafaelsen, and E.J. Sachar. Marcel-Dekker, Inc., New York.

60. Post, R.M., Ballenger, J.C., Goodwin, F.K. (1980): In: Neurobiology of Cerebrospinal Fluid, Vol. I, edited by J.H. Wood, pp. 685–717. Plenum Press, New York.

61. Post, R.M., Jimerson, D.C., Bunney, W.E., Jr., Goodwin, F.K.: Psychopharmacology 67:297–305.

62. Post, R.M., Ballenger, J.C., Rey, A.C., Bunney, W.E., Jr. (In press, 1981): Psychiatry Res.

63. Pradhan, S.N. (1980): Personal communication.

64. Randrup, A., Munkvad, I., Fog, R., Gerlach, J., Molander, L., Kjellberg, B., Scheel-Kruger, J. (1975): Curr. Dev. Psychopharmacol. 2:205–248.

65. Robertson, H.A. (1980): Eur. J. Pharmacol. 61:209–211.

66. Rondot, P., Bathien, N., Ribadeau-Dumas, J.L. (1975): In: Advances in Neurology, Vol. 9, edited by D.B. Calne, T.N. Chase, A. Barbeau, pp. 373–381. Raven Press, New York.

67. Schwartz, J.C., Costentin, J., Martres, M.P., Protais, P., Baudry, M. (1978): Neuropharmacology 17:665-685.
68. Segal, D.S., Mandell, A.J. (1974): Pharmacol. Biochem. Behav. 2: 249-255.
69. Serra, G., Argiolas, A., Klimek, V., Fadda, F., Gessa, G.L. (1979): Life Sci. 25:415-424.
70. Shopsin, B., Gershon, S. (1978): Neuropsychobiology 4:1-14.
71. Sweet, R.D., Wasterlain, C.G., McDowell, F.H. (1974): Clin. Pharmacol. Ther. 15:1077-1082.
72. Tarsy, D., Baldessarini, R.J. (1973): Nature 245:262-263.
73. Taylor, D.L., Ho, B.T., Fagan, J.D. (1979): Commun. Psychopharmacol. 3:137-142.
74. Tepper, S.J., Haas, J.F. (1979): J. Clin. Psychiatr. 40:21-29.
75. van Praag, H.M.S., Korf, J. (1975): Pharmakopsychiatrie 8:322-326.
76. Van Scheyen, J.D., van Praag, H.M., Korf, J. (1977): Br. J. Clin. Pharmacol. 4:179-184.
77. Walters, J.R., Bunney, B.S., Roth, R.H. (1975): In: Advances in Neurology, Vol. 9, edited by D.B. Calne, T.N. Chase, A. Barbeau, pp. 273-284. Raven Press, New York.
78. Wilner, K.D., Butler, I.J., Seifert, W.E., Clement-Cormier, Y.C. (1980): Society for Neuroscience Abstracts, Vol. 6, p. 800, Abstract #271.5.

Apomorphine and Other Dopaminomimetics,
Vol. 2: Clinical Pharmacology, edited by
G. U. Corsini and G. L. Gessa, Raven Press,
New York © 1981.

Treatment of Parkinsonism with Artificial Dopaminomimetics: Pharmacokinetic Considerations

Richard S. Burns and Donald B. Calne

Experimental Therapeutics Branch, National Institute of Neurological and Communicative Disorders and Stroke, National Institutes of Health, Bethesda, Maryland 20205

INTRODUCTION

The first artificial dopaminomimetic to be employed for the treatment of Parkinson's disease was apomorphine. Before its pharmacological properties were known, Schwab et al. (59) gave apomorphine to Parkinsonian patients because the drug was known to reduce decerebrate rigidity in animals, and increased muscle tone is a feature of Parkinsonism. Following the recognition of the dopaminergic activity of apomorphine, Cotzias et al. (12) repeated and extended Schwab's observation, noting that the major problems limiting the use of the drug were emesis and impairment of renal function. The emesis was subsequently ameliorated by concomitant administration of domperidone, a dopamine receptor blocking agent which does not readily cross the blood-brain barrier (11). In 1976 Cotzias et al. (13) found that a derivative of apomorphine, N-propylnoraporphine, alleviated Parkinsonism with fewer adverse reactions, but still the unwanted effects were sufficiently troublesome to dispel any enthusiasm for developing this drug as a routine therapeutic agent.

Piribedil, a piperazine derivative, was another dopaminergic agonist to be studied for the treatment of Parkinsonism: it was shown to possess therapeutic activity, but the high incidence of psychiatric reactions precluded its widespread use (8,45,68).

The discovery that certain ergot derivatives have dopaminomimetic properties derived from the observation, by Shelesnyak (60), that ergotoxine (a mixture of ergocornine, ergocristine, and ergocryptine) interferes with deciduoma formation in rodents, through a mechanism dependent on an intact hypothalamo-pituitary axis. Since certain aspects of pituitary function are under the control of dopamine released by the hypothalamus, it was reasonable to ask whether any of the ergots achieved their effects via an action on dopamine receptors. When the ergots were tested in screening procedures designed to detect dopaminomimetic properties in vitro and in vivo, it soon became apparent that certain of the ergots were powerful dopamine agonists. Consequently, it was a logical step to investigate the therapeutic potential of these drugs in Parkinson's disease. Artificial dopaminomimetics possess theoretical advantages over levodopa in having greater specificity for dopamine receptors, and in bypassing the need for dopa decarboxylase, an enzyme which is depleted in the brain of Parkinsonian patients.

Bromocriptine was the first ergot derivative to be studied for the treatment of Parkinson's disease. It was shown to alleviate all the major motor deficits of

Parkinsonism (7,14,20,39,54).   Lergotrile is another ergot derivative which has therapeutic actions in Parkinsonism (38,65); unfortunately it causes hepatic dysfunction in a high proportion of patients, so its use has been abandoned (63).

The advantages of bromocriptine are: (a) it causes less dyskinesia than levodopa; (b) it has a more prolonged action than levodopa; and (c) it induces less prominent early morning dystonia than levodopa.   The drawbacks of bromocriptine are: (a) it induces psychiatric reactions more frequently than levodopa, and these tend to be more severe, taking longer to clear after stopping the drug; (b) in high doses it can produce a vasculopathy characterized by erythema, edema and tenderness of the feet, ankles and lower legs; (c) rarely, it has been reported to induce bilateral pulmonary infiltration with pleural effusions (53).   Another ergot, CF 25-397 has been investigated because it is active in certain behavioral screening tests which are thought to denote dopaminergic activity (31); clinical observations with this agent have, however, failed to reveal any significant efficacy (64).   Most recently, two new dopaminomimetic ergots, lisuride (25,37) and pergolide (37) are undergoing evaluation.   These drugs seem promising, but experience with them is limited and more extensive studies will have to be carried out before any firm conclusion can be drawn concerning their long term efficacy and toxicity.

With the establishment of a role for the dopaminergic ergot derivatives in the treatment of Parkinsonism, their clinical pharmacology has become important. The development of specific and sensitive radioimmunoassay methods for bromocriptine and lisuride has made pharmacokinetic studies possible.

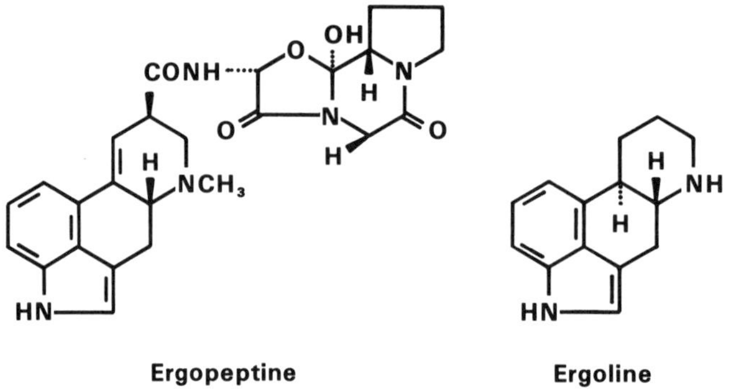

Ergopeptine   Ergoline

FIG. 1. Structure of ergolines and ergopeptines.

Structural Features of the Dopaminomimetic Ergot Derivatives

Ergot derivatives with marked central dopaminergic activity belong to two structural groups of the ergot derivatives which differ in their extent of absorption, bioavailability, major sites of metabolism, and excretion pattern. The basic structure of the ergopeptines, like bromocriptine, consists of the naturally occurring D-lysergic acid linked to a tricyclic peptide moiety by a peptide bond (FIG. 1). The simpler ergolines, which include lergotrile, lisuride and pergolide, contain the unsubstituted tetracyclic structure of lysergic acid (FIG. 1). Buried in the ergoline nucleus, which is common to both groups, is the structure of dopamine (FIG. 2). Unlike most other dopamine agonists, ergot derivatives do not possess a catechol moiety. The substituents appear to be important in the intensity and profile of the central dopaminergic activity of the ergots. Small changes in the stereochemistry or the substituents can increase one dopaminergic effect and decrease another (27).

Tricyclic structures representing the rigid pyrroleethlyamine moiety of the ergolines (FIG. 2) show dopaminergic activity, so the benzene ring of the ergots does not appear to be essential for dopaminergic activity (3).

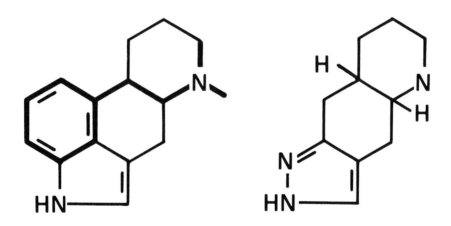

FIG. 2. The tetracyclic structure of ergot derivatives, with a possible fit for the dopamine moiety in heavy lines (left). The tricyclic component (right) also has dopaminergic properties. The relative contribution of these various structural elements to dopaminergic activity is not known.

ASSAYS FOR ERGOT DERIVATIVES

Measurement of the concentration of the ergot derivatives in body fluids is difficult because of their biological and physical properties. These compounds are highly potent with therapeutic doses in the range of 100 µg to 30mg (7,37). Incomplete absorption, extensive first pass metabolism, and widespread binding to tissues result in concentrations in plasma in the picogram $(10^{-12}$ gm)/ml to nanogram $(10^{-9}$ gm)/ml range. Thermal instability and low volatility prevent the application of gas chromatography-mass spectrometry which is chemically specific and has sensitivities in this range. The measurement of total radioactivity and following the administration of radiolabeled drug is a highly sensitive method of assay, but does not distinguish between parent compound and metabolites; it is of limited value with the ergot derivatives that undergo rapid and extensive biotransformation into multiple metabolites.

Specific and sensitive radioimmunoassay methods have been developed for bromocriptine and lisuride. The bromocriptine assay has a sensitivity of 100-150 pg/ml; it utilizes an antiserum directed against dihydroergocriptine conjugated with serum albumin at the indol nitrogen that is distal to the major site of metabolism on the peptide moiety. The antiserum is highly specific for the peptide portion of the intact ergopeptine structure and does not show significant cross reactivity with lysergic acid and peptide aminocyclol metabolites (58). The radioimmunoassay for lisuride (28) has a sensitivity of 25 pg/ml; it involves the use of an antiserum with high specificity for the diethylurea portion of the molecule where metabolism is thought to take place predominantly (66,70).

ABSORPTION AND EXCRETION

Molecular size, polarity, and undefined structural features are important in the biliary excretion of drugs and their metabolites. Like other substances that are excreted extensively in bile, the ergopeptines have a molecular weight greater than 400 and contain both polar and nonpolar groups (62). Most of the ergopeptines have molecular weights of about 600 (27), and over 80% of an absorbed dose of these compounds is excreted in the bile (19,35,57). Substances with molecular weights of 300 or less tend to be excreted in the urine, with not more than 5-10% of the dose appearing in the bile (62); ergolines, with a molecular weight of about 300, conform to the pattern of predominant excretion in urine (Table 1). Lergotrile is an exception to this rule.

TABLE 1

Pharmacokinetic Studies Using Radiolabeled Ergot Derivatives in Man

	Absorption	Excretion		Ref.
		Urine	Feces	
ERGOLINES				
[3]H-lisuride	>60%	60%	40%	70
[14]C-pergolide	>55%	55%	40%	55
[14]C-lergotrile	>20%	20%	60%	56
ERGOPEPTINES				
[14]C-bromocriptine		2%	98%	57
[3]H-bromocriptine		6%	94%	1
[3]H-ergotamine		4%	96%	1

Mass balance studies of oral ^{3}H-bromocriptine and ^{14}C-ergotamine, in monkeys with biliary fistulae or cannulated bile ducts, have shown that only 37% and 32% respectively, of the administered dose of these ergopeptines is absorbed (35,47). In this animal model, the extent of absorption can be calculated directly from the sum of the cumulative excretion of radioactivity in the bile and the urine. Seventy-seven percent of the absorbed dose of ^{3}H-bromocriptine and 81% of the absorbed dose of ^{14}C-ergotamine is excreted in bile (35,47). Similar results have been obtained in rats with cannulated bile ducts, where 29% of an oral dose of ^{3}H-bromocriptine is absorbed and 92% of this fraction is excreted in the bile (35). Approximately 2% of an oral dose of the ergopeptine ^{3}H-dihydroergocristine is reabsorbed from bile in the rat, suggesting that enterohepatic recirculation of the ergopeptines is not significant in the intact animal (47).

In rats with cannulated bile ducts, 15% of an intravenous dose of ^{14}C-lisuride is eliminated in urine, and in non-cannulated rats 18%; these findings suggest the existence of a small enterohepatic recirculation of lisuride or its metabolites (29).

By comparing the cumulative excretion of radioactivity in urine after oral and intravenous administration of ^{3}H-bromocriptine (1), the extent of the absorption of this drug in man has been claimed to be 95%. The low urinary excretion of the radiolabel (6%), limits the sensitivity of studying this route for information on absorption, so methodological problems may explain the unexpectedly high level of absorption that has been proposed as a consequence of these human studies.

The cumulative excretion of radioactivity in the urine following oral administration of ^{3}H-lisuride and ^{14}C-pergolide in man represents 60% and 55% of the original dose, respectively (55,70). These values provide us with a lower limit for the extent of absorption of lisuride and pergolide. However, the radiolabel of lisuride was metabolically unstable (^{3}H$_2$O) and complete absorption of lisuride was discussed on the basis of unchanged drug plasma levels (28).

In summary, ergopeptines and ergolines differ in their extent of absorption and pattern of excretion in bile and urine. Animal studies have demonstrated that ergolines are more readily absorbed than ergopeptines and they are excreted mainly in the urine. Ergopeptines show limited absorption and are excreted mainly in the bile.

Metabolism

Our knowledge of the biotransformation of the ergot derivatives is limited by the difficulties that exist in isolating and identifying their metabolites. The concentration of the metabolites in biological fluids is in the picogram to nanogram/ml range, with each of several products representing only a small fraction of the original dose. The pattern of metabolism of the ergolines and the ergopeptines differs. The major sites of metabolism of the ergolines include the 1-methyl, the 6-methyl, the 8-substituent, and the aromatic ring (19). Ergopeptines, although possessing the ergoline nucleus, undergo biotransformation almost exclusively in the proline fragment of the peptide moiety (19).

Metabolism by the liver determines the fate of ergot derivatives following oral administration, and is the key to understanding their pharmacokinetics. Following absorption, these compounds are extensively metabolized during the initial passsage through the liver prior to reaching the systemic circulation. Ninety-four percent of the absorbed fraction of bromocriptine, and 78-90% of an oral dose of lisuride are metabolized on first pass in the liver (28,57); only trace amounts of unchanged drug are excreted in the urine. The plasma clearance rates of bromocriptine (900 ml/min) and lisuride (740 ml/min) approach the rate of hepatic blood flow (29,57) (Table 2). However, a high degree of plasma protein binding and extensive distribution into tissues reduce the availability of these compounds to rapid degradation in the liver. Ninety to ninety-six percent of bromocriptine and 95-96% of pergolide are bound to plasma proteins (55,57). The apparent volumes of distribution of bromocriptine and lisuride in man are 240 liters and 144 liters, respectively (28,57). The elimination half-lives of bromocriptine and lisuride are 3 and 1.7 hours (28,57). The kinetics of bromocriptine in man appears to be linear in the therapeutic dose range (57).

TABLE 2

Pharmacokinetic Studies of Ergot Derivatives Using
Radioimmunoassay Methods

	Volume of Distribution	Plasma Clearance	Elimination Halflife	Bioavail-ability	Ref.
Lisuride	144 L	740 ml/min	1.7 h	10-22%*	28
Bromocriptine	240 L	900 ml/min	3.0 h	6.4%	57

*possibly dose dependent

BIOAVAILABILITY

The bioavailability of a drug is usually defined as the percentage of the dose which reaches the general circulation unchanged. In the case of drugs, which act on the central nervous system, but do not readily enter the brain, the significance of the classically defined bioavailability is clearly limited. Nevertheless, it is relevant to consider the fraction of the drug in the blood stream, since the systemic circulation is the sole route to the brain.

The bioavailability of the ergot derivatives in man is low. The fraction of an oral dose of bromocriptine which reaches the systemic circulation unchanged approximates to 6% of the absorbed dose, based upon comparison of the areas under the plasma concentration curve for bromocriptine and total radioactivity (57). The bioavailability of oral lisuride was found to be 10-22% on comparison of the areas under the curve following oral and intravenous administration of the drug (28). The bioavailability of the ergolines, in general, appears to be greater than that of the ergopeptines, and this difference may be reflected in the daily doses of the ergot derivatives required in Parkinsonism (with the exception of lergotrile, see Table 3).

Following oral administration in man, the bioavailability of bromocriptine and lisuride, as well as ergotamine, displays a large interindividual and relatively small intraindividual variation (2,5,57). A twelve-fold difference in the peak plasma concentration and a seven-fold difference in the area under the curve has been found following a 300 μg oral dose of lisuride in Parkinsonian patients. The times to reach peak concentration and the elimination half lives were similar in all patients. The peak concentration following a single dose was generally predictive of the steady state levels attained when multiple oral doses were administered (5). The large interindividual variation in the bioavailability of the ergot derivatives may explain the wide therapeutic dosage ranges of these compounds (Table 3).

TABLE 3

Doses of Ergot Derivatives Used in Parkinsonism

	Daily Starting Dose	Maximum Single Dose	Maximum Daily Dose	Usual Daily Dosage Range	Ref.
ERGOLINES					
Lisuride	200 µg	1.2 mg	10 mg	0.6-10 mg	25,26
Pergolide	100 µg	400 µg	5 mg	2-5 mg	37,40
Lergotrile*	6 mg	30 mg	160 mg	20-100 mg	36,40, 41,42
ERGOPEPTINES					
Bromocriptine	5 mg	100 mg	300 mg	30-100 mg	6,7, 44,49, 50,52

*no longer in clinical use because of hepatotoxicity.

TIME COURSE OF ACTION

Certain behavioral and biochemical measures of the activity of dopamine agonists are characterized by a delayed onset and a prolonged duration. Conversion of the parent drug to an active metabolite, distribution kinetics, and the intrinsic response of effector cells may contribute to these time courses.

Active Metabolites

The motor responses induced by intermediate doses of bromocriptine in rodents are thought to be secondary to agonist activity at dopamine receptors (21). Hyperactivity in the mouse is first observed 1-2 hours after intraperitoneal administration of 2.5-10 mg/kg bromocriptine and persists for up to 7 hours (17,32). Stereotyped behavior in the rat induced by 2.5-20 mg/kg of intraperitoneal bromocriptine appears at 2 hours and lasts for more than 7 hours (32). In rats with unilateral nigral lesions, 1-2 mg/kg of intraperitoneal bromocriptine produces contralateral turning after a delay of 1 hour; this persists for more than 8 hours (10,32). Following 5 mg/kg intraperitoneal bromocriptine, the turning behavior lasts 18-24 hours, and at higher doses for several days (21,22).

The time to reach equilibrium concentrations in the brain and the elimination half life of bromocriptine and its major metabolites are unknown. Conversion of bromocriptine into a metabolite that is active and has a relatively long half life could result in the delayed onset and prolonged duration of the motor responses observed in rodents. Alternatively, an extremely high potency of unchanged bromocriptine combined with a slow rate of distribution into brain tissue and slow dissociation from binding sites in the brain could also explain the observed time course of motor activity.

In man, up to 30% of an oral dose of lergotrile is converted to 13-hydroxy-lergotrile, which is 10 times as potent as the parent compound in its inhibition of prolactin release and its affinity for binding to dopamine receptors (56). 13-hydroxylergotrile is found in feces and is probably initially excreted in the bile. An enterohepatic circulation of 13-hydroxylergotrile could contribute to the observed effects of the parent drug.

Distribution

Tissue clearance studies of the ergot derivatives have been carried out in animals using radiolabeled drugs. The time to reach peak levels of radioactivity in brain appears to be shorter for lysergic acid derivatives and ergolines than for the ergopeptines. After intravenous administration in the rat, ^{3}H-lysergic acid diethylamide penetrates the brain within 5 minutes, reaching a peak in 15 minutes and disappearing by 1 hour (16). Intravenous lisuride generates maximum levels of the drug in the rat's brain by 15 minutes (28). In the cat, peak brain levels of radioactivity occur 1 hour after intravenous administration of 2 mg/kg of the ergopeptine ^{3}H-dihydroergocornine (30). Following intravenous ^{3}H-bromocriptine, the equilibration time of total radioactivity in the rat's brain is more than 2 hours (35).

The slower rate of brain equilibriation following administration of radio-labeled ergopeptines may result from a lower permeability at the blood brain barrier. The metabolites of ergopeptines may penetrate the brain more readily than the parent compound.

The relationship between total radioactivity in brain and the concentration of the parent drug versus metabolites has been studied in the rat for ^{14}C-lisuride (70). Lisuride crosses the blood brain barrier rapidly; the concentrations in brain and plasma are equal up to 30 minutes after injection. At 15 minutes, unchanged drug represents 80% of the radiolabeled material in brain; at 1 hour and 3 hours, lisuride accounts for 63% and 54% of the total radiolabel in brain, respectively.

In the cat, the clearance rate of the radiolabel from the caudate nucleus after intravenous administration of the ergopeptines of ^{3}H-dihydroergocornine and ^{3}H-dihydroergonine is slower than the clearance rate from the blood and the visceral organs (30). In the rat, the concentration of intravenously administered lisuride in the brain decreases more slowly than in the plasma; this results in higher levels of lisuride in brain compared to plasma, from 30 minutes to 8 hours after the injection (29).

The clearance rate of total radioactivity from the cat's pituitary following intravenous administration of ^{3}H-dihydroergocornine and ^{3}H-dihydroergonine is similar to that of the blood and well perfused organs, such as liver, kidney and lung (30). The early levels of radioactivity in the pituitary are 50 times greater than other brain regions including the caudate nucleus. In the monkey, radioactivity in the pituitary was found to be twice as high as that of other brain regions after intravenous administration of ^{82}Br-bromocriptine (43). The highest regional concentration of ^{14}C-lisuride in rat's brain is found in the pituitary (29).

The Plasma Prolactin Response

The time course of the changes in plasma prolactin that follow administration of ergot derivatives reflects the kinetics of the drug and of prolactin, and the intrinsic response of the lactotrophs to these compounds. A delay of 30 minutes in the reduction of plasma prolactin levels is observed following intravenous administration of 25 µg of lisuride (28). This occurs despite the fact that the pituitary is outside the blood brain barrier. Distribution of ergot derivatives within the pituitary to reach the lactotrophs is unlikely to be rate limiting.

The half life of prolactin in man is 40-50 minutes (9,61), which limits the temporal resolution of the initial decrease in plasma prolactin that marks the onset of the response. The inhibitory effect of 10^{-7}M bromocriptine on prolactin release from isolated rat pituitary cells becomes maximal after 30 minutes of perfusion (69). In contrast, the inhibition of prolactin release on exposure to 5×10^{-6}M dopamine is rapid, occurring within 7.5 minutes (69). The delay in onset of the decrease in plasma prolactin following administration of ergot derivatives may be related to the mechanism of the intrinsic response of pituitary cells to these compounds.

The plasma prolactin is reduced for up to 24 hours following a single 4 mg oral dose of bromocriptine (15), although the plasma half life of bromocriptine in man is only 3 hours (57), (Table 4). Suspended rat pituitary cells perfused with 10^{-7}M bromocriptine for 30 minutes, do not recover completely from the inhibitory effect on prolactin release during a subsequent period of washing in saline for 3 hours (69). Unchanged bromocriptine possesses greater affinity than its metabolites for displacing spiroperidol from binding sites on pituitary membranes; hence the parent compound is probably responsible for most of the dopaminergic activity at the anterior pituitary (46).

TABLE 4

The Plasma Prolactin Response to Ergot Derivatives, p.o.

	Earliest Recorded Decrease	Duration of Decrease	Ref.
ERGOLINES			
Pergolide 150 µg	1 h	> 36-40 h	37,40,41
Lisuride 300 µg	30 min	> 24-48 h	18,28
Lergotrile 2 mg	90 min	4-6 h	40,42
ERGOPEPTINES			
Bromocriptine 4 mg	2.5 h	> 24 h	15

Intrinsic Activity

The fraction of an orally administered dose of bromocriptine that gains entry to the brain unchanged is very low. If unchanged bromocriptine is responsible for the observed central dopaminergic activity of this compound, it is extremely potent. Following oral administration of 2.5 mg - 250 µCi of ^{14}C-bromocriptine in man, only 6% of the absorbed fraction of the dose reaches the systemic circulation unchanged (57). One two-thousandth of an injected dose of ^{82}Br-bromocriptine is detectable in whole rat's brain 2 hours after intravenous administration of 5 mg/kg; this represents a maximum bromocriptine concentration of 2.5 x 10^{-8}M in the brain (43).

The dopaminergic ergot derivatives used in the treatment of Parkinsonism interact with both D-1 and D-2 dopamine receptors. They all possess potent agonist properties at the D-2 receptor, but they have diverse actions at D-1 receptor sites. Lisuride and lergotrile inhibit D-1 receptors in homogenates of rat striatum (33,51), whereas pergolide is a partial agonist and bromocriptine may be a weak partial agonist (23,24,48,67). These properties are summarized in Table 5.

TABLE 5

Activity of Ergot Derivatives at Central Dopamine Receptors

	D-1	D-2
Lergotrile	Antagonist	Agonist
Lisuride	Antagonist	Agonist
Bromocriptine	Weak partial agonist	Agonist
Pergolide	Partial agonist	Agonist

SUMMARY

The pharmacokinetic properties of dopaminergic ergot derivatives are reviewed. These compounds are difficult to study biochemically, so some reference to non-dopaminergic ergots is included to provide a broader range of background information. The dopaminergic ergots fall into two groups, the ergolines and the ergopeptines. Ergolines are more readily absorbed than ergopeptines. Ergolines enter the brain more rapidly than ergopeptines. The tetracyclic ring structure is involved in metabolic transformation of ergolines, while the proline component of the peptide moiety is metabolized in ergopeptines. Although first passage through the liver leads to extensive breakdown of most ergot derivatives, this does not preclude the parent compound being the most active. The effects of ergot derivatives occur more slowly and persist for longer than would be anticipated from pharmacokinetic observations. Ergolines are excreted predominantly as metabolites in the urine, while ergopeptines are excreted mainly as metabolites via the bile and feces.

References

1   Aellig, W.H. and Nuesch, E. (1977): Int. J. Clin. Pharmacol., 15:106-112.

2.   Ala-Hurula, V., Mylly Lä, V.U., Arvela, P., Heikkila, J., Karki, N., and Hokkanen, E. (1979): Europ. J. Clin. Pharmacol., 15:51-55.

3.   Bach, N.J., Kornfeld, E.C., Jones, N.D., Chaney, M.O., Dorman, D.E., Paschal, J.W., Clemens, J.A., and Smalstig, E.B. (1980): J. Med. Chem., 23:481-491.

4.   Berde, B., and Stürmer, E. (1978): In: Ergot Alkaloids and Related Compounds, Handbook of Experimental Pharmacology, Vol. 49, edited by B. Berde, and H.O. Scheld, pp. 1-28. Springer-Verlag, Berlin.

5. Burns, R.S., Gopinathan, G., Hümpel, M., Dorow, R. (1981): In preparation for presentation at AAN Meeting.

6. Calne, D.B., Teychenne, P.F., Claveria, L.E., Eastman, R., Greenacre, J.K., and Petrie, A. (1976): Br. Med. J., 4:442.

7. Calne, D.B., Williams, A.C., Neophytides, A., Plotkin, C., Nutt, J.G., and Teychenne, P.F. (1978): Lancet 1:735-738.

8. Chase, T.N., and Shoulson, I. (1975): In: Advances in Neurology, Vol. 9: Dopaminergic Mechanisms, edited by D.B. Calne, T.N. Chase, and A. Barbeau, pp. 359-366. Raven, Press, New York.

9. Cooper, D.S., Ridgway, E.C., Kliman, B., Kjellberg, R.N., and Maloof, F. (1981): In press.

10. Corrodi, H., Fuxe, K., Hökfelt, T., Lidbrink, P., and Ungerstedt, U. (1973): J. Pharm. Pharmacol., 25:409-412.

11. Corsini, G.U., Gessa, G.L., Del Zompo, M., and Mangoni, A. (1979): Lancet, 1:954-956.

12. Cotzias, G.C., Lawrence, W.H., Duby, S.E., Ginos, J.Z., and Mena, I. (1972): Trans. Am. Neurol. Assoc., 97:156-158.

13. Cotzias, G.C., Papavasiliou, P.S., Tolosa, E.S., Mendez, J.S., and Bell-Midura, M. (1976): N. Engl. J. Med., 294:567-572.

14. Debono, A.G., Donaldson, I., Marsden, C.D., and Parkes, J.D. (1975): Lancet, 2:987-988.

15. Del Pozo, E. (1972): J. Clin. Endocrinol. Metab., 35:768-771.

16. Diab, I.M., Freedman, D.X., and Roth, L.J. (1971): Science, 173:1022-1024.

17. Dolphin, A.C., Jenner, P., Sawaya, M.C.B., Marsden, C.D., and Testa, B. (1977): J. Pharm. Pharmacol., 29:727-734.

18. Dorow, R., Gräf, K.J., Nieuweboer, B., and Horowski, R. (1980): Acta Endocrinol., 94:9.

19. Eckert, H., Kiechel, J.R., Rosenthaler, J., Schmidt, R., and Schreier, E. (1978): In: Ergot Alkaloids and Related Compounds, Handbook of Experimental Pharmacology, Vol. 49, edited by B. Bede and H.O. Schild, pp. 719-803. Springer-Verlag, Berlin.

20. Fahn, S., Cote, L.J., Snider, S.R., Barrett, R.E., and Isgreen, W.P. (1979): In: Dopaminergic Ergot Derivatives and Motor Function, edited by K. Fuxe and D.B. Calne, pp.303-312. Pergamon Press, Oxford.

21. Fuxe, K., Fredholm, B.B., Agnati, L.F., Ögren, S.O., Everitt, B.J., Jonsson, G., and Gustafsson, J.A. (1978): Pharmacology, 16:99-134.

22. Fuxe, K., Fredholm, B.B., Ögren, S.O., Agnati, L.F., Hökfelt, T., and Gustafsson, J.A. (1978): Fed. Proc., 37:2181-2190.

23.   Goldstein, M., Lieberman, A., Lew, J.Y., Asano, T., Rosenfeld, M.R., and Makman, M.H. (1980): Proc. Natl. Acad. Sci., 77:3725-3728.

24.   Goldstein, M., Lieberman, A., Lew, J.Y., Rosenfeld, M.R., and Makman, M.H. (1980): Fed. Proc., 39:529.

25.   Gopinathan, C., Teräväinen, H., Dambrosia, J., Ward, C., Sanes, J., Stuart, W., Evarts, E., and Calne, D.B. (1980): Neurology, 30:366.

26.   Gopinathan, G., Teräväinen, H., Dambrosia, J.M., Ward, C.D., Sanes, J.N., Stuart, W.K., Evarts, E.V., and Calne, D.B. (1980): Neurology, in press.

27.   Hauth, H. (1979): In: Dopaminergic Ergot Derivatives and Motor Function, edited by K. Fuxe and D.B. Calne, pp. 23-32. Pergamon Press, Oxford.

28.   Hümpel, M., Nieuweboer, B., Hasan, S.H., Wendt, H. (1981): Eur. J. Clin. Pharmacology, in press.

29.   Hümpel, M., Toda, T., Oshino, N., Pommerenke, G. (1981): Eur. J. Metabolism and Pharmacokinetics, in press.

30.   Iwangoff, P., Enz, A., and Meier-Ruge, W. (1978): Gerontology, 24:126-138.

31.   Jaton, A.L., Loew, D.M., and Vioguret, J.M. (1976): Br. J. Pharmacol., 56:371.

32.   Johnson, A.M., Loew, D.M., and Vigouret, J.M. (1976): Br. J. Pharmacol., 56:59-68.

33.   Kebabian, J.W., Calne, D.B., and Kebabian, P.R. (1976): Commun. Psychopharmacol., 1:311-318.

34.   Kebabian, J.W. and Kebabian, P.R. (1978): Life Sci., 23:2199-2204.

35.   Kiechel, J.R., Rosenthaler, J., and Schrier, E. (1980): Personal communication.

36.   Lieberman, A., Estey, E., Kupersmith, M., Gopinathan, G., and Goldstein, M. (1977): JAMA, 238(22):2380-2382.

37.   Lieberman, A., Leibowitz, M., Neophytides, A., Kupersmith, M., Pact, V., Walker, R., Zasorin, N., and Goldstein, M. (1980): Neurology, 30:366.

38.   Lieberman, A., Miyamoto, T., Battista, A.F., and Goldstein, M. (1975): Neurology, 25:459-462.

39.   Lieberman, A., Zolfaghari, M., Boal, D., Hassouri, H., Vogel, B., Battista, A., Fuxe, K., and Goldstein, M. (1976): Neurology, 26:405-409.

40.   Lemberger, L. and Crabtree, R.E. (1980): In: Ergot Compounds and Brain Function: Neuroendocrine and Neuropsychiatric Aspects, edited by M. Goldstein, D.B. Calne, A. Lieberman, M.O. Thorner, pp. 117-124. Raven Press, New York.

41. Lemberger, L. and Crabtree, R.E. (1979): Science, 205:1151-1153.

42. Lemberger, L., Rubin, A., and Crabtree, R.E. (1979): In: Dopaminergic Ergot Derivatives and Motor Function, edited by K. Fuxe. and D.B. Calne, pp. 263-269. Pergamon Press, Oxford.

43. Markey, S.P., Colburn, R.W., and Kopin, I.J.: In preparation.

44. Marsden, C.D., Jenner, P., Parkes, J.D., Price, P.A., and Reavill, C. (1979): In: Dopaminergic Ergot Derivatives and Motor Function, edited by K. Fuxe, and D.B. Calne, pp. 313-318. Pergamon Press, Oxford.

45. McDowell, F.H. and Sweet, R.(1975): In: Advances in Neurology, Vol. 9: Dopaminergic Mechanisms, edited by D.B. Calne, T.N. Chase, and A. Barbeau, pp. 367-371. Raven Press, New York.

46. Munemura, M., Eisler, T., Calne, D.B., and Kebabian, J.W. (1980): In preparation.

47. Nimmerfall, F. and Rosenthaler, J. (1976): J. Pharmacokinet. Biopharm., 4:57-66.

48. Pagnini, G., Camanni, F., Crispino., A., and Portaleone, P. (1978): J. Pharm. Pharmacol., 30:92-95.

49. Parkes, J.D. (1979): N. Eng. J. Med., 301:873-878.

50. Parkes, J.D., DeBono, A.G., and Marsden, C.D. (1976): J. Neurol. Neurosurg. Psychiatry, 39:1101-1108.

51. Pieri, L., Keller, H.H., Burkard, W., and Da Prada, M. (1978): Nature, 272-280.

52. Price, P., DeBono, A., Parkes, J.D., Marsden, C.D., and Rosenthaler, J. (1978): Br. J. Clin. Pharmacol., 6:303-309.

53. Rinne, U.K. (1981): Lancet, In press.

54. Rinne, U.K., Marttila, R., and Sonninen, V. (1979): In: Dopaminergic Ergot Derivatives and Motor Function, edited by K. Fuxe and D.B. Calne, pp. 319-324. Pergamon Press, Oxford.

55. Rubin, A., Lemberger, L., Dhahir, P., and Crabtree, R.E. (1980): Paper presented at World Conference on Clinical Pharmacology and Therapeutics, August, 1980, London.

56. Rubin, A., Lemberger, L., Dhahir, P., Warrick, P., Crabtree, R.E., Obermeyer, B.D., Wolen, R.L., and Rowe, H. (1978): Clin. Pharmacol. Ther., 23:272-280.

57. Schran, H.F., Bhuta, S.I., Schwartz, H.J., and Thorner, M.O. (1980): In: Ergot Compounds and Brain Function: Neuroendocrine and Neuropsychiatric Aspects, edited by M. Goldstein, D.B. Calne, A. Lieberman, and M.O. Thorner, pp. 125-139. Raven Press, New York.

58. Schran, H.F., Schwarz, H.J., Talbot, K.C., and Loeffler, L.J. (1979): <u>Clin. Chem.</u>, 25/11:1928-1933.

59. Schwab, R.S., Amador, L.V., and Lettvin, J.T. (1951): <u>Trans. Am. Neurol. Assoc.</u>, 76:251-253.

60. Shelesnyak, M.C. (1954): <u>Am. J. Physiol.</u>, 179:301-304.

61. Sieversten, G., Lim, U.S., Narawatase, C., and Fronman, L.A. (1979): <u>Clin. Res.</u>, 27:260A.

62. Smith, R.L. (1971): In: <u>Handbook of Experimental Pharmacology, Vol. 28</u>, edited by B.B. Brodie and J.R. Gillette, pp. 354-385. Springer-Verlag, Berlin.

63. Teychenne, P.F., Jones, E.A., Ishak, K.G., and Calne, D.B. (1979): <u>Gastroenterology</u>, 76:575-583.

64. Teychenne, P.F., Pfeiffer, R., Bern, S.M., and Calne, D.B. (1977): <u>Neurology</u>, 27:1140-1143.

65. Teychenne, P.F., Pfeiffer, R.F., Bern, S.M., McInturff, D., and Calne, D.B. (1978): <u>Ann. Neurol.</u>, 3:319-324.

66. Toda, T., Oshino, N. (1981).

67. Trabucchi, M., Spano, P.F., Tonon, G.C., and Frattola, L. (1976): <u>Life Sci.</u>, 19:225-231.

68. Vakil, S.D., Calne, D.B., Reid, J.L., and Seymour, C.A. (1973): In: <u>Advances in Neurology, Vol. 3., Progress in the Treatment of Parkinsonism.</u>, edited by D.B. Calne, pp. 121-130. Raven Press, New York.

69. Yeo, T., Thorner, M.O., Jones, A., Lowry, P.J., and Besser, G.M. (1979): <u>Clin. Endocrinol.</u>, 10:123-130.

70. Internal Reports of Schering.

*Apomorphine and Other Dopaminomimetics,
Vol. 2: Clinical Pharmacology*, edited by
G. U. Corsini and G. L. Gessa, Raven Press,
New York © 1981.

The Treatment of Parkinson's Disease with Dopaminergic Agonists in Combination with Domperidone

Y. Agid, *N. Quinn, **P. Pollak, †A. Illas, ‡A. Destee, J. L. Signoret, and F. Lhermitte

*Clinique de Neurologie et Neuropsychologie, Hôpital de la Salpêtriere, 75634 Paris, Cedex 13 France; *Department of Neurology, Institute of Psychiatry, London SE5 8AF, United Kingdom; **Clinique de Neurologie, CHU, Grenoble, France; †Department of Neurology, Faculty of Medicine, Athens, Greece; ‡Clinique de Neurologie, CHU, Lille, France*

INTRODUCTION

The advent of L-DOPA and the increase in its efficacy obtained through combination with a peripheral decarboxylase inhibitor (PDI) revolutionized the treatment of Parkinson's disease. The use of dopaminergic (DA) substances acting directly at post-synaptic level, such as piribedil (5), bromocriptine (22) or N-propyl-apomorphine (8) holds out the prospect of further advances in therapy. Bromocriptine, because of its long duration of action (12), has been used with some success for several years. However, its application has been limited mainly because of undesired side effects (9). Among these, dizziness and psychic disturbance are the most striking particularly when high doses are employed (4). The other complications are similar in nature and frequency to those of L-DOPA, particularly gastrointestinal intolerance and orthostatic hypotension which can arise even at the very start of treatment (4).

How can these side effects be avoided? To develop a rational treatment plan, it is necessary to examine the actions of bromocriptine in the brain (Fig.1). Bromocriptine stimulates DA receptors throughout the brain, in particular in the striatum which is situated inside the blood brain barrier but also in the area postrema which probably constitutes the chemoreceptor trigger zone of the vomiting center, and is located outside the blood brain barrier (Fig.1). Thus, the amelioration of parkinsonian symptoms achieved through stimulation of central DA receptors may be accompanied by nausea

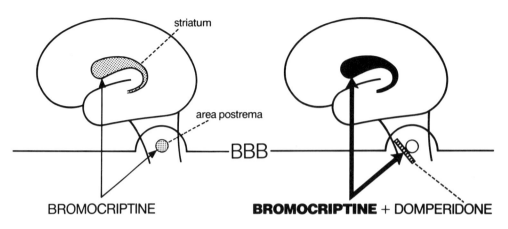

FIGURE 1.

and vomiting caused by stimulation of DA receptors in the
area postrema. Neuroleptics (21) or substituted benzamides
(14,15) can reduce the incidence of nausea by blocking DA
receptors in the area postrema, but only at the expense of
limiting the beneficial actions of L-DOPA or bromocriptine
by blocking striatal DA receptors as well. In order to pre-
serve the central effects of DA agonists whilst at the same
time suppressing the peripheral effects, it would be necessary to block only the peripheral DA receptors, leaving central
receptors unaffected. In other words, one should administer
bromocriptine together with a DA receptor blocker which does
not cross the blood brain barrier. Such a drug exists: domperidone. This substance is a butyrophenone with great affinity for DA receptors, but which does not cross the blood brain
barrier even at high doses (13). If bromocriptine is given
together with domperidone (Fig.1), the peripheral side effects of treatment such as nausea and vomiting, and perhaps
hypotension, caused by stimulation of receptors in the region
of the area postrema should be diminished or abolished without any reduction of central antiparkinsonian effect. Following this hypothesis, one could hope that domperidone might
be to bromocriptine what a PDI has become to L-DOPA, although
clearly acting through a different mechanism.

The Use of Domperidone in tne Treatment of Parkinson's
Disease by Bromocriptine.

Acute, subacute and chronic studies have been undertaken.
In an initial double blind trial in 17 patients treated
with bromocriptine, we postulated that the prevention of
nausea and vomiting by domperidone (20 mg t.d.s.) would

allow increased daily doses of bromocriptine, resulting in improved antiparkinsonian efficacy (2). The 8 patients treated by domperidone plus bromocriptine did not experience vomiting; the mean daily dose of bromocriptine reached 148 mg; the therapeutic benefit was at least as good as that obtained with L-DOPA plus PDI, the mean clinical score improving by 76% over baseline score on no treatment. Among the 9 patients taking placebo instead of domperidone, it was not possible to raise the mean daily dosage of bromocriptine above 92 mg, with a mean clinical improvement of only 48%. In 5 of these 9 subjects, the dose of bromocriptine could not be increased because of nausea and vomiting. Prior to the trial we had confirmed that domperidone did not inhibit bromocriptine induced clinical improvement and therfore was not crossing the blood brain barrier (2).

A second study (17) was undertaken to confirm the findings of the initial study after more prolonged treatment. This was a single blind study in 20 patients receiving bromocriptine in total dose increments of 22.5 mg per day. In one group of patients, domperidone was given from the outset in association with bromocriptine, in the other group, the patients initially received bromocriptine and placebo. This study enabled us: 1) to confirm that patients could be improved by an average of 71% over baseline with a mean daily bromocriptine dose of 148 mg as a result of the reduction in intensity and frequency of nausea caused by domperidone; 2) to establish the advantage of introducing domperidone from the outset of treatment, which allowed effective doses of bromocriptine to be attained in 3 to 8 days; 3) to demonstrate the need to continue domperidone in more than half the patients (13/20). In this series the beneficial results of the association of bromocriptine with domperidone were still present after two months of treatment, with no significant change in parkinsonian score or dose of bromocriptine (17).

A total of 42 patients treated with bromocriptine ± domperidone alone at the beginning of follow-up have been reviewed after longer periods (3) (Table 1). They fell into three groups: those who were still on the same treatment, those who were taking additional L-DOPA plus PDI, and those in whom bromocriptine had been discontinued. Fifteen patients were still taking bromocriptine ± domperidone after 18 months: the mean daily dosage of bromocriptine was 146 mg and almost half of these patients were still taking domperidone (Table 1). In 12 patients, L-DOPA plus PDI was added to treatment most commonly in order to compensate for an unacceptable delay before the first morning dose of bromocriptine took effect:

TABLE 1. Long term results of bromocriptine plus domperidone treatment in Parkinson's disease.

Treatment	Number of patients	Duration of treatment (months)	Daily dose of bromocriptine (mg)	Number of patients taking domperidone	Daily dose of L-DOPA + PDI (mg)
Parlodel $\pm$ Domperidone	15	18.5 (10 - 33)	146 (50 - 240)	7[++]	0
Parlodel $\pm$ Domperidone and L-DOPA + PDI	12	20.8[+] (10 - 34)	85 (10 - 180)	3	454 (100 - 1125)

+ Treatment with Parlodel $\pm$ Domperidone alone had been continued for 11.4 months

++ The daily dose was 150 mg in 2 patients and 60 mg in 5 patients respectively

in these subjects, the mean daily dosage of bromocriptine
was accordingly lower than in the first group (85 mg) (Table
1). Finally, treatment with bromocriptine ± domperidone had
to be abandoned in 15 patients. Of these, 2 died of inter-
current illness and 3 were lost to follow up. Of the remaining 10, 3 preferred the control of symptoms obtained with
their previous regime, and 1 patient who had previously responded well to L-DOPA obtained no therapeutic response with
bromocriptine even at a dose of 240 mg per day. The other 6
patients were obliged to stop bromocriptine because of severe
side effects : 1 patient developed continuous headache, and
1, intractable hiccough; 1 patient with a past history of
orthostatic hypotension developed severe hypotension; 3 developed confusional states with hallucinations necessitating
immediate withdrawal of bromocriptine; in 2 of these, this
side effect persisted long after the resumption of treatment
with a minimal dose of L-DOPA plus PDI; in the other patient,
replacement of bromocriptine with small doses of L-DOPA was
associated with a rapid disappearance of confusion. It is
important to note that the last 3 patients all had antecedents
of intellectual deterioration, and two of them had previously
experienced acute mental disturbance.

Particular attention was paid to the incidence of hypotension (18) considering the following questions. 1) Does a dose-
dependent hypotension occur with bromocriptine? 2) What is
the frequency of episodes of significant postural hypotension
(SPH)? 3) Is the hypotension produced of central or peripheral
origin? The hypotensive action of bromocriptine has been previously described after acute administration of single variable doses (10) and with subacute treatment at relatively low
doses (47 mg per day) (11). But what happens to blood pressure
in patients treated with dosages of bromocriptine of the order
of 150 mg per day? The comparison of blood pressure and pulse
in 20 parkinsonian patients receiving a mean dose of bromocriptine of 148 mg per day with the values in the same patients
on no treatment showed a significant and dose-dependent fall
in erect systolic and diastolic, and supine systolic blood
pressure, and an increase in erect pulse rate (Table 2) (18).
Episodes of SPH have also been observed with bromocriptine
treatment, sometimes occurring with single doses as low as 2.
5 mg (4). What is their frequency with high doses of bromocriptine? In our study (18), episodes of SPH were recorded in 13
of the 20 patients occurring on 33 occasions out of a total
of 234 series of blood pressure readings, with a maximal frequency corresponding to individual doses of 40 to 50 mg. These
episodes were usually asymptomatic, appearing immediately on

rising or after one minute standing and disappearing after
5 minutes standing. In all patients these episodes of SPH
were a transitory phenomenon and never caused us to stop treatment or slow down the rate of dose increase. The mechanism
of hypotension induced by bromocriptine is unclear. Since
bromocriptine is first and foremost a DA agonist (1), the mechanism would seem most likely to be a dopaminergic one, although the drug may in addition have some α-stimulant effect
(6). But is this effect centrally or peripherally mediated?
We were able to compare the same patients under different treatments i.e with both central and peripheral DA receptors
stimulated (Bromocriptine plus Placebo) and with central receptor stimulation only (equivalent dose of bromocriptine
plus domperidone) (18). Figure 2 shows that systolic and diastolic blood pressure and pulse on a constant high dose of
bromocriptine were not affected by the addition or discontinuation of domperidone, suggesting that the mechanism by which
bromocriptine produces an overall lowering of blood pressure
is principally a central one. However these results should
not be regarded as conclusive, particularly in view of the
recent finding in an acute study (16) that orthostatic hypotension caused by the administration of a single dose of 20
mg of bromocriptine in parkinsonian patients could be diminished or prevented by pretreatment with domperidone. Such apparently differing findings may nevertheless be compatible

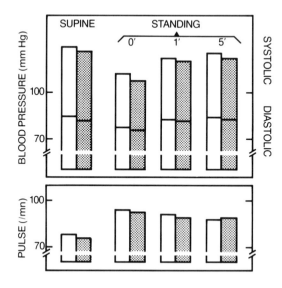

FIGURE 2. Blood pressure and pulse in 20 Parkinsonian
        patients treated with bromocriptine (134-142
        mg daily) with (white column) and without
        (shaded column) domperidone.

since, as has been suggested for L-DOPA (19), the smooth dose-dependent lowering of blood pressure seen with bromocriptine may be mediated through a different mechanism than episodic postural hypotension.

The Use of Domperidone in the Treatment of Parkinson's Disease by other Dopaminergic Agonists.

Parallel to our initial study, Corsini et al (7) were able to show that apomorphine-induced nausea and vomiting could be abolished by previous administration of domperidone. Domperidone has also been used in combination with the potent ergolene derivative, lisuride (20). We have recently tested a putative DA receptor stimulating agent (CQ 3284, SANDOZ, another ergolene derivative) in 5 parkinsonian patients receiving domperidone as well. During a mean period of time of 12 days, CQ 3284 was progressively increased to a mean daily dose of 68 mg (10 to 150 mg). Nausea observed at the beginning of treatment disappeared following increase in the daily dose of domperidone (150 mg per day). Parkinsonian score was reduced by 57% but treatment had to be discontinued in 2 patients because of the occurrence of delusions and hallucinations and no therapeutic benefit was obtained in 2 others.

CONCLUSION

The association of domperidone with a direct DA receptor agonist is of value in the treatment of Parkinson's disease. This has been demonstrated in patients studied over a period of days (2,17) and on review after two months (17) and twenty months (3). This drug combination is useful wherever bromocriptine treatment is indicated, but particularly when end-of-dose wearing off effect in Parkinson's disease is a troublesome problem (12). The degree of clinical benefit obtained, at least equal to that with L-DOPA plus PDI, probably depends on the attainment of sufficiently high doses levels (on the order of 120 to 140 mg per day in our patients). In our experience with 37 patients followed-up, this treatment has not led to significant problems, other than the usual minor undesirable effects (mainly somnolence, but also abnormal involuntary movements, headache, conjunctivitis, hot flushes and subjective palpitations) on condition that patients with a previous history of orthostatic hypotension or autonomic failure, or with evidence of intellectual deterioration or

past mental disturbance were excluded. It should also be noted that this treatment regime was always commenced under
hospitalization. The addition of domperidone has a marked effect in reducing nausea and vomiting without influencing dose-
dependent lowering of blood pressure or SPH. The postural hypotension seen was always transitory, and was not therfore a
contraindication to continuing treatment or further increasing the dose of bromocriptine. In summary, we have found domperidone useful in two respects: firstly, it permits bromocriptine doses to be rapidly increased and, secondly, the
higher daily dose levels achieved allow optimum therapeutic
benefit to be obtained. The systematic association of domperidone with new DA agonists used in Parkinson's disease is a
promising development.

REFERENCES

1. Agid,Y., Bonnet,A.M.,Javoy-Agid,F.,Kato,G.,Lhermitte,F.,
    Pollak,P.,Signoret,J.L.,(1979): Biomedicine,30: 67-71.

2. Agid,Y.,Pollak,P.,Bonnet,A.M.,Signoret,J.L.,Lhermitte,F.
    (1979): Lancet, i: 570-572.

3. Agid,Y.,Quinn,N.,Lhermitte,F.(in press)

4. Calne,D.B.,Plotkin,C.,Williams,A.C.,Nutt,J.G.,Neophytides,
    A.,Teychenne,P.F.(1978): Lancet, i: 735-738.

5. Chase,T.N.,Woods,A.C.,Glaubiger,G.A.,(1974): Arch.Neurol.
    30: 383-386.

6. Clark,B.J.,Scholtysik,G.,Fluckiger,E.(1978): Acta Endo-
    crinologica , suppl 216: 88: 75-81.

7. Corsini,G.U.,Del Zompo,M.,Gessa,G.L.,Mangoni,A.(1979):
    Lancet, i: 954-956.

8. Cotzias,G.C.,Papavasiliou,P.S.,Tolosa,E.S.,Mendez,J.S.,
    Bell-Midura,M.(1976): New Engl.J.Med.,294: 567-572.

9. Fahn,S.,Cote,L.J.,Snider,S.R.,Barret,R.E.,Isgreen,W.P.
    (1979): Neurology,29: 1077-1083.

10. Galea Debono,A.,Marsden,C.D.,Asselman,P.,Parkes,J.D.(1976)
    : Brit.J.Clin.Pharm.,3: 977-982.

11. Greenacre,J.K.,Teychenne,P.F.,Petrie,A.,Calne,D.B.,Leigh,
    P.N.,Reid,J.L.(1976): Brit.J.Clin.Pharm.,3: 571-574.

12. Kartzinel,R.,Calne,D.B.(1976): Neurology,26: 508-510.

13. Laduron,P.M.,Leysen,J.E.(1979): Biochem.Pharmacol.,
    8: 2151-2155.

14. Lhermitte,F.,Signoret,J.L.,Agid,Y.(1977): Sem.Hop.Paris, 53: 9-15.

15. Parkes,J.D.,Debono,A.G.,Marsden,C.D.(1976): J.Neurol. Neurosurg.Psy.,39: 1101-1108.

16. Pollak,P.,Gaio,J.M.,Hommel,M.,Pellat,J.,Chateau.(in press)

17. Quinn,N.,Illas,A.,Lhermitte,F.,Agid,Y.(1981): Neurology, (in press).

18. Quinn,N.,Illas,A.,Lhermitte,F.,Agid,Y.(1981):(submitted for publication).

19. Reid,J.L.,Calne,D.B.,George,C.F.,Vakil,S.D.,(1972):Clin. Sci.,43: 851-859.

20. Schachter,M.,Blackstock,J.,Dick,J.P.R.,George,R.J.,Marsden,C.D.,Parkes,J.D.(1979): Lancet,ii: 1129.

21. Tarsy,D.,Parkes,J.D.,Marsden,C.D.(1975): J.Neurol.Neurosurg.Psy., 38: 331-335.

22. Teychenne,P.F.,Calne,D.B.,Leigh,P.N.,Greenacre,J.K.,Reid, J.L.,Petrie,A.,Bamji,A.N.(1975): Lancet, ii: 473-476.

Apomorphine and Other Dopaminomimetics,
Vol. 2: Clinical Pharmacology, edited by
G. U. Corsini and G. L. Gessa, Raven Press,
New York © 1981.

Piribedil and Parkinson's Disease: Protection of Peripheral Side-Effects by Domperidone

*A. Agnoli, M. Baldassarre, S. Del Roscio, N. Palesse, and S. Ruggieri

Clinica Neurologica, Università di Roma, 00100 Roma, Italy; Clinica Neurologica, Istituto Universitario di Medicina, 67100 L'Aquila, Italy

INTRODUCTION

Dopaminergic (DA) agonists revealed interesting therapeutic applications in Parkinson's disease. Their use allowed: a) to delay l-dopa treatment in early stages of this disease, thus prolonging the period of therapeutic effectiveness of l-dopa (7), b) to reduce dosage of l-dopa in patients affected by l-dopa long-term syndrome, c) to reduce some side effects in long-term syndrome (9), d) and finally, to improve the progression of the disease, since they stimulate directly dopamine receptors without affecting dopaminergic neurons.

Moreover, DA agonists improve tremor, which is the symptom less influenced by l-dopa treatment.

Among DA agonists, the ergolinic derivatives such as bromocriptine, lisuride and pergolide and the piperidin derivatives such as piribedil have been successfully employed.

Unfortunately these drugs exert many side effects which are the result of a stimulation of peripheral (nausea, vomiting, hypotension) and central dopamine receptors (confusion, delusion).

The arising of these side effects limits the possibility of reaching effective doses of DA agonists in the combined treatment with l-dopa or l-dopa + decarboxylase inhibitors (DI).

Actually the use of decarboxylase inhibitors in combination with l-dopa did not completely overcome the problems connected with the use of the inhibitors alone.

Benserazide, in fact, induces hyperprolactinemia, either alone or in combination with l-dopa (2,10). Carbidopa does not completely abolish gastric side-effects induced by l-dopa (11), moreover, both inhibitors reduce the oxidative metabolism of tryptophan (3).

Recently in order to prevent the side-effects induced by DA agonists, a peripheral DA antagonist, domperidone, a benzimidazolinic deriviative that does not cross the blood-brain barrier (6), has been used.

The combination of domperidone with bromocriptine (1) or with apomorphine (5) in Parkinson's disease revealed a better control of some side-effects, of the latter, resulting in a therapeutic improvement.

The aim of this study was to evaluate the combination of piribedil with domperidone in Parkinson's disease.

Piribedil has been used in the present study since, besides stimulating DA receptors like the ergolinics, it also releases DA from the neuronal extragranular pool (4). Further a relevant number of clinical studies on the efficacy of piribedil in Parkinson's disease is available (TAB. 1).

TABLE 1. <u>Piribedil in Parkinson's disease: review of literature data</u>
<u>(mod. by Lieberman et al. '75 -8-)</u>

AUTHORS	Nr. Patients	Nr. Showing Anti-park. Effect	Predominant Sign (Ameliorated)	Piribedil Maximum (Mg/day)
Vakil '73	16	4	Tremor	240
Shaw & Stern '74	17	0	0	120
Mc Lellan '74	9	3	Tremor	200
Fieschi '74	18	13	Tremor and rigidity	180
Emile & Chanelet '74	10	6	Tremor and bradikinesia	240
Chase '74	16	12	Tremor, bradikinesia and rigidity	540
Lieberman '74	8	3	Tremor	280
Engel '74	10	6	Tremor	240
Mc Dowell '75	15	6	Tremor, bradikinesia and rigidity	300
Truelle '77	60	39	Tremor	450
Balzer & Stauton '78	10	9	Bradikinesia	120-200

See for references Lieberman '75 (8).

MATERIALS AND METHODS

15 subjects, 8 men and 7 women, with a mean age of 66 years, affected by Parkinson's disease from 1 to 5 years have been studied. Disability rank was between the I and V stage of the Hoehn-Yahr scale.

The clinical forms were as follows: complete form (7 cases), hyperkinetic form (5 cases) and akinetic-hypertonic form (3).

All subjects already under treatment (8 with l-dopa + D.I. associated with an anticholinergic, 4 only with anticholinergics) and those not treated (3 cases), underwent a drug washout period of 10 days. After the wash-out period (FIG.1), domperidone was administered (15 mg/os/day in 3 doses).

After 4 days of treatment, piribedil was added in 3 daily doses. The administration was progressively increased (50 mg every 3 days) until the highest tolerated dose or up to a maximum dose of 500 mg/day. At this time the treatment continued for 30 days at least.

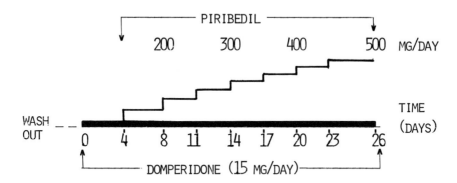

FIG. 1. Methodology of the study.

Evaluation of the severity of the disease has been performed by means of the Webster rating scale, including 10 items with a score that varied from 1 (minimum) to 4 (maximum).

Tremor, bradikynesia and rigidity were evaluated with a semiquantitative scale scored from 1 (min.) to 4 (max. disability). The baseline was evaluated at the end of the wash-out period and repeated until reaching the doses of 200, 300, 400, and 500 mg of piribedil.

Side-effects were assessed with a side-effects rating scale. The routine laboratory and instrumental tests were performed at baseline time and at the end of the study. Statistical analyses have been performed using the Student's "t" test for unpaired data.

RESULTS

The maximum dose of 500 mg/day was not achieved in 3 subjects, because of the upcoming of serious hypotension (1 case), hallucination (1 case) and diskinesia (1 case) at the dose of 350-400 mg/day. These side-effects regressed with the reduction of the dosage. The other patients did not present disabling side-effects (TAB. 2).

The improvement induced by piribedil seems to be correlated to the dosage. In fact (FIG. 2), the overall improvement of Webster rating scale was 3.5% at 200 mg/day and 29% at 500 mg/day. Bradikynesia and rigidity show a similar course but rigidity showed more improvement than bradikynesia that appears to be the less influenced symptom (maximum improvement 18.7% to 400 and to 500 mg/day). However, even if the improvement of rigidity is more evident (31% to 500 mg/day), it does not achieve statistical significance.

On the contrary, the improvement of tremor is statistically significant (32%) at the dose of 300-400 mg/day and is of higher significance at 500 mg/day.

TAB. 2.   Side-effects of piribedil + domperidone in 15 patients with
          Parkinson's disease.

SYMPTOMS	MILD nr. patients	SEVERE nr. patients
Hypotension	3	1
Confusion	3	0
Allucination	0	1
Abnormal involuntary movements (A.I.M.)	1	1
Drowsiness	2	0
Nausea or vomiting	6	0

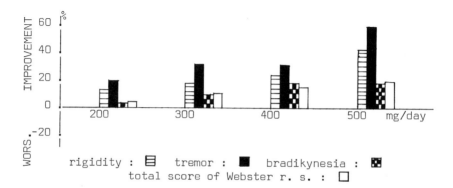

rigidity : ▤   tremor : ■   bradikynesia : ▥
          total score of Webster r. s. : ☐

FIG. 2.   Modification of symptomatology after piribedil + domperidone at
          different doses in 15 parkinsonian patients.

    Regarding the drug effectiveness in relationship to the clinical
forms, the treatment with piribedil + domperidone improves mostly the
complete form (FIG. 3), than the akinetic -hypertonic form (FIG. 4).

    This finding, also considering the improvement induced by piribedil
in the hyperkinetic form (FIG. 5) indicates that the drug is effective
mainly on tremor, less on rigidity and least on bradikynesia.

                        DISCUSSION AND CONCLUSION.

    The treatment of Parkinson's disease with a DA agonist, such as
piribedil, in combination with a peripheral dopaminergic blocker, such
as domperidone, showed that this combined treatment has an undoubtedly
therapeutic effectiveness along with a decrease of the side-effects.
    Piribedil, at the doses used, specifically affects tremor, a symp-
tom significantly improved by the combined treatment, thus confirming
the previous observations (TAB. 1).
    On the contrary, the improvement is less evident and sometimes ab-

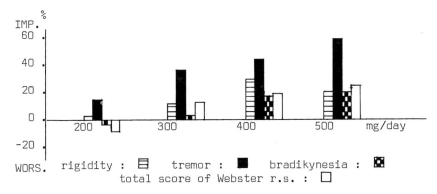

FIG. 3. Modification of symptomatology after piribedil + domperidone at different doses in 7 parkinsonian patients with complete form.

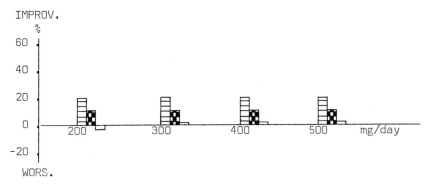

FIG. 4. Modification of symptomatology after piribedil + domperidone at different doses in 3 parkinsonian patients with akinetic-hyper-tonic form.

sent on bradikynesia and rigidity.

The therapeutic use of piribedil alone or in combination with 1-dopa might be helpful in the clinical forms of Parkinson's disease in which tremor represents a dominant sign.

The efficacy of piribedil alone is ranging between 25-36% improvement in the total score of Parkinson's disease severity (TAB. 1); maximal efficacy has been shown on tremor.

It should be emphasized that the most effective dose seems to range between 400 and 500 mg/day, much higher than most of the effective doses reported in the literature (TAB. 1). At this dosage however it is necessary to combine domperidone in order to avoid unpleasant side-effects of piribedil.

The use of piribedil + domperidone, at the doses employed, showed to induce few side-effects, mainly on cardiovascular and gastric apparatus, and to be of great value in the treatment of Parkinson's disease with an hyperkinetic symptomatology that is less sensitive to 1-dopa treatment.

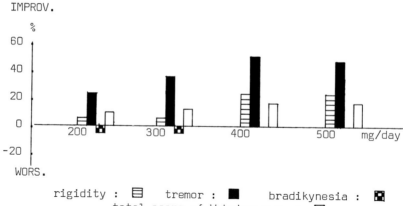

FIG. 5. Modification of symptomatology after piribedil + domperidone at different doses in 5 parkinsonian patients with hyperkinetic form.

REFERENCES

1. Agid, Y., Pollack, P., Bonnet, A.M., Signoret, J.L., Lhermitte, F. (1979): Lancet, March 17, 570-572.
2. Agnoli, A., Ruggieri, S., Baldassarre, M., Rocco, A., Del Roscio, S., D'Urso, R., Mearelli, S., Falaschi, P., Frajese, G. (1980): Neurochemistry and Clinical Neurology, edited by L. Battistin, G.A. Hashim, A. Lajtha, pp. 154-162, Alan Liss, New York.
3. Bender, D.A. (1980): Biochemical Pharmacol., 29: 707-712.
4. Corrodi, H., Fuxe, K., Ungerstedt, U. (1971): J.Pharm.Pharmac., 23: 989-991.
5. Corsini, G.U., Del Zompo, M., Gessa, G.L., Mangoni, A. (1979): Lancet, May 5: 954-956.
6. Costall, B., Fortune, D.H., Naylor, R.J. (1979): J.Pharm.Pharmacol., 31: 344-347.
7. Fahn, S., Calne, D.B. (1978): Neurology, Jan. 78: 5-7.
8. Lieberman, A.N., Shopsin, B., Lebrun, Y., Boal, D., Zolfaghari, M. (1975): Adv. in Neurology, Vol. 9, edited by Calne, D.B., Chase, T.N., Barbeau, A., pp.399-405, Raven Press, New York.
9. Lieberman, A.N., Liebowitz, M., Neophytides, A., Kupersmith, M., Mehl, S., Kleinberg, D., Serby, M., Goldstein, M. (1979): Lancet, Nov.24: 1129-1130.
10. Pontiroli, A.E., Castegnaro, E., Vettaro, M.P., Viberti, G.C., Pozza, G. (1977): Acta Endocrinol., 84: 36-44.
11. Rinne, U.K., Mölsä, P. (1979): Neurology, 29: 1584-1589.
12. Sweet, R.O., Warterlain, C.G., McDowell, F.H. (1974): Clin.Pharm & Ther., 16: 1077-1082.
13. Vakil, S.D., Calne, D.B., Reid, J.L., Seymour, C.A. (1973): In: Adv. in Neurology, Vol. 3, edited by Calne, D.B., pp. 121-125, Raven Press, New York.

*Apomorphine and Other Dopaminomimetics,
Vol. 2: Clinical Pharmacology*, edited by
G. U. Corsini and G. L. Gessa, Raven Press,
New York © 1981.

Animal Models for the Prediction and Prevention of Dyskinesias Induced by Dopaminergic Drugs

K. G. Lloyd, C. L. E. Broekkamp, F. Cathala, P. Worms, *M. Goldstein, and T. Asano

*Biology Department, LERS, Synthélabo, F75013 Paris, France; *Department of Neurochemistry, New York University Medical Center, New York, New York 10016*

INTRODUCTION

Dopamine mimetics have several therapeutic uses in man, including the therapy of Parkinson's disease (e.g. L-DOPA, bromocriptine, piribedil, cf. 4, 8, 21, 28), depression (nomifensine, cf. 18), various neuro-endocrine disorders (e.g. bromocryptine, cf. 32, 33) and have potential use as diuretics (17) and antipsychotics (apomorphine, but possibly not other DA mimetics, cf. 10, 40, 42). Dopamine mimetics can act via various mechanisms, including metabolism to dopamine itself (L-DOPA), direct receptor activation (apomorphine, piribedil), inhibition of metabolism of dopamine (MAO inhibitors), inhibition of reuptake (nomifensine) or induction of release (amphetamine). However, no matter which mechanism of activity is involved, all the dopamine mimetics presently used chronically in clinical situations induce stereotyped behaviours or abnormal-involuntary movements (AIMs) as secondary effects. In some instances these effects force the reduction or cessation of therapy, especially in the treatment of Parkinson's disease (1, 3, 28, 34). These stereotyped behaviours can be blocked by the administration of neuroleptic drugs (cf. 44), but this has two inherent disadvantages : (i) dopamine receptor blockade often reduces in parallel the therapeutic effect of the dopamine mimetic (5, 11), (ii) after cessation of the neuroleptic there is a supersensitivity to dopamine mimetics, resulting in a pronounciation of their stereotypic effect (13, 16, 39).

It would be of considerable benefit if an index of the stereotypic potential of new dopamine mimetic compounds could be assessed, at an early stage of their development. An obvious method is the induction of stereotyped behaviours in laboratory animals. However, such stereotyped behaviours are not necessarily the same as dyskinetic movements, and such behaviours can be species specific. Furthermore, the rating scales used to quantify stereotyped behaviours varies considerably between investigators. The present study had the following goals : (i) to find a simple behavioural test to predict the potential of a compound to induce stereotypies or abnormal involuntary movements ; (ii) to further

develop the hypothesis that stereotyped behaviours can be effectively
reduced by compounds other than those which block dopamine receptors
(ie neuroleptics), specifically GABA agonists, as these compounds have
been shown to reduce both presynaptic and postsynaptic indices of
dopamine neuron function (cf. ref. 31) as well as decreasing DA-mimetic
induced stereotypies (5, 15, 31). Such a compound is progabide
(SL 76 002), a non-toxic GABA agonist (12, 30). Several prototypic
dopamine mimetics were used : apomorphine, which is a direct dopamine
receptor agonist, activating the dopamine sensitive adenylate cyclase
(22, 25), piribedil, also a dopamine agonist, but which has at most a
marginal effect on adenylate cyclase but whose catechol metabolite
activates adenylate cyclase (22) ; amphetamine, which both stimulates
dopamine release and inhibits its uptake into nerve terminals (9),
nomifensine, an inhibitor of dopamine uptake (20, 27) and L-DOPA, the
immediate precursor of dopamine in its synthetic pathway.

METHODS

Measurement of Stereotyped Behaviours and Dyskinesias

For the induction of stereotyped movements in the rat, drugs were
injected either subcutaneously (apomorphine, nomifensine) or intraperitoneally (d-amphetamine, piribedil), and the animals were then
observed for 4 hours post-administration. The presence or absence of
the following stereotyped movements were noted on an "all-or-none"
basis : licking, sniffing, gnawing and/or biting.

In mice, a climbing behaviour on a wire mesh is induced by some
dopamine mimetics and is considered by some authors to be a variant of
stereotyped behaviour (35). The test compounds were administered either
subcutaneously (apomorphine) or intraperitoneally, the mice were then
placed in individual cages, and the climbing behaviour assessed as
previously described (44).

In cats, the stereotyped behaviours and dyskinetic-movements were
monitored by a remote television camera, as the physical presence of
an observer was found to greatly alter the behaviour of the animals.
Stereotypies were defined as purposeless patterned elements of behaviour, pre-existing in the behavioural repertoire. Oral-buccal movements were excluded. Many of these behaviours persisted in the face of
a distraction (e.g. the presence of an observer). Dyskinesias were
defined as movements that are not (or at most sporadically) observed in
untreated cats. These included sudden limb extensions or limb flicks,
shaking, or athetoid movements. These behaviours are rather easily
suppressed by distractions.

The abnormal movements induced by dopamine mimetics in the monkey
were grouped into three categories : (i) AIMs Type I included increased
aggressiveness and threatening posture, restlessness, chattering, irra-
tability, hypersensitivity and increased water intake ; (ii) AIMS
Type II were comprised of repetitive movements of mouth, tongue and
face, hyperkinesias, increased prolonged repetitive grooming of the
same body area, monotonous side-to-side swaying, repetitive purposeless
hand movements, and unusual posturing ; and (iii) choreas.

Other Behaviours

Emetic episodes in Beagle dogs were counted over a 1-hour period after a slow (2 min) intraveinous infusion of the compound to be studied. the effect of compounds on the initial exploratory phase of locomotor activity in mice was assessed as previously described (44). The antagonism of haloperidol-induced catalepsy was studied in rats previously (30 min) injected with haloperidol (1.0 mg/kg, ip). The test compounds were administered subcutaneously (apomorphine) or intraperitoneally and the catalepsy assessed on a "all-or-none" basis by means of the four-cork test (44).

RESULTS

Models Predictive of AIMs Production

Of the four different dopamine mimetics studied (Table 1) in the rat, apomorphine was the most potent in producing a high incidence of stereotyped movements (gnawing, sniffing, grooming, etc...), whereas piribedil was the least effective. However, at doses which induced stereotypies in all of the animals, piribedil had the longest duration of action whereas that of apomorphine was the shortest.

Apomorphine was the only compound to induce a horizontal mesh-climbing behaviour in the mouse. The other compounds used were inactive at doses equal to (amphetamine, piribedil) or greater than (nomifensine) those which induced stereotyped behaviour. However, the other compounds potentiated this effect of apomorphine (data not shown). In contrast only amphetamine and nomifensine increased the exploratory phase of locomotor behaviour of mice placed in a novel environment. Piribedil and apomorphine actually decreased this exploratory phase, although the latter compound greatly increased locomotion once the animals were habituated to their surroundings (data not shown).

The ability of different compounds to reverse the cataleptic state induced by haloperidol in the rat seemed to be closely related to their stereotypic potential. Thus, apomorphine and amphetamine were very active in reversing catalepsy, nomifensine was equally active in both stereotypy and catalepsy tests and piribedil was the least active in either test.

The emetic activity of a large series of dopamine mimetics was tested and compared with their ability to induce stereotyped behaviour (Table 2). Pergolide, hydergine and apomorphine were very active in this test, whereas d-amphetamine and nomifensine were inactive. Thus, the ability of different dopaminergic compounds to provoke vomiting in the dog does not appear to be related to their induction of stereotypies in the rat. However, the cat may be more susceptible to the emetic effects of these latter compounds (unpublished results).

The differentiation of dopamine mimetic-induced stereotyped behaviours from dyskinesias was assessed in the cat (Fig. 1). Apomorphine provoked dyskinetic movements at relatively low doses whereas stereotyped behaviours were seen only at the highest dose used. In contrast, nomifensine and d-amphetamine readily induced stereotyped

Table 1. Induction by different dopamine mimetics of stereotypies and related behaviour in rodents

Compound	Stereotyped Movements		Induction of Mesh-Climbing	Increase in Exploratory Motor Activity	Reversal of Haloperidol Catalepsy
	ED_{100}, mg/kg	Duration of action (min)	ED_{50}, mg/kg	ED_{100}, mg/kg	ED_{50}, mg/kg
Apomorphine	0.5 sc	45	1.0 sc	> 2.0 (↗) sc	1.8 sc
d-Amphetamine	5.0 ip	90	> 5.0 ip	2.0 ip	0.9 ip
Nomifensine	5.0 sc	90	> 30 ip	10 ip	5.5 ip
Piribedil	60 ip	180	> 60 ip	> 60 (↗) ip	47 ip

[1]. Dose inducing stereotyped movements in 100 percent of the animals (rats)
[2]. Dose inducing mesh-climbing in 50 percent of the mice.
[3]. Dose increasing by 100 percent the motor activity during the exploratory phase (mice).
[4]. Dose reversing haloperidol induced catalepsy in 50 percent of the rats.

FIG. 1., Induction of stereotypies and dyskinesias by dopamine mimetics in the Cat.

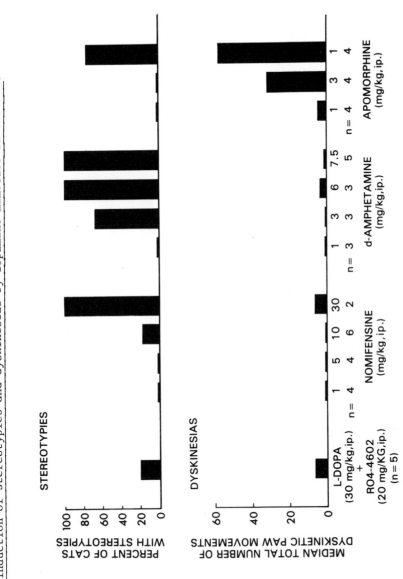

Stereotypies and dyskinesias were assessed as described in the text, with observation times of 40 min post-injection for nomifensine, d-amphetamine, and apomorphine and 80 min for L-DOPA.

Table 2. The emetic activity of dopamine mimetics in the Beagle-Dog : comparison with stereotypy potential in the Rat.

Compound	Emetic Effect ED_{50}, g/mg, iv	Stereotypy Potential (Rat)
Pergolide	3.9	nt
Hydergine	5.2	nt
Apomorphine	12.5	++++
Bromocryptine	15.1	nt
Piribedil	45	++
6,7 ADTN	60	nt
5,6 ADTN	82	nt
n-dipropyldopamine	194	nt
L-DOPA	1492	+
d-Amphetamine	> 2500	++++
Nomifensine	> 2000	++++
Amantadine	> 2000	nt

The ED_{50} is the dose which induces vomiting in 50 percent of the dogs. Drugs were administered in saline on a cumulative dose-response curve, 3-8 doses per dose-response curve, 4-6 dogs per compound.
nt : not tested ; +   slight ; ++ mild ; +++ strong ; ++++ very strong.

Table 3. Apomorphine-induced stereotypies in rats after repeated treatment with haloperidol or haloperidol plus progabide

Chronic treatments (10 days, daily injections)	Accumulated stereotypy scores (mean ± SEM) after a challenge dose of apomorphine (mg/kg, sc)		
	0.125	0.25	0.50
Vehicle	8.2 ± 0.3	16.3 ± 0.5	23.5 ± 0.7
Haloperidol (2 mg/kg, ip)	13.9 ± 0.8*	23.6 ± 0.7*	30.7 ± 0.6*
Haloperidol (2 mg/kg, ip) + Progabide (400 mg/kg, ip)	11.3 ± 0.7*+	19.8 ± 0.6*+	26.6 ± 0.9++

*p < 0.01 vs vehicle treated ;
+p < 0.05 ; ++p < 0.001 vs halop. treated.
n = 18 rats per treatment group per dose of apomorphine.

behaviours but were associated with the appearance of dyskinetic movements in most of the animals. L-DOPA was relatively ineffective in the induction of either dyskinetic or stereotyped movements.

Reduction of Dopamine Mimetic-Induced AIMs by GABAergic Mechanims

The reduction of dopamine-receptor related stereotyped behaviours has been assessed in two animal models related to different clinical situations. The first concerns the stereotypies which appear after chronic neuroleptic treatment. The model is the hypersensitivity to the stereotypic effects of apomorphine after withdrawal from a 10-day daily treatment schedule with haloperidol, in the rat (Table 3). Coadministration of progabide, a GABA agonist, with haloperidol throughout the administration period, resulted in a marked diminution of the supersensitivity to apomorphine, over a range of doses.

The effect of progabide on the frequency of dopamine mimetic-induced AIMs in a primate model of Parkinson's disease, was also studied. Preliminary results (Table 4) show that progabide completely blocked the mild oral dyskinesies (AIMs Type 2) and chorea induced by either L-DOPA or piribedil and at somewhat higher doses markedly reduced the Type 1 AIMs, especially those due to piribedil.

Table 4. Effect of progabide on L-DOPA and piribedil-induced abnormal involuntary movements (AIMs) in a monkey model of Parkinson's disease

Compounds	AIM Type I (Chattering)	AIM Type II (Oral Dyskinesia)	Chorea
L-DOPA			
50 mg/kg, ip	+-++	+	+-++
L-DOPA + Progabide			
25 mg/kg, po	±-+	absent	absent
50 mg/kg, po	+-++	absent	absent
Piribedil			
3 mg/kg, ip	+++	+	+
Piribedil + Progabide			
25 mg/kg, po	++-+++	absent	absent
50 mg/kg, po	-+	absent	absent
100 mg/kg, po	±-+	absent	absent

Rating scale : ± at limit of detection ; + slight ; ++ moderate ; +++ marked.

DISCUSSION

Drugs which are reputed to be dopamine mimetics induce a wide range of behavioral effects. These differ between mimetics and likely depend not only on which type of dopamine receptor is activated and whether the compounds work by primarily pre- or post synaptic mechanisms, but also on any non-dopaminergic effects induced by the different dopaminergic agents. In this regard, for the compounds presently used, apomorphine and piribedil are relatively specific for dopamine receptors, but amphetamine (9) and nomifensine (27) increase the synaptic concentrations of noradrenaline in addition to dopamine. Despite their different mechanisms of action, these compounds all induced stereotyped behaviours and reversed haloperidol catalepsy in the rat. The similar activities in these two tests together with the potent antistereotypic effect of haloperidol (23, 44) would suggest that the same dopamine receptor is responsible for both effects. Furthermore, manipulation of GABA receptors has parallel, opposite effects on stereotyped behaviours and catalepsy (31). It is also possible that the receptor involved is linked to an adenylate cyclase, as those neuroleptics which do not block dopamine-sensitive adenylate cyclase (e.g. sulpiride, 41) are much less effective in blocking stereotyped behaviours (43). What is clear from Tables 1 and 2 is that the ability of different dopamine mimetics to induce stereotyped movements (at least in laboratory animals) is not related to their ability to induce other behavioral effects such a mesh-climbing, increased exploratory activity, or emesis. For the later behaviour, the lack of effect of amphetamine and nomifensine, and the weak activity of L-DOPA is not surprising, as there are not many dopamine terminals in the area postrema (7, 14) at which these compounds could act.

The ability of these dopamine mimetics to induce stereotyped behaviours is not limited to the rat. Stereotypies are also noted in the cat (Fig. 1), the guinea-pig (26), the monkey (Table 4, ref. 38) and several other species, including man (36, 37). In the cat and the monkey it is possible to differentiate between stereotypies and dyskinetic movements. In cats, the compounds acting by releasing endogenous dopamine or blocking its reuptake (amphetamine, nomifensine) were more effective in inducing stereotypies (excluding oro-facial AIMs) than dyskinetic movements. Conversely, direct stimulation of dopamine receptors by apomorphine preferentially resulted in dyskinesias. This could be interpreted as meaning that stimulation of all forms of DA receptors (as occurs by greatly augmenting release and the synaptic levels of endogenous dopamine) results in stereotypies whereas selective activation of the apomorphine-sensitive receptors produces dyskinesias. Preliminary results indicate that piribedil has the same effect as apomorphine.

The present results confirm and extend previous observations that GABA agonists diminish stereotyped behaviours due to dopamine receptor stimulation both in the acute situation (5, 15, 31) and after cessation of chronic neuroleptic administration (29). Thus, in the rat, the hypersensitivity to apomorphine, three days after the end of a ten day haloperidol administration period, was significantly decreased by administration of progabide throughout the haloperidol treatment period. Furthermore, in monkeys with lesions of the nigrostriatal dopamine pathway, progabide completely blocked the chorea and oral dyskinesias (AIMs Type II) induced by either L-DOPA or piribedil and greatly reduced the AIMs Type I.

The mechanism of action of this antistereotypic effect of progabide is unclear. The reduction of dopamine neuron action, and dopamine release by progabide and other GABA agonists and the blockade of neuroleptic-induced dopamine neuron activation (2, 5, 19, 24, 31) may at least partially account for the reduction of the AIMs provoked by L-DOPA and withdrawal from repeated neuroleptic administration. However, this cannot explain the decrease in stereotypies due to apomorphine in the rat, or to piribedil in the monkey with nigrostriatal lesions, as these effects are not dependent upon the release of dopamine from nigrostriatal nerve terminals. These effects must be exercised post-synaptically to the dopamine receptor, either at the level of the dopamine neuron target cell, or in the neuronal chain responsible for the expression of dopamine receptor stimulation. GABA agonists do not antagonize all of the effects of dopamine receptor stimulation. Thus the emetic effects of apomorphine in the dog are not altered by doses of progabide as high as 500 mg/kg, po (F. Cathala, unpublished results). Thus, the effect of GABA agonists on dopamine-receptor mediated events is dependent on the neuronal interconnections associated with the different dopamine target cells.

CONCLUSIONS

Stereotyped behaviours or dyskinetic movements are induced by dopamine mimetics active via a wide variety of mechanisms. Of the other dopamine receptor mediated events studied, only the antihaloperidol-catalepsy effect of dopamine mimetics seems to parallel the induction of stereotyped behaviours. In the cat and monkey stereotypies can be distinguished from dyskinetic movements. In the former species, increased synaptic concentrations of endogenous dopamine appear to have a greater stereotypic than dyskinetic effect. Stereotypies due to either increased dopamine release (L-DOPA) or direct dopamine receptor stimulation (apomorphine, piribedil) in the monkey were completely reversed or greatly diminished by progabide, a GABA receptor agonist.

REFERENCES

1. Agid, Y., Bonnet, A. M., Signoret, J. L. and Lhermitte, F. (1979) : In : The Extrapyramidal System and Its Disorders, edited by L. J. Poirier, T. L. Sourkes and P. J. Bédard, pp. 401-410, Raven Press, New York.
2. Andén, N. E. and Stock, G. (1973) : Naunyn Schmiedeberg's Arch. Pharmac. 279 : 89-92.
3. Barbeau, A. (1976) : Pharmac. Therap. CI : 475-494.
4. Barbeau, A., Roy, M., Gonce, M. and Labrecque, R. (1979) : In : The Extrapyramidal System and Its Disorders, edited by L. J. Poirier, T. L. Sourkes and P. Bédard, pp. 433-450, Raven Press, New York.
5. Bartholini, G., Lloyd, K. G., Worms, P., Constantinidis, J. and Tissot, R. (1979) : In : The Extrapyramidal System and Its Disorders, edited by L. J. Poirier, T. L. Sourkes and P. Bédard, pp. 253-257. Raven Press, New York.
6. Bédard, P., Parkes, J. D. and Marsden, C. S. (1978) : Br. Med. J. 1 : 954-956.
7. Borison, H. L. (1974) : Life Sci. 14 : 1807-1817.
8. Calne, D. B. (1978) : In : Clinical Neuropharmacology, vol. 3, edited by H. L. Klawans, pp. 153-166, Raven Press, New York.
9. Carlsson, A. (1970) : In : Amphetamines and Related Compounds, edited by E. Costa and S. Garattini, pp. 289-300. Raven Press, New York.
10. Corsini, G. U. (1981) : In : Clinical Pharmacology of Apomorphine and Other Dopaminomimetics, edited by G. L. Gessa and G. U. Corsini, in press, Raven Press, New York.
11. Corsini, G. U., Del Zompo, M., Cianchetti, C., Mangini, A. and Gessa, G. L. (1976) : Psychopharmacology 47 : 169-173.
12. Desarmenien, M., Feltz, P., Headley, P. M. and Santangelo, M. (1981) : Br. J. Pharmac., in press.
13. Fjalland, B. and Nielsen, I. M. (1974) : Psychopharmacologia 34 : 105-109.
14. Fuxe, K. and Owman, C. (1965) : J. Comp. Neurol., 125 : 337-344.
15. Fuxe, K., Ogren, S. O., Perez de la Mora, M., Schwarcz, R., Hokfelt, T., Eneroth, P., Gustafsson, J. A. and Skett, P. (1979) : In : GABA-Neurotransmitters, edited by P. Krogsgaard-Larsen, J. Scheel-Kruger and H. Kofod, pp. 74-94. Munksgaard, Copenhagen.
16. Gianutsos, G., Drawbough, R. B., Hyres, M. D. and Lal, H. (1974) : Life Sci. 14 : 887-898.

17. Goldberg, L. (1981) : In   Clinical Pharmacology of Apomorphine and Other Dopaminomimetics, edited by G. L. Gessa and G. U. Corsini, in press, Raven Press, New York.

18. Grof, P., Saxena, B., Daigle, L. and Mahutte, G. (1977) : Br. J. Clin. Pharmac. 4 : 2219-2259.

19. Guidotti, A. and Gale, K. (1977): In : Nonstriatal Dopaminergic Neurons, edited by E. Costa and G. L. Gessa, pp. 455-460. Raven Press, New York.

20. Horn. A. S., (1978) : In : Dopamine, edited by P. J. Roberts, G. N. Woodrugg and L. L. Iversen, pp. 25-34, Raven Press, New York.

21. Hornykiewicz, O. (1975) : Biochem. Pharmacol. 24 : 1061-1065.

22. Iversen, L. L., Horn, A. S. and Miller, R. J. (1979) : In : Pre- and Postsynaptic Receptors, edited by E. Usdin and W. E. Bunney, pp. 207-241. Marcel Dekker, New York.

23. Janssen, P. A., Niemegeers, C. J. E. and Schellekens, K. H. L. (1965) : Arznein. Forsch. 15 : 104-117.

24. Kaariainen, I. (1976) : Acta Pharmac. Toxic. 39 : 393-400.

25. Kebabian, J. W., Petzold, G. L. and Greengard, P. (1972) : Proc. Natl. Acad. Sci. USA, 69 : 2145-2149.

26. Klawans, H. L. and Margolin, D. I. (1975) : Arch. Gen. Psychiat. 32 : 725-732.

27. Koe, B. K. (1976) : J. Pharmacol. Exp. Therap. 199 : 649-661.

28. Lieberman, A. N., Kupersmith, M., Casson, I., Dierso, R., Foo, S. H., Khayali, M., Tartaro, T. and Goldstein, M. (1979) : In : The Extrapyramidal System and Its Disorders, edited by L. J. Poirier, T. L. Sourkes and P. Bédard, pp. 461-474. Raven Press, New York.

29. Lloyd, K. G. and Worms, P. (1980) : In : Long Term Effects of Neuroleptics, edited by F. Cattabeni, G. Racagni, P. F. Spano and E. Costa, pp. 253-258. Raven Press, New York.

30. Lloyd, K. G., Worms, P., Depoortere, H. and Bartholini, G. (1979) : In : GABA-Neurotransmitters, edited by P. Krogsgaard-Larsen, J. Scheel-Kruger and H. Kofod, pp. 326-339, Munksgaard, Copenhagen.

31. Lloyd, K. G., Worms, P., Zivkovic, B., Scatton, B. and Bartholini, G. (1980) : Brain Res. Bull. 5, Suppl. 2 : 439-445.

32. Lotti, G., Delitala, G., Masala, A., Alagna, S. and Devilla, L. (1979) : In : Neuroendocrinology : Biological and Clinical Aspects, edited by A. Polleri, and R. M. Mac Leod, pp. 233-256. Academic Press, London.

33. Muller, E. E., Cocchi, D., Locatelli, V., Frigerio, C. and Mantegazza, P. (1979) : In : Neuroendocrine Correlates in Neurology and Psychiatry, edited by E. E. Muller and A. Agnoli, pp. 57-70. Elsevier, Amsterdam.

34. Price, A., Debono, A., Jenner, P., Parkes, J. S. and Marsden, C. D. (1979) : In : The Extrapyramidal System and Its Disorders, edited by L. J. Poirier, T. L. Sourkes and P. J. Bédard, pp. 423-432, Raven Press, New York.

35. Protais, P., Gostentin, J. and Schwartz, J. C. (1976) : Psychopharmacology 50 : 1-6.

36. Randrup, A. and Munkvad, I. (1967) : Psychopharmacologia 11 : 300-310.

37. Randrup, A. and Munkvad, I. (1974) : J. Psychiat. Res. 11 : 1-10.

38. Sassin, J. F., Taub, S. and Weitzman, E. D. (1972) : Neurology, 22 : 1122-1125.

39. Smith, R. C. and Davis, J. M. (1975) : Psychopharm. Comm. 1 : 285-293.

40. Taminga, C. (1981) : In : Clinical Pharmacology of Apomorphine and
    Other Dopaminomimetics, edited by G. L. Gessa and G. U. Corsini,
    in press, Raven Press, New York.
41. Trabucci, M., Longoni, R., Fresia, P. and Spano, P. F. (1976) :
    Life Sci. 17 : 1551-1556.
42. Trabucci, M., Andreoli , V. M., Fraltola, L. and Spano, P. F. (1977)
    In : Nonstriatal Dopaminergic Neurons, edited by E. Costa and G. L.
    Gessa, pp. 661-665, Raven Press, New York.
43. Worms, P. (1981) : In : Benzamides, edited by M. Stanley and J.
    Rotrosen, In Press. Raven Press, New York.
44. Worms, P. and Lloyd, K. G. (1979) : Pharmac. Therap. 5 : 445-450.

Apomorphine and Other Dopaminomimetics,
Vol. 2: Clinical Pharmacology, edited by
G. U. Corsini and G. L. Gessa, Raven Press,
New York © 1981.

Estrogen Control of DA-Receptor Related Dyskinesias

Catherine Euvrard and Jacques R. Boissier

Centre de Recherches Roussel-Uclaf 102, 93230 Romainville, France

The demonstration of an antidopaminergic action of estrogens on prolactin release at the anterior pituitary level (12,22) opened the way to studies on the interactions between steroids and brain dopaminergic (DAergic) systems (11).Furthermore the recent observation of a beneficial effect of estrogens on DA-receptor related dyskinesias (neuroleptic-induced dyskinesias and L-dopa-induced dyskinesias) (3,4,25,26) led us to investigate the effect of estrogens on DAergic transmission in the extrapyramidal system (9-11).

The strategy of our experiments has consisted of measuring the changes in striatal acetylcholine (ACh) levels induced by DAergic drugs (apomorphine or haloperidol) after various modifications of the hormonal status. Indeed, striatal cholinergic interneurons have been demonstrated to be the principal target cells of the nigrostriatal DA pathway (18) and striatal ACh content represents a valid index for the estimation of the state of DAergic transmission in the extrapyramidal system (15).

METHODS

Intact, castrated or hypophysectomized male and castrated female Sprague-Dawley rats (obtained from Iffa Credo, les Oncins, France) weighing 200-225 g were used. The animals were kept in a controlled temperature environment (22 + 2°C) on a 12 h-light 12-dark cycle (lights on at 07.00h) for at least one week before use. High serum prolactin levels in rats were induced by transplantation of three additional pituitaries from male donor under the kidney capsule. In sham operated rats, the kidney was dislocated and the capsule split. Animals were used ten days later for drug experiments. Since drug effects on striatal ACh levels were similar in decapitated or microwave-irradiated animals (11,16) decapitation was used to sacrifice the rats.

ACh was assayed according to the radioenzymatic method of Guyenet et al. (15).

In the present experiments, the following steroids were used : moxestrol, a potent synthetic estrogen (23) ; 2-OH- moxestrol, a catechol estrogen derivative ; RU 16117, a weak synthetic estrogen (5) ; promegestone, a potent synthetic progestin (24), testosterone, 5-α-dihydrotestosterone and corticosterone. These compounds were dissolved in a minimal volume of ethanol before being diluted in 0.9% saline.

Statistical significance of the results was calculated according to the multiple-range test of Duncan-Kramer.

RESULTS

Hormonal pretreatments and striatal ACh levels : interaction with
apomorphine.

   Repeated administration of the synthetic estrogens (moxestrol
(R 2858), 2-OH moxestrol and RU 16117), at a dose of 20 µg/kg s.c.
daily for 7 days, significantly reduced (60 to 80%) the enhancement
of striatal ACh levels produced by apomorphine (Fig. 1). In contrast
a progestin (promegestone (R 5020)), androgens (testosterone and
5-α dihydrotestosterone) or a glucocorticoid (corticosterone) were
without effect on the apomorphine-induced increase in striatal ACh
concentrations (Fig.1). These results suggest that estrogens and not
other steroids exert a potent antidopaminergic effect at the striatal
level.

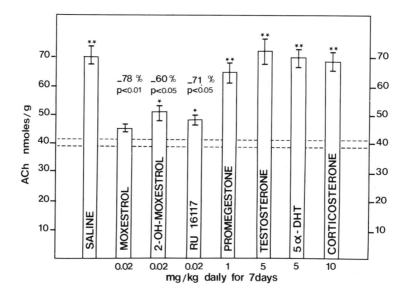

Fig. 1 Effect of hormonal pretreatments on the apomorphine-induced
        increase in striatal ACh levels.

   Apomorphine (2.5 mg/kg i.p.) was injected 24 hrs after the last
administration of saline or hormone and the animals were killed 45
min later. The range of striatal ACh contents in non-apomorphine
treated rats are represented by the two dotted lines. The data represent the mean ± SEM for 7 rats per treatment group. The indicated
percentages and p values are for apomorphine versus apomorphine +
hormone treatment ; * and ** represent the significance for apomorphine versus saline treatment at the level of $p < 0.05$ and $p < 0.01$
respectively.

Modification of the haloperidol-induced decrease in striatal ACh
levels by estrogen pretreatment.

Pretreatment with moxestrol (20 µg/kg s.c. daily for 5 days) led
to a marked potentiation of the decrease in striatal ACh levels induced by haloperidol (Fig.2). In rats pretreated with this synthetic
estrogen, an enhanced reduction in striatal ACh levels was found
after administration of low doses of haloperidol (0.05 mg/kg and 0.10
mg/kg i.p.). When this neuroleptic was injected at a higher dose
(0.25 mg/kg i.p.) the increase in the activity of striatal cholinergic neurons was maximal and no potentiation by moxestrol was observed.

These data give further support to the hypothesis of an antidopaminergic effect of estrogens at the striatal level.

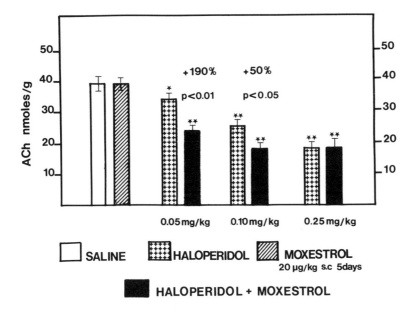

Fig. 2   Effect of moxestrol on the haloperidol-induced decrease
in striatal ACh levels.

Saline or haloperidol was injected 24 hrs after the last administration of moxestrol and the animals were killed 45 min later. The
data represent the mean $\pm$ SEM for 7 rats per treatment group. The
indicated percentages and p values are for haloperidol versus haloperidol + moxestrol treatments.   * and ** represent the significance
for haloperidol versus saline treatment at the level of $p < 0.05$ and
$p < 0.01$ respectively.

Interaction of estrogen pretreatment with striatal ACh increase
induced by chronic haloperidol.

      As an experimental model of neuroleptic-induced tardive dyskine-
sias, the following procedure was used. Three days after the last
injection of a repeated administration of haloperidol (1 mg/kg, daily
for 12 days), a large increase in striatal ACh content is detected,
probably due to a rebound hyperactivity of striatal DAergic transmission following its blockade (Fig. 3). When moxestrol (20 µg/kg daily
for 5 days) was injected into rats receiving such a chronic treatment
with haloperidol,three days after the withdrawal of haloperidol,
striatal ACh levels were significantly lower than with chronic haloperidol alone (-54%), suggesting that moxestrol has antagonized the
compensatory hyperfunction of the striatal DAergic transmission which
has developed.

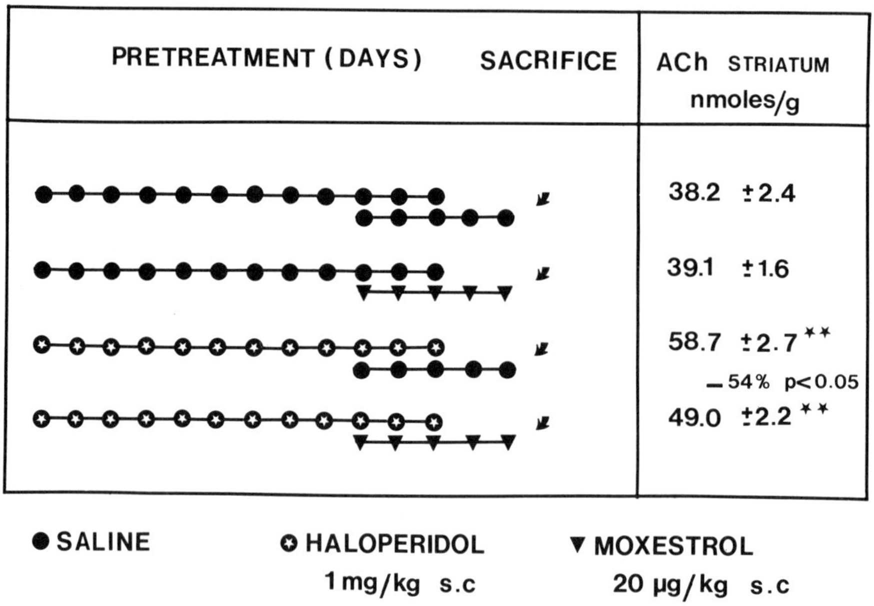

PRETREATMENT (DAYS)	SACRIFICE	ACh STRIATUM nmoles/g
•-•-•-•-•-•-•-•-•-•-•-• •-•-•-•	↙	38.2 ±2.4
•-•-•-•-•-•-•-•-•-•-•-• ▼-▼-▼-▼	↙	39.1 ±1.6
⊘-⊘-⊘-⊘-⊘-⊘-⊘-⊘-⊘-⊘-⊘-⊘ •-•-•-•	↙	58.7 ±2.7 ** —54% p<0.05
⊘-⊘-⊘-⊘-⊘-⊘-⊘-⊘-⊘-⊘-⊘-⊘ ▼-▼-▼-▼	↙	49.0 ±2.2 **

● SALINE   ⊘ HALOPERIDOL   ▼ MOXESTROL
                     1 mg/kg s.c   20 µg/kg s.c

Fig. 3 Effect of moxestrol on the striatal ACh increase observed
after withdrawal from chronic haloperidol administration.

Saline, haloperidol or moxestrol was injected according to the schedule indicated and rats were killed 3 days after the last administration of haloperidol. Results are the mean ± SEM for 7 rats per treatment group. The indicated percentage and p values are for haloperidol
versus haloperidol + moxestrol treatments ; ** represents the significance for haloperidol versus saline treatment at the level of
p < 0.01.

Pituitary mediation of the antidopaminergic effect of estrogens.

In hypophysectomized rats, moxestrol was completely ineffective in blocking the apomorphine-induced increase in striatal ACh levels (Fig. 4) indicating that the pituitary gland is directly involved in the antidopaminergic effect of estrogens. Such an interlocutary effect of the pituitary gland is also supported by data obtained from hyperprolactinaemic pituitary transplanted rats. Indeed, in such rats, in which serum prolactin levels are very high (serum PRL levels 22 $\pm$ 3 ng/ml in sham operated rats and 318 $\pm$ 45 ng/ml in pituitary transplanted rats), the apomorphine effect on striatal ACh levels was significantly reduced as compared to sham operated animals (Fig. 4).

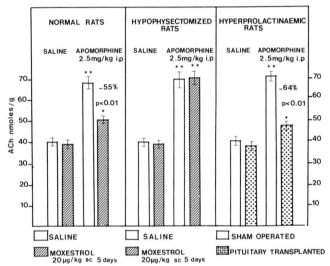

Fig. 4   Effect of apomorphine on striatal ACh levels in rats following modifications of their hormonal status.

Saline or apomorphine was injected into intact, hypophysectomized or hyperprolactineamic pituitary transplanted male rats and the animals were killed 45 min later. Values are expressed as the mean $\pm$ SEM of results obtained with groups of 7 rats. The indicated percentages and p values are for apomorphine versus apomorphine in pretreated (moxestrol or pituitary transplanted) rats ; * and ** represent the significance for apomorphine versus saline treatment at the level of $p < 0.05$ and $p < 0.01$ respectively.

Similar results have been observed when measuring the haloperidol induced decrease in striatal ACh levels.
As represented in Fig. 5, hypophysectomy completely abolished the effect of moxestrol found in normal rats, whereas in the hyperprolactinaemic pituitary transplanted rats (serum prolactin levels : 25 $\pm$ 3 ng/ml in sham operated rats and 490 $\pm$ 28 ng/ml in pituitary transplanted rats), the decrease in striatal ACh levels observed after haloperidol injection was significantly enhanced (Fig. 5).

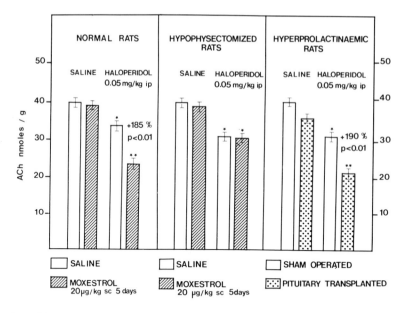

Fig. 5   Effect of haloperidol on striatal ACh levels in rats
         following modifications of their hormonal status.

Saline or haloperidol was injected into intact, hypophysectomized or
hyperprolactinaemic pituitary transplanted male rats and the animals
were killed 45 min later. Values are expressed as the mean $\pm$ SEM of
results obtained with groups of 7 rats. The indicated percentages and
p values are for haloperidol in pretreated (moxestrol or pituitary
transplanted) rats ; * and ** represent the significance for
haloperidol versus saline treatment at the level of $p < 0.05$ and
$p < 0.01$ respectively.

                              DISCUSSION

     The present results clearly show that estrogens impair the
DAergic control of striatal cholinergic neurons since the alterations
produced by DAergic drugs on these neurons are markedly modified
after repeated estrogen administration. Thus in rats pretreated with
estrogens, the increase in striatal ACh levels induced by the DA
agonist apomorphine is significantly reduced, while the decrease in
this biochemical parameter produced by the DA antagonist haloperidol
is enhanced (Fig. 1 and Fig. 2). This effect seems to be specific for
estrogens as only those steroids having estrogenic properties are
able to exert such an antidopaminergic activity at the striatal
level. Since moxestrol treatment alone does not alter baseline
striatal ACh levels nor does it affect choline acetyltransferase or
acetylcholinesterase activities (11), its effect on the changes in
striatal ACh levels induced by apomorphine or haloperidol is unlikely
to be due to an inhibition of ACh synthesis or an enhancement of ACh
degradation. However, we cannot rule out the possibility of a change
in striatal ACh turn-over induced by moxestrol (6).

The interaction between estrogens and the DAergic control of striatal cholinergic function is also supported by the results obtained using an experimental model for neuroleptic-induced tardive dyskinesia. After repeated administration of haloperidol, a large increase in striatal ACh content is detected three days after the last injection of the drug. This is probably due to the compensatory hyperactivity of striatal DAergic transmission which develops during the long-term blockade of DA receptors (Fig. 3). Moxestrol, administered to rats receiving a chronic treatment with haloperidol, reduces the increase in striatal ACh levels observed after the withdrawal of the neuroleptic. This result demonstrates that moxestrol is able to antagonize the compensatory hyperfunction of the striatal DAergic transmission. In accordance with these findings, estradiol benzoate attenuated the enhanced stereotypic response to apomorphine observed after the cessation of repeated neuroleptic administration (14).

The lack of effect of moxestrol in hypophysectomized rats (Fig. 4 and Fig. 5) demonstrates that the pituitary gland is directly involved in the antidopaminergic activity of moxestrol observed at the striatal level. The interlocutory effect of the pituitary gland for the antidopaminergic effect of estrogens may possibly be explained by the following proposals : (1) a biotransformation of estrogens to catechol estrogens in the pituitary is a necessary step for their action on the brain. Thus, recent evidence indicates that catechol estrogens are major constituents of brain estrogenic compounds, occuring in high concentrations in the pituitary gland and hypothalamus and possessing potent biological and endocrine activities similar to their parent compounds (7,13,19,21). As catechol estrogen-forming enzymes are present in the pituitary gland (2), it can be assumed that estrogens are partially biotransformed at this level and perhaps this enzymatic step is an essential link in the brain steroid-DAergic interaction. (2) A pituitary factor, released by estrogen administration, acts as the mediator of the antidopaminergic estrogenic activity. A likely candidate for a pituitary mediator of estrogenic effects on DAergic neurotransmission could be PRL, since estrogens are known to markedly stimulate its secretion and synthesis. Indeed repeated administration of moxestrol increases serum PRL levels with a time-course which closely parallels that of the antidopaminergic effect of moxestrol (11). A similar effect on serum PRL levels has already been described with the other synthetic estrogen RU 16117 (17). Furthermore, the results obtained with hyperprolactinaemic rats bearing pituitary transplants under the renal capsule support such an hypothesis but do not exclude the involvement of another pituitary hormone.

The present results clearly show that after estrogen administration, the DAergic control of striatal cholinergic neurons is strongly impaired since the biochemical alterations produced by DA agonists or antagonists in striatal cholinergic neurons are markedly modified. Tardive dyskinesias following chronic treatment with neuroleptics or L-dopa-induced dyskinesias have been related to the development of an overactivity of DAergic transmission in the extrapyramidal system (1,8). This compensatory hyperactivity of the DAergic system produces a dysfunction of striatal cholinergic neurons and an imbalance between DAergic and cholinergic function. As estrogens are able to reduce such neurological disorders, one possible interpretation of these clinical observations is that estrogens, by blocking striatal DAergic transmission normalize the imbalance between DA and ACh neurons which is probably involved in the appearance of these dyskinesias.

REFERENCES

1. Baldessarini, R.J. (1979) : Trends in Neuro Sci., 2 : 133-135.
2. Ball, P., and Knuppen, R. (1978) : J. Clin. Endocrinol. Metab., 47 : 732-736.
3. Bédard, P., Langelier, P., and Villeneuve, A. (1977) : Lancet, 2 : 1367-1368.
4. Bédard, P., Langelier, P. Dankova, J., Villeneuve , A., Di Paolo, T., Barden, N., Labrie, F., Boissier, J.R., and Euvrard, C. (1979) :In: Extrapyramidal system and its disorders,edited by L.J Poirier T.L. Sourkes and P. Bedard, pp. 411-422.Raven Press, New York.
5. Bouton, M.M., and Raynaud, J.P., (1979) : Endocrinology, 105 : 509-517.
6. Cheney, D.L., and Costa, E. (1977) : Ann. Rev. Pharmacol. Toxicol 17 : 369-386.
7. Davies, I.J., Naftolin, F., Ryan, K.J., Fishmann, J., and Siu, J. (1975):Endocrinology, 97 : 554-557.
8. De Silva, L. (1977) : Drugs, 14 : 300-310.
9. Euvrard, C., Labrie, F., and Boissier, J.R. (1979) : Brain Res., 169 : 215-220.
10. Euvrard, C., Labrie, F., and Boissier, J.R. (1980) : Comm. in Psychopharmacology, 3 : 329-334.
11. Euvrard, C., Oberlander, C., and Boissier J.R. (1980) : J. Pharm. Exp. Ther., 214 : 179-185.
12. Ferland, L., Labrie, F., Euvrard, C., and Raynaud J.P. (1979) : Mol. Cell. Endocrinol., 14 : 199-204.
13. Fishmann, J. (1977) : Neuroendocrinology, 22 : 363-374.
14. Gordon, J.H., Borison, R.L., and Diamond, B.I. (1980) : Neurology 30 : 551-554.
15. Guyenet, P., Agid, Y., Javoy, F., Beaujouan, J.C., Rossier, J., and Glowinski, J. (1975) : Brain Res., 84 : 227-244.
16. Guyenet, P., Javoy, F., Euvrard, C., and Glowinski, J. (1977) : Neuropharmacology, 16 : 385-390.
17. Kelly, P.A., Asselin, J., Caron, M.G., Labrie, F., and Raynaud, J.P. (1977) : J. Natl. Cancer Inst., 58 : 623-628.
18. Lloyd, K.G. (1978) : In : Essays in Neurochemistry and Neuropharmacology, Vol. 3, edited by N.B.H. Youdim, W. Lowenberg D.F. Sharmann and J.R. Lagnado pp 131-207, Wiley, New York.
19. Naftolin, F., Morishita, H., Davies, I.J., Todd, R., and Ryan K.J. (1975) : Biochem. Biophys. Res. Commun, 64 : 905-910.
20. Parvizi, N., and Ellendorff, F. (1975) : Nature (London) 256 : 59-60.
21. Paul, S.M. and Axelrod, J. (1977) : Science (Washington), 197 : 657-659.
22. Raymond, V., Beaulieu, M., Labrie, F., and Boissier, J.R. (1978) Science (Washington), 200 : 1173-1175.

23. Raynaud, J.P., Bouton, M.M., Gallet-Bourquin, D., Philibert, D., Tournemine, C., and Azadian-Boulanger, G. (1973) : Molec. Pharmacol., 9 : 520-533.

24. Raynaud, J.P. (1977) : In : Progesterone Receptors in normal and neoplastic tissues, edited by W.L.M. Mc Guire, J.P. Raynaud and E.E. Beaulieu, pp. 9-21. Raven Press, New York.

25. Villeneuve, A., Langelier, P., and Bédard, P. (1978) : Can. Psychiat. Ass. J., 23 : 68-70.

26. Villeneuve, A., Cazejust, T., and Côté, M. (1980) : Neuropsycho-biology, 6 : 145-151.

Apomorphine and Other Dopaminomimetics,
Vol. 2: Clinical Pharmacology, edited by
G. U. Corsini and G. L. Gessa, Raven Press,
New York © 1981.

Dyskinesia, Dystonia, and Dopaminergic System: Effect of Apomorphine and Ergot Alkaloids

L. Frattola, M. G. Albizzati, S. Bassi, and M. Trabucchi

Department of Neurology and Pharmacology, University of Milan, Bassini Hospital,
20092 Cinisello Balsamo, Italy

Hyperkinetic involuntary movements are a common symptom, present in several neurological diseases. Given the different ethiopathogenesis and lesional characteristics of the various diseases, the pathophysiological bases underlying motor disorder are different and not always well defined.

Usually they are ascribed to a predominance of the dopaminergic over cholinergic transmission at the striatal level, but increasing evidence suggests that other neurotransmitter systems could be involved in their pathogenesis (1,4,6,7,10,13,16,17).

As a result of this incomplete knowledge, the pharmacological indications for the treatment of these motor disorders are often empirical and inconsistent with the simple hypothesis of a dopaminergic hyperactivity. In fact apomorphine, a direct stimulant of dopamine receptors, improves the dyskinesias of different origins (5,15,17); furthermore bromocriptine, an ergot derivative with dopamine-agonist properties, is able to reduce the gravity of hyperkinetic movements present in Huntington's chorea (3,12).

Recently another ergot derivative, namely CF 25-397, has been used in the treatment of dyskinesias with discordant results (9,13).

The positive effect of apomorphine and bromocriptine in dyskinesias treatment can be explained in the following way: at low doses the two drugs -by a specific mechanism- reduce the activity of dopamine neurons by a stimulation of the presynaptic dopamine receptors, that in turn inhibit the dopamine turnover and the impulse flow in dopamine neurons.

The action of CF 25-397, on the other hand, is more complex and not yet well defined. In fact this drug acts on the dopaminergic system but also as a serotonergic and noradrenergic agonist properties (3,13).

In this paper we will show the results of our studies on the clinical effects of bromocriptine and CF 25-397 on dyskinesias of various origins. Most of these data have been previously reported (9).

MATERIALS AND METHODS

Our study was carried out on two groups of patients suffering from hyperkinetic involuntary movements.

Group 1 consisted of three men and three women with Huntington's chorea (mean age 46.2 years; range 28-56). None of them had rigid akinetic

Huntington's chorea.

Group 2 included sixteen patients suffering from different neurological disorders characterized by involuntary movements with a dystonic component of varying degree: three patients with Wilson's disease (mean age, 26.6 years; range 22-31); three patients with idiopatic torsion dystonia (mean age, 30.3 years; range 9-45); four patients with congenital cerebral palsy with athetoid dyskinesia (mean age, 31.1 years; range 25-43); six patients suffering from tardive dyskinesia (mean age, 38.4 years; range 29-53), which occurred in the course of long-term treatment with neuroleptic drugs. These six patients had stable tardive dyskinesia for at least six months before the beginning of the study and none of them showed neurological or physical illness.

The nature and purpose of the investigation was explained to the patients and their consent was obtained. Fifteen of these patients were admitted to the Department of Neurology of the University of Milan, the others lived at home.

TRIAL DESIGN

Preparations of identical appearance each containing 2.50 mg of bromocriptine or 2.50 mg of CF 25-397 were used.
Similar preparations filled with lactose served as placebo. Neither the patients nor their next of kind were informed of the nature of the drugs during the trial.

The treatment previously given was withdrawn at least ten days before the beginning of the trial and, at the end of this period, the patients were examined to obtain the baseline values. A double-blind crossover study was performed with placebo, bromocriptine or CF 25-397, and three different phases of the trial were carried out with an interval of ten days between each phase.

Bromocriptine was given in three different ways consisting subsequently of 10, 15, 20 mg days, each period of dosage lasting ten days. CF 25-397 was administered following the same system but with 10,20, 30 mg / day of drug. These doses were chosen on the basis of our previous studies (8,9).

Both the patients living at home and those hospitalized were visited at least twice weekly during the trial to report the evolution of the motor disorders and the presence of unwanted effects. Routine tests were performed at the end of each treatment, together with the evaluation of the neurological function.

CLINICAL EXAMINATION

Neurological functions were rated every five days by two persons in charge of the study and by one independent observer.

Chorea severity, finger dexterity, gait, speech and severity of the disease of huntingtonian patients were evaluated and recorded as indicated by Frattola et al. (8).

After various pilot studies, the method of Bedard et al.(2) with some modifications was chosen for the clinical examination of group 2 patients.

Dystonic movements were assessed separately in the arms and legs, in the face, neck and trunk and severity was rated as follows: 0 = absence of involuntary movements; 1 = mild; 2 = moderate; 3 = severe gravity of dyskinesia (maximum severity score = 15).

Furthermore, considering that the intensity of dystonic movements is considerably influenced by physiological movements and by the various postures, the patients were examined under three different conditions: a) resting in bed; b) while walking; c) sitting with upper limbs forward and the palms up. In the last position the evaluation lasted for two minutes, while for the other positions the observational rating period lasted for three-five minutes and was repeated after fifteen minutes.

The score made up of the sum of all these observations produces a total dyskinesia score with a maximum level of 45.

The patients of group 2 were also evaluated for the symptoms of parkinsonism using the Webster rating scale.

Statistical analysis was performed with the paired t-test.

RESULTS

Table 1 shows the effects of bromocriptine and CF 25-397 in Huntington's patients.

TABLE 1. Effects of bromocriptine and CF 25-397 in Huntington's chorea

	Chorea severity	Finger dexterity	Gait	Speech	Disease severity
Baseline	7.1±0.4	2.7±0.4	2.2±0.3	2.1±0.2	14.1±1.3
Bromocriptine	3.6±0.5*	1.9±0.4	1.6±0.3	1.5±0.3	8.6±1.1*
Δ X %	− 49	− 30	− 27	− 28	− 39
CF 25-397	4.9±0.4**	2.4±0.4	1.7±0.2	2.4±0.3	11.5±1.3
Δ X %	− 31	− 11	− 22	+ 14	− 18
Placebo	7.1±1.1	2.5±0.5	2.2±0.3	2.1±0.4	13.9±2.3

Each value represents the mean ± S.E.M.

Δ X % = percent change in the treatment score.

The score for bromocriptine was recorded after a 10 days of treatment with 15 mg/day of drug. The csore for CF 25-397 was recorded after a 10 days of treatment with either 10 or 15 mg/day of drug depending on the best clinical response observed.

* = P < 0.005; ** = P < 0.01 (versus baseline score). Other differences were not statistically significant.

Bromocriptine significantly improves chorea and disease severity; also the scores for finger dexterity, gait and speech are decreased in comparison to baseline scores, but these differences were not of statistical significance.

The results with CF 25-397, at the optimal doses, are less indicative. In fact, the drug demonstrates a mild effectiveness only in the reduction of the chorea severity score.

The doses of the drugs indicated in the Table 1 are those which have given the best results. Higher doses of both drugs fail to induce further positive results.

On the contrary, bromocriptine at the dose of 20 mg/day, and CF 25-397 at the dose of 30 mg/day, induced a sudden increase of hyperkinesias in two patients, which forced their withdrawal from the study.

The results of our study on the dyskinetic-dystonic syndromes of different ethiology are summarized in Table 2.

TABLE 2.   Effects of placebo, bromocriptine and CF 25-397
           on dystonic symptoms of different ethiology

	Total dyskinesia score			
	Baseline	CF 25-397 (20 mg/day)	Bromocriptine (15 mg/day)	Placebo
Wilson's disease	5.3±0.9	3.1±0.7* (− 41)	4.1±1.1 (− 22)	5.7±1.1
Idhiopatic torsion dystonia	3.7±0.6	2.4±0.5 (− 32)	3.5±0.9 (− 5)	3.5±0.5
Congenital cerebral palsy	4.2±0.7	1.8±0.4* (− 56)	3.6±0.8 (− 14)	4.1±0.7
Tardive dyskinesia	10.4±1.8	7.7±1.1 (− 26)	9.1±1.7 (− 12)	10.8±1.8

Each number represents the mean ± S.E.M.
The number in brackets are the percent changes in treatment score versus the baseline score.
* = $P < 0.01$ in comparison to baseline values.

Bromocriptine administration induced only a very slight reduction, not significant, of the total dyskinesia score. None of the patients showed a development of parkinsonian symptoms, but for three of them (one with Wilson's disease and two with torsion dystonia) the trial was stopped at the doses of 15 mg/day due to the worsening of involuntary movements.

In another patient with tardive dyskinesia the study was stopped because of psychosis exacerbation.

More convincing results were obtained with CF 25-397 therapy. In patients suffering from Wilson's disease and cerebral palsy a significant improvement in their motor disturbances was observed.

The maximum drug effect is achieved at the dose of 20 mg/day, where the mean total dyskinesia score decreases from 5.3 to 3.1 and from 4.2 to 1.8 respectively for Wilson's disease and for congenital cerebral palsy with athetoid dyskinesia. A reduction in the total dyskinesia score was observed also in other patients, but with an improvement of the motor disturbances that was not statistically significant.

From an individual analysis of the patients reported in Table 2, two showed a worsening of dyskinesia (one suffering from tardive dyskinesia and the other from idhiopatic torsion dystonia), and two failed to show any symptoms variation following the various experimental procedures.

The treatment with CF 25-397 did not produce parkinsonian symptoms. However, at the dose of 20 or 30 mg/day, four patients (two with congeni tal cerebral palsy and two with idhiopatic torsion dystonia) experienced a subjective reduction of motor performance.

The most important side effects with CF 25-397 were headaches and hy- potension (five subjects), nausea and paresthesias.

DISCUSSION

Our study indicates that bromocriptine and CF 25-397 have somewhat different clinical profiles, both of which are different again from apo- morphine.

Regarding this last drug, several reports confirm its effectiveness in the treatment of dyskinesias of any origin, such as in Huntington's cho- rea, in tardive dyskinesia, in spasmodic torticollis, in Meige's disease. In Parkinson's disease this drug is able to reduce both the tremor and the dyskinesias induced by L-Dopa treatment. However, apomorphine cannot be used in clinical practice because of its short-term action and its side-effects.

Bromocriptine shows a clinical effectiveness only in Huntington's cho rea. The beneficial action is evident only when the drug is used in low doses (8,12).

In contrast, as is well known, bromocriptine in higher doses increases the severity of chorea (11), but lessens tremor, hypokinesia and rigidi- ty of the parkinsonian patients.

On dyskinesias of other origins, bromocriptine has no therapeutic effect. Recently Delwaide and Hurlet (6) reported that buccolinguofacial dyskine sias in patients with senile dementia are lower during bromocriptine the rapy.

CF 25-397 is not particularly useful in controlling dyskinesias. Although an improvement of the severity of involuntary movements with a dystonic component has been observed, it is of poor clinical relevance and achieves statistical significance only in patients with athetoid dyskinesia. In tardive dyskinesia results similar to ours have been re- ported by Tamminga and Chase (13).

Despite these negative clinical results, the use of CF 25-397 may sug gest some speculation.

In Parkinson's disease this drug tends to ameliorate tremor slightly and to reduce dyskinetic movements of the "on-off" syndrome, but this improvement was accompained by a worsening of hypokinesia and rigidity (14, 18); on the contrary, in the patients with dyskinetic-dystonic syndromes CF 25-397 tends to reduce the severity of their motor disorders without inducing the appearance of parkinsonian symptoms.

This observation may suggest that the clinical effects of the studied drugs are not dependent only on their action in a specific neuronal system, but also on the biological substrates involved in the disease, which are not limited to the basal ganglia.

Several recent studies (4,6,10,13,17) have been carried out with the aim to observe if the use of drugs acting on a specific neuronal structure may give some insight to the understanding of the mechanisms of neurotransmission that underlie the different motor disturbances in man. Unfortunately this approach is limited by the complexity of the biological substrates involved in the diseases, and by the fact that the biochemical properties of the various drugs are often not completely known.

REFERENCES

1. Barbeau,A.,and Ando,K.(1975): Lancet, i:987.
2. Bédard,P.,Parkes,J.D.,and Marsden,C.D.(1978): Brit.Med.J., 1:954-956.
3. Burki,H.R.,Asper,H,Ruck,W.,and Zuger,P.E.(1978): Psychopharmacology, 57:227-235.
4. Chasey,D.E.(1980): Neurology, 30:690-695.
5. Corsini,G.U.,Onali,P.L.,Masala,C.,Cianchetti,C.,Mangoni,A.,and Gessa G.L.(1978): Arch.Neurol., 35:27-30.
6. Delwaide,P.J.,and Hurlet,A.(1980): Arch.Neurol., 37:441-443.
7. Divac,I.(1977): Acta Neurol.Scandinav., 56:357-360.
8. Frattola,L.,Albizzati,M.G.,Spano,P.F.,and Trabucchi,M.(1977): Acta Neurol.Scandinav., 56:37-45.
9. Frattola,L.,Albizzati,M.G.,Bassi,S.,Spano,P.F.and Trabucchi,M.(1980): In: Ergot Compounds and Brain Function,edited by M.Goldstein, D.B. Calne, A.Lieberman, and M.O.Thorner, pp.381-386. Raven Press, New York.
10. Juntunen,J.,Kaste,M.,Iivanainen,M.,Ranta,T.,and Seppala,M.(1979): Arch.Neurol., 36:449-450.
11. Kartzinel,R.D.,Hunt,R.D.,and Calne,D.B.(1976): Arch.Neurol., 33:517-518.
12. Loeb,C.,Roccatagliata,G.,Albano,C.,and Besio,G.(1979): Neurology, 29:730-733.
13. Tamminga,C.A.,and Chase,T.N.(1980): Arch.Neurol., 37:204-205.
14. Teychenne,P.F.,Pfeiffer,R.,Bern,S.M.,and Calne,D.B.(1977): Neurology 27:1140-1143.
15. Tolosa,E.S.,and Sparber,S.B.(1974): Life Sci., 15:1371-1380.
16. Tolosa,E.S.,and Lai,C.(1979): Neurology, 29:1126-1130.
17. Trabucchi,M.,Albizzati,M.G.,Spano,P.F.,Tonon,G.C.,and Frattola,L.

(1979): In: Dopaminergic Ergot Derivatives and Motor Function, edited by K.Fuxe and D.B.Calne, pp.361-369, Pergamon Press, Oxford.

Apomorphine and Other Dopaminomimetics,
Vol. 2: Clinical Pharmacology, edited by
G. U. Corsini and G. L. Gessa, Raven Press,
New York © 1981.

Dopamine and Sleep—A Neurophysiologist's Introduction

Michel Jouvet

Department of Experimental Medicine, Université Claude-Bernard, Lyon, France

Although Dopamine (DA) is the most widely studied monoamine in the Brain, it was the latest to enter the monoamine game in sleep physiology, long after serotonin and noradrenaline (NA). In fact DA has a good right to belong to the club of sleep modulators since apomorphine –a DA agonist with a sleep enhancing effect –is the only one to bear the name of Morpheus, the God of Sleep, among the numerous DA agonists or antagonists.

For such a distinguished audience of DA experts who may sleep well or not, but who are not obligatory experts in sleep mechanisms, let me summarize briefly some specific problems of the physiology and pharmacology of sleep.

I –As in the field of binding, in which everything seems to bind to everything, the pharmacologist studying sleep should remember that almost anything can alter some parameter of the sleep waking cycle Aspirin or alcohol, feeding or sexual activity, heat or cold, rest or exercise, learning or even placebo (in man) may significantly alter some parameter of sleep. The unbalance between waking and sleep mechanisms may secondarily affect sleep, either by delaying sleep onset or by increasing a state of subwakefulness which looks like sleep, but in fact is only a state of sedation.

II –Then, how can we be sure that a drug or a transmitter facilitates sleep mechanisms? First, we should remember that sleep is not a homogenous state, but that it is composed of the periodical succession of slow wave sleep (SWS) (with 2 stages : I and II) and paradoxical sleep (PS) with low voltage cortical activity (desynchronized or REM sleep). A simple but very efficient way to observe the facilitation of hypnogenic mechanisms consists in depriving rats or cats, either from total sleep or from entering PS. Such suppression is followed by a rebound during which either both SWS and PS, or only PS increase significantly.

Then, if we observe a significant increase of PS after any pharmacological alteration, we can be sure that the drug has some specific sleep inducing effect.

III —Now, what is the evidence that DA acts upon the sleep - waking cycle?

A -Let us consider first the role of DA in behavioural and electrophysiological alertness : the well-known arousing effect of amphetamine can be suppressed by pretreatment with alpha methyl P. tyrosine, an inhibitor of catecholamine (CA) synthesis. This fact led to the hypothesis that CA, either DA or NA, were involved either in behavioural and/or electrophysiological alertness. Subsequent studies with local destruction of the main NA system in the locus coeruleus region or in the dorsal NA pathway or of the main DA system in the substantia nigra led to the conclusion that NA was mainly involved in electrophysiological alertness while DA was responsible for behavioural arousal (6). However, more recent experiments have shown that DA mechanisms could also be involved in EEG alertness. Thus, the local administration of haloperidol in n.accumbens may block the cortical activation of amphetamine in the rat (4). Thus the participation of DA in waking mechanism may explain why, on the one hand, high doses of apomorphine, a stimulator of brain DA receptors, increase waking, and why, on the other hand, spiroperidol, which is considered as a specific DA antagonist, produces a dose dependant increase of cortical synchronization and a decrease of PS (8). In this latter case, it is safe to assume that spiroperidol induces a state of subwakefulness (or sedation) by altering waking mechanisms, but does not directly increase sleep since PS is suppressed.

B -However, the role of DA in controlling PS should also be considered since low doses of apomorphine increase PS in the rat (11). Does apomorphine at low doses act only upon DA autoreceptors and then decrease DA liberation? In such cases, this would imply that DA plays an inhibitory role upon PS. On the other hand, apomorphine might act upon some special kind of postsynaptic receptor, then some DA system might facilitate PS. What do we know about PS mechanism which could help to solve this riddle?

First, whatever might be the precise localization of the nervous structures responsible for PS, they should be localized in the lower brain stem, since a pontine cat whose brain stem is transected below the substantia nigra and A10 group of mesolimbic DA neurons still present periodical PS episodes (7). Then, if there is a direct control of DA mechanisms upon PS executive structures, there should be some DA perikarya located below the A9 or A10 groups. Immunofluorescent techniques have permitted to describe tyrosine hydroxylase positive and DBH negative neurons in the raphe dorsalis (12).

This putative group of DA perikarya located in the rostral raphe could project to the locus coeruleus complex which is involved in both permissive and executive mechanisms of PS. Since it is possible that there exists DA presynaptic inhibitory receptor on NA neurons.

The activity of DA neurons could suppress the release of NA from the locus coeruleus. Indeed, the locus coeruleus is one of the principal gating mechanisms for PS (a total cessation of unitary activity in the locus coeruleus is a prerequisite for PS to appear)(3). Then a putative DA agonist mechanism could increase PS via a presynaptic mechanism, by decreasing NA liberation from some terminals of the locus coeruleus which control PS mechanism.

Secondly, what is the pharmacological evidence that putative DA mechanisms located in the lower brain stem may control PS? This evidence comes from the effect of gamma-hydroxybutyrate (γOH). γOH (and its precursor gamma-butyrolactone) is able to induce PS in the pontine cat (7). Since numerous studies have shown that γOH could either inhibit DA release in the striatum of the rat (14) or increase DA release in the striatum of the cat (2). There is a possibility that the PS facilitatory or inducing mechanism of γOH in the pontine cat could be produced also through lower brain stem DA mechanisms. But whatever might be the selective effect of γOH upon DA mechanisms, a word of caution is necessary since not only γOH but also butyrate, valerate and caproate are even more effective for PS inducing effect in the mesencephalic cat (9) and unfortunately there has yet been no study relating the effect of C^4, C^5 or C^6 fatty acids upon DA mechanisms

Finally, the DA putative PS facilitating or suppressing effects disclosed by low dose of apomorphine may not act directly upon PS ponto-bulbar executive mechanisms since there is also evidence of supraponti-ne studies facilitating or inhibiting PS mechanisms. Thus the lesion of the preoptic area decreases PS (10) while lesion of the isthmus area increases PS (13). Interestingly enough, the striking hypersomnia which follows lesion of the isthmus is accompanied by a significant decrease of DA in the locus coeruleus area (1). Since HVA or DOPAC were not determined, this decrease of DA presumably located in some terminals could have been provoked either by a decrease or an increase turnover of DA. The use of polarographic microelectrodes permitting the in vivo determination of DOPAC (5) in the Pons, after the lesion of the isthmus could solve this problem.

All these results, among many others, show that there is still some room for DA in controlling the sleep-waking mechanisms and I am anxious to learn more about the experiments which will be reported in this session. They will certainly contribute to solve (or to compli-cate) a little more the puzzle of sleep mechanisms.

REFERENCES

1)   Blondaux C.,Buda M.,Petitjean F.,Pujol J.F. (1975): Brain Res. 88:425-437.

2)   Cheramy A.,Nieoullon A.,Glowinski J. (1977): J.Pharmacol. Exp. Ther., 203: 283-293.

3)   Chu N.S.,Bloom F.E. (1974): J.Neurobiol., 5: 544-577.

4)   Dzoljic M.R.,Godschalk M. (1978): Waking and Sleeping, 2: 153-155.

5)   Gonon F.,Buda M.,Cespuglio R.,Jouvet M.,Pujol J.F. (1980): Nature,
     286: 902-904.

6)   Jones B.E.,Bobillier P.,Pin C.,Jouvet M. (1973): Brain Res., 58:
     157-177.

7)   Jouvet M. (1972): Ergebn. der Physiol., 64: 166-307.

8)   Kafi S.,Gaillard J.M. (1976): Europ.J.Pharmacol., 38: 357-363.

9)   Matsuzaki M.,Takagi H.,Tokizane T. (1964): Science, 146: 1328-
     1330.

10) McGinty D.J.,Sterman M.B. (1968): Science, 160: 1253-1255.

11) Mereu G.P.,Scarnati E.,Paglietti E.,Pellegrini Quarantotti B.,
     Wadman S.K. (1979): Electroencephalogr. clin.Neuro., 46: 214-219.

12) Nagatsu I.,Inagaki S.,Kondo Y.,Karasawa N.,Nagatsu T. (1979):
     Acta Histochem. Cytochem., 12: 20-37.

13) Petitjean F.,Sakai K.,Blondaux C.,Jouvet M. (1975): Brain Res.,
     88: 439-453.

14) Roth R.H.,Suhr Y. (1970): Biochem.Pharmacol., 19: 3001-3012.

*Apomorphine and Other Dopaminomimetics,
Vol. 2: Clinical Pharmacology*, edited by
G. U. Corsini and G. L. Gessa, Raven Press,
New York © 1981.

What is the Role of Dopamine in the Regulation of Sleep–Wake Activity?

†J. Christian Gillin, *D. P. van Kammen, *R. M. Post, *N. Sitaram,
† R. J. Wyatt, and *W. E. Bunney, Jr.

*Biological Psychiatry Branch, IRP, National Institute of Mental Health, Bethesda, Maryland
20205; †Adult Psychiatry Branch, IRP, National Institute of Mental Health,
St. Elizabeths Hospital, Washington, D.C. 20032*

The role of dopaminergic neurons in the regulation of circadian rhythms of sleep–wake activity and of sleep remains enigmatical. These relationships have been investigated by means of lesions, especially in brain areas containing dopaminergic neurons, by administration of pharmacological agents which affect dopaminergic neurotransmission, by correlating between dopamine and its metabolites and sleep–wake activity, and by measuring the changes in dopamine metabolism induced by alterations in sleep–wake activity.

In an attempt to study the role of significant dopamine-containing neurons, Jones et al. (17) lesioned the substantial nigra (A9, A10) in cats. They suggested that these dopaminergic neurons within the ventral tegmentum might be essential for behavioral arousal. They observed akinesia, hypertonus, normal waking EEG patterns, diminished dopamine levels in striatum, and marked absence of behavioral arousal. Kovacevic and Radulovacki (24) later supported this hypothesis. They biopsied the brains of cats during NonREM sleep. Compared with those obtained during wakefulness, samples from striatum and thalamus showed significantly reduced concentrations of dopamine, and, especially, homovanillic acid (HVA), (a major metabolite of dopamine), which actually fell to undetectable levels. In contrast, however, the dopamine concentration within the hippocampus increased during NonREM sleep, which the authors suggested would be consistent with the hypothesis that catecholamines prime REM sleep.

Jones et al. (17) did not present EEG sleep data in any detail following the lesions of the substantia nigra. Corsi-Cabrera et al. (6), however, lesioned the caudate nucleus of the rat, and reported a significant increase in both time spent on paradoxical (REM) sleep and in the number of episodes of paradoxical sleep, especially in relation to lesions of the medio-medial portion of the caudate-putamen. This study has apparently not been replicated and is uninterpretable in terms of a dopamine hypothesis for the control of sleep or of REM sleep.

Studies of the sleep of Parkinsonian patients have yielded variable results, with reports of decreased delta sleep (22), a mild reduction in REM sleep (36), and prolonged sleep latency (22, 23) in some but not all investigations. Two studies have reported persistent EMG activity during

REM sleep (31,36), which may reflect involvement of the locus coeruleus, lesions of which have abolished the atonia of REM sleep in cats (18). Persistent oculo-palpebral signs and blepharaspasm preceding REM sleep have also been reported as has reduced spindle activity and the occurrence of eye movements in all sleep stages (31). Reduced nighttime sleep and increased daytime sleepiness are said to be common complaints of patients with Parkinson's disease.

Since the cyclic alteration of NonREM and REM sleep persists in cats whose brains have been transected at the level of the mesencephalon, the major regulatory systems for sleep architecture appear to be located in the area of the pons, where few intrinsic dopaminergic neurons apparently lie. If more rostral dopaminergic neurons are involved in the regulation of sleep architecture, they may act as regulators or modulators rather than as executive systems. It also appears that the role of aminergic neurons, in general, and dopaminergic neurons, in particular, may vary with age. Laguzzi et al. (26) showed that intraventricular injections of 6-hydroxydopamine (6-OH-DA), which decreases concentrations of catecholamines and serotonin, had no effect in the one- to two-week-old kitten on active or quiet sleep, the ontogentic precursors of REM and NonREM sleep, respectively. In contrast, 6-OH-DA administration, with or without pretreatment with chlorimipramine (to protect serotonergic neurons), decreased both REM and, to a lesser extent, NonREM sleep when given at 5 weeks of age.

In the study of Laguzzi et al. (26), as in so many others, it has been virtually impossible to separate out the relative roles of dopamine and norepinephrine systems. This has been a special problem in the interpretation of pharmacological studies, such as those involving administration of alpha-methyl-para-tyrosine (AMPT), which inhibits tyrosine hydroxylase, the rate limiting enzymatic step in the synthesis of dopamine and norepinephrine. The results of the AMPT studies have been inconsistent, with reports that it increases, decreases, or leaves unaltered the amounts of REM sleep (see ref. 8,13,20,28,42). It is of interest, however, that drowsiness is a major side effect of AMPT with its clinical use in hypertensive patients and EEG determined total sleep time increases significantly in normal volunteers given AMPT (3 gr/day) for three days in an experimental situation which permits them to sleep as long as they wish (Sitaram, Gillin, Bunney; unpublished data). Furthermore, once AMPT is discontinued, patients and volunteers experience a period of significant hyposomnia compared with the pre-AMPT period; these findings have been shown both with nurses' estimates of total sleep (2) and with EEG monitored sleep measures (Sitaram, Gillin, Bunney; unpublished data). It is perhaps entirely consistent with this observation that marked hypersomnia accompanies withdrawal in amphetamine addicts (40). Tolerance probably develops to the hypersomnia induced by chronic administration of AMPT (42) and to the hyposomnia induced by chronic administration of amphetamine (40). These findings suggest that adaptational changes in monoaminergic pathways, such as, for example, alterations in dopaminergic receptor sensitivity, could underlie changes in sleep-wake behavior produced by administration and withdrawal of certain drugs.

In light of the hypothesis that dopaminergic neurons are involved in behavioral arousal, it is perhaps inconsistent that the major tranquilizers, which are known for their antagonism of post-synaptic dopaminergic receptors, do not in general increase total sleep time to any great extent in normal subjects (13,15,28); in patients, however, changes in clinical status confound interpretation regarding changes in total sleep. In the case of pimozide, for example, Sagales and Erill (35) found that it had little effect on the sleep of normal volunteers, whereas we (11) found that it increased total sleep time and sleep efficiency to a small but significant degree during a clinical trial in psychiatric patients. The apparent greater effect in patients than normal volunteers could reflect a higher dose, longer duration of administration, or the clinical improvement of the patients with a secondary normalization of sleep. As shown in a rat study, very high doses of chlorpromazine may be required to increase total sleep time (21).

On the other hand, the hypothesis that dopaminergic neurons maintain arousal receives some support from studies with other pharmacological agents which affect dopaminergic neurotransmission. As reported extensively elsewhere in this book, apomorphine may act as a dopamine agonist at either pre- or post-synaptic sites depending upon the dose, and has dose dependent effects on sleep. Corsini, Gessa and their collaborators (3,4, 5,29) and others (1,19) have shown that apomorphine induces sleep at low doses and delays sleep onset at high doses both in man and animals. High doses also delay and reduce REM sleep. These effects can be blocked by pretreatment with a variety of neuroleptics, such as pimozide, sulpiride, benzperidol, or haloperidol. Consistent findings were also reported by Radulovacki, et al. (34), who showed that bromocriptine, which may also act as a dopamine agonist, increases wakefulness, and reduced REM sleep in rats who had been previously REM deprived. Alpha-flupenthixol, a dopamine receptor blocker, increases NonREM sleep and decreased wakefulness and blocked bromocriptine induced wakefulness and loss of REM sleep in REM deprived animals.

Piribedil (ET 495), another somewhat specific dopaminergic agonist, has been given to man (33). It increased REM Latency and decreased REM sleep in psychiatric patients, most of whom were depressed. L-DOPA, which may also act as an indirect dopamine agonist, has been reported to have similar effects on REM sleep in man in some studies, but not all. Wyatt et al. (41) showed that it decreased REM sleep in Parkinsonian patients when administered orally over long periods of time. In addition, a small dose (50 mg), administered intravenously during the first NonREM period, increased REM Latency in depressed patients (10). A similar dose, administered at the onset of the first REM period, curtailed the first REM period; interestingly, the second REM period increased to the same extent as the first one was shortened, suggesting that compensation for the loss of REM sleep was taking place. Since a shortened REM Latency and a long first REM period are now well established findings in certain types of depression, the normalization of REM Latency and duration of the first REM period by L-DOPA in depressed patients is of interest. While this finding could be consistent with the catecholamine hypothesis of affective illness, it may also be consistent with the hypothesis of an increased ratio of cholinergic to noradrenergic activity in depression.

Interpretation of the L–DOPA results, as well as those of other agents presumably sharing properties as dopamine agonists, are difficult because of pre- and postsynaptic receptors and their possible influence upon dopamine, noradrenergic, serotonergic and possible other sites of action. As also mentioned previously, the effects of L–DOPA on human sleep have been inconsistent in various studies and may depend upon dose, route and duration of administration, and type of subjects (10, 14,22,28,41). Parkinsonian patients who improve on L–DOPA, for example, may show an increase in REM sleep compared to those who show no clinical change (23).

Vardi et al. (39) reported similar sleep patterns in Parkinsonian patients treated with bromocriptine and L–DOPA. In addition, patients who developed nocturnal myoclonus while on prolonged L–DOPA therapy continued to show these symptoms when switched to bromocriptine (38). These sleep studies provide some validation, therefore, that L–DOPA and bromocriptine share similar pharmacological effects. In a similar fashion, Bassi et al. (1) have used the sleep effects of apomorphine to support the hypothesis that prolonged administration of L–DOPA "down regulates" dopamine receptors (27). They showed that Parkinsonian patients who had been treated with L–DOPA failed to vomit or sleep in response to apomorphine, in contrast to normal volunteers or Parkinsonian patients without specific treatment.

Amphetamine-induced arousal and insomnia appear to be mediated by dopaminergic mechanism rather than norepinephrine. Many investigators have shown that amphetamine prolongs sleep latency and REM Latency, and reduces total sleep time and REM sleep. These effects are greater for dextroamphetamine than for levo-amphetamine (12,16). Pretreatment with pimozide (13) but not with lithium (12) completely blocks the effects of d-amphetamine on human sleep, suggesting a dopaminergic mediation for amphetamine-induced sleep-wakefulness. In addition, Jones et al. (18) reported that lesions of the locus coeruleus, a noradrenaline containing nucleus, did not alter the effect of amphetamine on feline sleep. It should be noted, however, that Monti (30) claimed that d-amphetamine-induced wakefulness in the rat was not blocked by doses of pimozide which were reported to block dopamine receptors exclusively, only by higher doses which were also reported to block noradrenaline receptors; spiroperidol, which was said to be devoid of noradrenaline-blocking properties, was ineffectual in reversing the effects of amphetamine. Since he presented no direct data on the relative effects of these neuroleptics on dopamine and noradrenergic receptors, further studies are needed to settle these questions.

Because of evidence suggesting that dopamine is involved both in amphetamine-induced sleep changes and in the pathophysiology of schizophrenia, we compared the effects of amphetamine upon EEG monitored sleep in schizophrenic and nonschizophrenic psychiatric patients (Gillin, van Kammen, Post, Bunney, unpublished data). A bolus infusion of amphetamine (20 mg base) was administered at 8 am to 15 schizophrenic patients and 6 depressed patients. The patients were unmedicated, hospitalized, and moderately to severely ill at the time of the study. All night EEG sleep recordings were obtained before, during, and after the study. The results indicate that amphetamine affected sleep similarly in both schizophrenics and controls. It reduced total sleep time, NonREM sleep and REM sleep. No significant differences between schizophrenics and depressives were found in either absolute values before, during, or after amphetamine, or in changes from baseline. In so far as amphetamine-induced sleep changes are mediated by dopamine and are related to the pathophysiological mechanisms of schizophrenia, these findings offer no support for the dopamine theory of schizophrenia. In addition, no consistent sleep abnormalities in schizophrenic patients have yet been convincingly described (28).

In contrast to the sleep changes induced by experimental alterations in dopamine transmission, alterations of sleep, principally deprivation of REM sleep, may change dopamine activity. Ghosh et al. (9) reported that REM deprivation, achieved by the "island" technique in rats, elevated striatal dopamine content at the end of 4 and 10 days. REM deprivation has also been reported to potentiate the behavioral response to amphetamine in animals. Ferguson and Dement (7) found that amphetamine elicited fighting and sexual behavior in REM deprived rats, but not in controls. Tufik et al. (37) reported that apomorphine induced greater aggressive and stereotyped behavior and lowered body temperature more in REM deprived animals than controls; this suggested to the authors that REM deprivation "sensitized" dopamine receptors.

It may also be possible that the REM rebound, which normally follows a period of REM deprivation, involves dopaminergic neurons. In a study of the effects of phenelzine (a monoamine oxidase inhibitor) in depressed patients, Kupfer and Bowers (25) found that it depressed both REM sleep and CSF concentrations of HVA. During the withdrawal period, the REM rebound correlated with increased concentrations of CSF HVA. Two other studies suggest that administration of dopamine agonists following REM deprivation may prevent the REM rebound. Nakazawa et al. (32) found that small doses of L-DOPA, which has no effect on sleep itself, prevented the REM rebound in man. In the study previously mentioned, Radulovacki et al. (34) reported that administration of bromocriptine attenuated the REM rebound in rats who had been previously deprived of REM sleep. Since REM deprivation may induce dopaminergic receptor supersensitivity, the REM suppressing effects of L-DOPA and bromocriptine may have been potentiated in the last two studies. The absence of REM rebound may not prove, therefore, that dopamine has an intrinsic role in REM sleep or in the REM rebound.

It is difficult to summarize these diverse and often inconsistent results with any clear, simple statement relating dopamine activity to sleep-wakeful behavior. It is almost preparadigmatic to state that dopaminergic mechanisms are involved in behavioral arousal and in the alerting effects of certain stimulants, such as amphetamine. Considerable evidence is suggestive of this hypothesis, but that data is not entirely clear and arousal mechanisms needs to be clarified. Likewise, the apparent role of dopaminergic mechanisms in REM sleep needs to be viewed in the context of other systems. The recent growth of knowledge about dopaminergic mechanisms, anatomical localization, pre- and post-synaptic sites, and new pharmacological agents affecting dopamine should stimulate further research in this area.

References

1. Bassi, S., Albizzati, M.G., Frattola, L., Passerini, D., and Tra-
    bucchi, M. (1979): J. Neurol. Neurosurg. Psychiatry, 42:458-460.

2. Bunney, W.E. Jr., Kopanda, R.T., and Murphy, D.L. (1977): Acta
    Psychiat. Scand. 56:189-203.

3. Chiara, G.D., Corsini, G. U., Mekey, G.P., Tissari, A., and Gessa,
    G.L. (1978): Adv. Biochem. Psychopharmacol, 19:275-292.

4. Cianchetti, C., Masala, C., Corsini, G.U., Mangoni, A., Gessa, G.L.
    (1978): Life Sci., 23:403-408.

5. Cianchetti, C., Masala, C., Mangoni, A., Gessa, G.L. (1980): Psy-
    chopharmacology, 67:61-65.

6. Corsi-Cabrera, M., Gunberg-Zylberbaum, Arditti, L.S. (1975): Phys-
    iol. Behav., 14:7-11.

7. Ferguson, J. and Dement, W. (1969): J. Psychiat. Res., 7:111-118.

8. Gaillard, J.M., and Kafi, S. (1979): Europ. J. Clin. Pharmacol.,
    15:83-89.

9. Ghosh, P.K., Hrdina, P.O., and Ling, G.M. (1976): Pharm. Biochem.
    Behav., 4:401-405.

10. Gillin, J.C., Post, R.M., Wyatt, R.J., Goodwin, F.K., Snyder, F.,
    and Bunney, W.E. Jr. (1973): EEG Clin. Neurophysiol., 35:181-186.

11. Gillin, J.C., van Kammen, D.P., Post, R.M., and Bunney, W.E., Jr.
    (1977): Commun. Psychopharmacol., 1:225-232.

12. Gillin, J.C., van Kammen, D.P., Graves, J., and Murphy, D.L.
    (1975): Life Sci., 17:1233-1240.

13. Gillin, J.C., van Kammen, D.P., and Bunney, W.E., Jr. (1978): Life
    Sci., 22:1805-1810.

14. Gillin, J.C., Mendelson, W.B., Sitaram, N., and Wyatt, R.J. (1978):
    Ann. Rev. Pharmacol. Toxicol., 18:563-569.

15. Hartmann, E., and Cravens, J. (1976): Psychopharmacologia 33:203-
    218.

16. Hartmann, E., and Cravens, J. (1976): Psychopharmacology, 50:171-
    175.

17. Jones, B.E., Bobillier, P., Pin, C., and Jouvet, M. (1973): Brain
    Res. 58:157-1977.

18. Jones, B.E., Harper, S.T., and Halaris, A.E. (1977): Brain Res., 124:273- 496.

19. Kafi, S., and Gaillard, J.M. (1976): Eur. J. Pharmacol., 38:357-363.

20. Kafi, S., Bourkas, C., Constantinides, J., and Gaillard J.M. (1977): Brain Res., 135:123-133, 1977.

21. Kafi, S., and Gaillard, J.M. (1978): Eur. J. Pharmacol., 49:251-257.

22. Kales, A., Ansel, R.D., Markham, C.H., Scharf, M.B., and Tan, T.L. (1971): Clin. Pharmacol. Ther., 12:397-406.

23. Kendel, K., Beck, U., Wita, C., Hohneck, E., and Zimmermann, H. (1972): Arch. Psychiat. Nervenkr., 216:82-100.

24. Kovacevic, R., and Radulovacki, M. (1976): Science, 193:1025-1027.

25. Kupfer, D.J., and Bowers, M.B. (1972): Psychopharmacologia, 27:183-190.

26. Laguzzi, R.F., Adrien, J., Bourgoin, S., and Hamon, M. (1979): Brain Res., 160:445-459.

27. Lee, T., Seeman, P., Pajput, A., Tarley, I., and Hornykiewicz, O. (1978): Nature, 273:113-121.

28. Mendelson, W.B., Gillin, J.C., and Wyatt, R.J. (1977): Human Sleep and its Disorders, Plenum Press, New York.

29. Mereu, G.P., Scarrati, E., Puglietti, E., Quarantotti, B.P., Chessa, P., (1979): Electroencephalogr. Clin. Neurophysiol. 46:214-219.

30. Monti, J.M. (1979): Brit. J. Pharmacol., 67:87-91.

31. Mouret, J. (1975): Electroencephalog. Clin. Neurophysiol., 38:675-657.

32. Nakazawa, Y., Tachibana, H., Kotorii, M., and Ogata, M. (1973): Folia Psychiatr. Neurol. Jpn., 27(3):223-230.

33. Post, R.M., Gerner, R.H., Carman, J.S., Gillin, J.C., Jimerson, D.C., Goodwin, F.K., Bunney, W.E., Jr. (1978): Arch. Gen. Psychiatry, 35:609-615.

34. Radulovacki, M., Wojcik, W.J., and Fornal, C. (1979): Life Sci., 24:1705-1712.

35. Sagales, T., and Erill, S. (1975): Psychopharmacologia, 41:53-56.

36. Traczynska-Kubin, D., Atzef, E., and Petre-Quadens, O. (1969): Acta. Neurol. Belg., 69:727-733.

37. Tufik,S.,Lindsey,C.J.,and Carlini,E.A. (1978): <u>Pharmacology</u>, 16:98–105.

38. Vardi,J.,Glaubman,H.,Rabey,J.,and Streifter,M. (1978): <u>J. Neurol.</u>, 218:35–42.

39. Vardi,J.,Glaubman,H.,Rabey,J.,and Streifter,M. (1979): <u>J. Neurol.Transmission</u>, 45:307–316.

40. Watson,R.,Hartmann,E.,Schildkraut,J.J. (1972): <u>Am.J.Psychiat.</u>, 129:263–269.

41. Wyatt,R.J.,Chase,T.N.,Scott,J.,Snyder,F.,and Engelman,K. (1970): <u>Nature</u>, 228:999–1001.

42. Wyatt,R.J.,Chase,T.N.,Kupfer,D.J.,Scott,J.,Snyder,F.,Sjoerdsma, A. (1971): <u>Nature</u>, 233:63–65.

Apomorphine and Other Dopaminomimetics,
Vol. 2: Clinical Pharmacology, edited by
G. U. Corsini and G. L. Gessa, Raven Press,
New York © 1981.

Effect of Sleep on Dopaminergic Agonists

P. Passouant

Service de Physiopathogie des Maladies Nerveuses, Montpellier, France

The influence of dopaminergic systems on the sleep of human is unclear. REM sleep would be decreased by about 50 percent in patients with
Parkinson's disease (Mouret 1975). Administration of L. Dopa in depressed
subjects or in subjects with Parkinson's disease would lead to a decrease
of REM sleep (Wyatt et al. 1970) whereas in normals it would lead to an
increase of this type of sleep (Azumi et al. 1972).

In an attempt to clarify this issue, we investigated the effects on
sleep patterns of two agonists of dopaminergic receptors: Piribedil and
Bromocriptine. The former in normals, the latter in subjects with
Parkinson's disease, together with the study of the 24 hour GH and PRL
secretory patterns.

PIRIBEDIL

Piribedil at a daily dosage of 100 mg (50 mg after lunch and 50 mg
after dinner) was given to 5 male normal volunteers, aged from 23 to
35 (mean: 28.4 years). All night polygraphic recordings were conducted
according to our usual technique, from 10:30 p.m. to 7:30 a.m. Subjective
evaluation of sleep was checked by means of a morning questionnaire.

Polygraphic recordings were scored according to Rechtschaffen and
Kales's criteria (1968). Statistical analysis used the Mann and Whitney
U test and the Fischer-Yates-Terry test.

The design of the 31 day experiment was as follows:

1. Adaptation to the laboratory: 2 nights with polygraphic monitoring.
2. Placebo: 7 days with polygraphic monitoring on nights 1,2, and 3.
3. Piribedil: 15 days with polygraphic monitoring on nights 1,2,3,8, and
   15.
4. Placebo: 7 days with polygraphic monitoring on nights 1,2,3 and 7
   (withdrawal period).

Placebo and Piribedil were taken in a similar way.

Results

Effect of Piribedil has been assessed according to several criteria:
sleep latency, total time spent asleep, NREM and REM sleep features,
subjective evaluation.

1. Sleep latency (scored from lights out to the first appearance of
NREM sleep stage 1 was not significantly modified: mean:5.8 min on placebo,

7.4 min on Piribedil, 12.4 during the withdrawal period.
      2. Total time spent asleep. No variation has been: mean = 512 min.
On placebo, 511 min, on Piribedil, 511 min during the withdrawal period.
      3. NREM sleep. A slight increase of stage 2 has been observed
during the first 2 nights. Afterwards NREM sleep percentage was quite
normal. During the withdrawal period, a 12 percent decrease has been
observed on the 1st night and a return to normal on the 3rd night. NREM
sleep stages 3 and 4 percentage did not show any significant variation.
      4. REM sleep. Piribedil led to modifications of this sleep:

TABLE 1. Effects of Piribedil on REM measures

	PLACEBO				
	Night 1	Night 2	Night 3		
REM %	26.3	26.2	25		
REM Latency (min)	69	58	50		
Length Period (min)	27	26	22		
REM efficiency	.89	.88	.87		
	PIRIBEDIL				
	Night 1	Night 2	Night 3	Night 8	Night 15
REM %	21.6	21.3	29.7	26.9	27.8
REM Latency (min)	86	61	69	77	86
Length Period (min)	25	22	29	28	32
REM efficiency	.92	.92	.91	.90	.96
	PLACEBO				
	Night 1	Night 2	Night 3	Night 7	
REM %	31.2	29.4	24.4	24.5	
REM Latency (min)	46	63	63	64	
Length Period (min)	29	30	25	23	
REM efficiency	.95	.93	.94	.88	

      Effects of Piribedil on REM Measures: (a) Significant decrease by
about 17 percent (p=0.05) on nights 1 and 2. (b) Significant increase
by about 15 percent (p=0.05) from night 3, up to 29 percent in one subject (G.E.). (c) A rebound effect during the withdrawal period with a
mean 14 percent increase in comparison with the last night on Piribedil
and a mean 23 percent increase in comparison with the baseline period.
This effect was observed in all subjects during the first night of the
withdrawal period, in 2 subjects during the first 2 nights, and in the
subject who showed the highest increase of REM sleep on Piribedil during
7 nights.
      The number of shifts into REM sleep was significantly decreased in
2 subjects, who, when on placebo, presented a high number of shifts into
REM sleep. It was not modified in the 3 other subjects.
      REM efficiency, which was a little less than 0.90 in all the subjects
(0.88) was slightly improved with Piribedil (0.92). This effect persisted
during the first three days of the withdrawal period.
      REM density and REM latency did not show any variation.
      5. Subjective evaluation of sleep:
      Sleep latency appeared shorter in 38 percent of the cases on
Piribedil and unmodified in 45 percent of the cases.

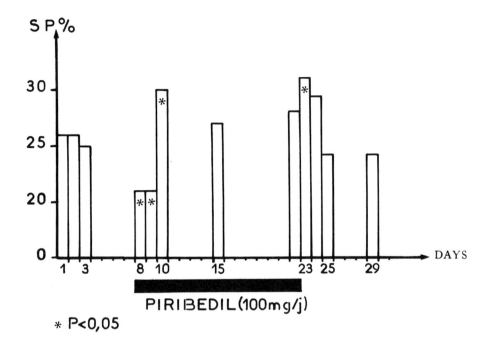

Figure 1. Effect of 100 mg of Piribedil on P.S. A significant reduction is seen during the first 2 days (days 8 and 9), an increase is noted on the 3rd day (day 10), and a rebound effect is present on the day treatment was stopped (day 23).

Sleep quality was similar though a better sleep quality was observed in 13 percent of the cases on Piribedil and in 30 percent of the cases during the withdrawal period.

Dream recollection was diminished on Piribedil. On placebo a dream report was obtained in 53 percent of the cases whereas on Piribedil it was obtained in only 28 percent of the cases.

BROMOCRIPTINE

This study was performed in 6 subjects with Parkinson's disease, aged from 50 to 67, (mean: 61 ± 2.9 years), 4 women and 2 men, who had not received any treatment before. Sleep related pituitary hormones, GH and PRL, as well as sleep architecture before and after Bromocriptine, were studied.

Design

Two 36 hour polygraphic recordings were performed, each starting with an adaptation night after which an indwelling catheter was inserted into an antecubital vein at 7:00 a.m. and left for the next 24 hours. The first recording was without drugs, the second with Bromocriptine, in dosages of 10 to 20 mg per day for a 3 to 4 week period, and in a single case for a 6 month period.

Plasma GH and PRL were measured in triplicate by radioimmunoassay using the CEA IRE SORIN double antibody unmodified method. Usual statistics were used.

Effects on sleep patterns were only studied during the adaptation night. Therefore this data is only of comparative value.

Results

A. 24-Hour GH and PRL secretory patterns.
1. Untreated patients with Parkinson's disease. The modifications were minor. They depended on sex and age.
PRL secretion was normal in the 4 women.

Table II. Mean 24 hour (day and night) PRL value in 6 subjects with Parkinson's disease before and after Bromocriptine.

Subject	Age	Sex	PRL Mean Without Treatment			PRL Mean Bromocriptine	
			Day	Night	dose mg/1	Day	Night
B...M.	67		5.34+0.18	10.79+1.7	15	0	0
Br..E.	66		3.32+0.18	5.23+0.6	10	3.07+0.1	2.28+0.1
E...G.	66		7.83+0.3	11.70+0.6	10	1.65+0.1	2.25+0.2
G...J.	54		8.82+0.38	9.47+0.05	15	2.82+0.8	2.87+0.12
A...J.	50		0.37+0.1	0.88+0.16	10	0	0
G...E.	63		9.61+0.9	9.18+0.3	20	0.73+0.1	0.76+0.1
Mean			5.88+1.4	7.87+1.6		1.37+0.5	1.36+0.51

Mean diurnal concentration ranged from 3.32 ng/ml to 8.82 ng/ml and mean nocturnal concentration from 5.23 to 11.70. In the 2 men, concentrations were either low or similar during day and night. TRH test induced a sharp secretory rise ranging from 60 to 100 ng/ml.

GH secretion was not associated with the onset of sleep in the 4 women. The maximum peak, up to 9 ng/ml occurred either during daytime or during the second part of the night. In the 2 men a moderately elevated secretory peak (2.5 ng/ml and 5 ng/ml) was found at the beginning of night sleep.

2. Patients with Parkinson's disease, after treatment with Bromocriptine: effects were clearcut on PRL secretion and practically nonexistent on GH secretion.

24-Hour PRL secretion was nonexistent in 2 subjects, daytime PRL secretion was very much decreased with the exception of a single subject and nocturnal PRL was very much decreased with the exception of a single subject. TRH test resulted in a very low response ranging from 5 to 7 ng/ml. In one subject there was no response at all.
Mean diurnal GH concentration was not modified (1.05 ng/ml before Bromocriptine, 1.10 ng after), and mean nocturnal GH concentration was slightly increased (1.31 ng/ml before Bromocriptine, 1.81 ng/ml after). No modification of the relationship GH/sleep was identified when compared to controls.

B. Sleep architecture.
The results only concern the adaptation night.
Before Bromocriptine sleep was unstable with frequent awakenings. REM sleep percentage was slightly reduced in 4 out of 6 subjects (14.3 to

Table III. <u>Mean 24 hour (day and night) GH value in 6 subjects with Parkinson's disease before and after Bromocriptine.</u>

Subject	Age	Sex	GH Mean Without Treatment		dose mg/1	GH Mean Bromocriptine	
			Day	Night		Day	Night
B...M.	67		2.63+0.5	2.42+0.2	15	1.58+0.2	1.79+0.2
Br..E.	66		0.66+0.09	1.08+0.02	10	0.31+0.1	1.64+0.2
E...G.	66		0.65+0.1	1.03+0.2	10	1.55+0.01	2.82+1.2
G...J.	54		0.92+0.1	0.84+0.2	15	1.43+0.2	1.81+0.1
A...J.	50		0.85+0.1	1.12+0.1	10	0.69+0.06	1.32+0.2
G...F.	63		0.60+0.13	1.31+0.2	20	1.04+0.1	1.52+0.1
Mean			1.05+0.3	1.31+0.23		1.10+21.1	1.81+0.2

18 percent), nonexistent in one subject, and normal in the last subject. NREM sleep stage 2 percentage was increased in 4 subjects (60.5 to 82.2 percent). NREM sleep stages 3 and 4 were absent in one subject, decreased in another one (5.8 percent), and normal in the final 4 (15.6 to 29 percent).

After Bromocriptine, NREM sleep was slightly modified, whereas REM sleep was slightly increased in 5 out of the 6 subjects.

DISCUSSION

Piribedil at a daily dosage of 100 mg modifies the sleep architecture. The most conspicuous effect is on REM sleep with at first a decrease of the duration of this type of sleep and then an increase further amplified during the withdrawal period.

Bromocriptine, at a daily dosage of 10-20 mg, during several weeks, increases REM sleep duration. This result is not of great value, because of the conditions of our experiment, but is tentatively paralleled with that obtained with Piribedil.

A few drugs only increase REM sleep and it is these drugs which lead particularly to a decrease of the catecholamines through a different mechanism. Reserpine (Hartmann 1966), AMPT in man (Wyatt et al. 1971), in animal (Rondouin et al. 1980), and methyldopa (Baekeland and Lundwall 1971) have this kind of effect.

The influence of dopaminergic systems on REM sleep in humans has been investigated by administration of L-Dopa. Among patients with Parkinson's disease, those who benefit the most by L-Dopa would be the ones whose REM sleep percentage would be reduced (Mouret 1975) or the ones whose REM sleep duration would increase with this treatment (Kendel et al. 1972). Results vary according to the administered dosage. At dosages of 28 to 80 mg/kg L-Dopa increases the duration of REM sleep in the subject with Parkinson's disease (Bricolo et al. 1970, Kendel et al. 1972), in the depressed (Zarcone et al. 1970), and in the normal subject (Azumi et al. 1972). On the other hand, a lack of effect has been pointed out in Parkinson's disease, with a similar dosage (Greenberg et al. 1970, Kales et al. 1971). At high dosages of 180 mg/kg in the depressed subject (Fram et al. 1970) and in the subject with Parkinson's disease (Wyatt et al. 1970) L-Dopa induces an important reduction of

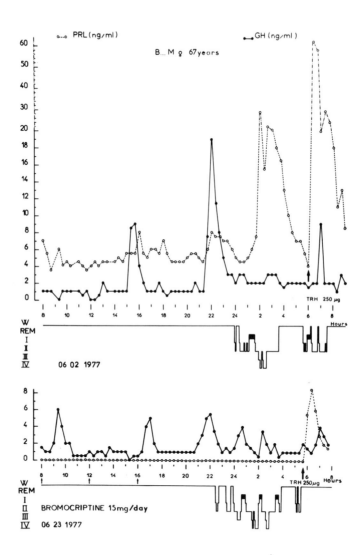

Figure 2.   24-Hour PRL (open circles) and GH (closed circles) secretion before and after Bromocriptine in a 67 year old woman with Parkinson's disease.   TRH test towards the end of the night.   Diagram of the
states of alertness at the bottom of each part of the figure.

REM sleep.

The two types of effects induced by Piribedil on REM sleep are rather surprising as the time of administration and the dosages remained identical. A modification of plasma concentration or a variation of the receptor sensitivity could be responsible. On the other hand, REM sleep rebound following the interruption of treatment - a rather surprising phenomenon as the duration of this type of sleep is increased by the medication - could depend on a particular effect at the receptor level.

Variations of the effects of Piribedil on REM sleep are associated with a prolonged administration of this medication and the difference of action between a unique dose and an administration of long duration could be retained.

In this sense the action of Bromocriptine on GH secretion is different with a unique dose which increases this secretions (Camanni et al. 1975) and a prolonged administration which has no effect. A somewhat similar result has been obtained in Parkinson's disease with Lergotril (Bell et al. 1978) and with L-Dopa (Galea-Debono 1977).

On the other hand PRL secretion, the regulation of which is dopaminergic, remains suppressed or very diminished by Bromocriptine after several weeks or months of administration.

The differences of effect of Piribedil on REM sleep as well as those of Bromocriptine on GH secretion, after a prolonged administration of these drugs suggest a competitiveness between several receptors or several monoaminergic mediators. However, complementary research will be necessary to clarify this effect and therefore the relationships between dopaminergic systems and the mechanisms of sleep.

CONCLUSION

In the normal subject, Piribedil at a daily dosage of 10 mg, slightly modifies REM sleep, with a decrease at first, and a secondary increase which is maintained during the withdrawal period.

In the subject with Parkinson's disease, Bromocriptine increases REM sleep duration. It has no effect on GH secretion and suppresses or decreases PRL secretion.

REFERENCES

1) Azumi K., Jinnai A. and Takahashi S.(1972): Eleventh Annual Meeting, Association for the Psychophysiology Study of Sleep (APSS), 4.
2) Baekland F. and Lundwall L. (1971): Electroenceph.Clin.Neurophysiol., 31:173-269.
3) Bell, R.D., Carruth A., Rosemberg, R.N., and Boyar, R.M. (1978): J. Clin.Endocrinol.Metabl., 47:807-811.
4) Bricolo A., Tutella, G., Mazza, C.A., Buffati, P., and Grosslercher, J.C. (1970): Sist.Nerv., 22:170-181.
5) Camanni, F., Massara, C.A., Belforte, L., Molinatti, G.M. (1975): J.Clin.Endocrinol.Metab., 40:363-366.
6) Fram, D.H., Murphy, D.L. Goodwin, F.K., Brodie, H.K.H., Bunney, W.E., Snyder, F. (1970): Psychophysiology, 7:316-317.
7) Galea-Debono, A., Jenner, P., Marsden, C.D., Parkes, J.D., Tarsy, D., Walters, J. (1977): J.Neurol.Neurosurg.Psychiat., 40:162-167.
8) Greenberg, R., and Perlman, C.A. (1970): Psychophysiology, 7:314.
9) Hartmann, E.L. (1966): Psychopharmacologia, 9:242-247.

10) Kales A., Ansel, R.D., Marhkam, C.H., Scharf, M.B., and Tan, T.L. (1971): Clin.Psychopharmacol.Ther., 12:397-406.
11) Kendel, K., Beck, U., Wita, C., Hohneck, E., and Zimmermann, H. (1972): Arch.Psychiat.Nervenkr., 216:82-100.
12) Mouret, J. (1975): Electroenceph.Clin.Neurophysiol., 38:653-654.
13) Rechtschaffen, A., and Kales, A., editors (1968): A manual of standardized terminology, techniques and scoring system for sleep stages of human subjects., N.I.H. Publ., 204, Washington, D.C., U.S. Government Printing Office.
14) Rondouin, G., Baldy-Moulinier, M., and Passouant, P. (1980): Brain Res., 181:413-424.
15) Wyatt, R.J., Chase, T.N., Scott, J., and Snyder, F. (1970): Nature, 228:999-1001.
16) Wyatt, R.J., Thomas, N.C., Kupper, D.J., Scott, J., Snyder, F., Sjoedsma, A., and Engelman, K. (1971): Nature, 223:63-65.
17) Zarcone, V., Hollister, L., and Dement, W.C. (1970): Psychophysiology 7:314-315.

Apomorphine and Other Dopaminomimetics, Vol. 2: Clinical Pharmacology, edited by G. U. Corsini and G. L. Gessa, Raven Press, New York © 1981.

Sleep Pattern Modifications by Dopamine Agonists in Man

C. Cianchetti, *C. Masala, P. Olivari, G. Marrosu, and **G. L. Gessa

*Department of Child Neurology and Psychiatry, *Clinic of Neurology, and **Institute of Pharmacology, University of Cagliari, 09100 Cagliari, Italy*

Several studies have been performed to ascertain the role of the dopamine (DA) system on human sleep. Oral administration of l-DOPA, the immediate precursor of DA, decreased rapid eye movement (REM) sleep in psychiatric (10) and neurologic (18) patients and, at high doses, in parkinsonians (2). However, this effect was not observed in normal subjects by Azumi et al.(1) and by Nakazawa et al.(14). Intravenous infusion of l-DOPA during non-REM (NREM)sleep delayed the onset of REM sleep, while its infusion at REM onset shortened the length of this stage (12).

However, the results of these studies do not permit differentiations of the relative roles of DA and norepinephrine (NE), since l-DOPA is metabolized both to DA and NE; moreover, it also affects serotonin metabolism (9). We thought that more information about the specific effects of DA on sleep could be obtained by using two direct stimulants of DA receptors, namely apomorphine (AP) and piribedil (PRB).

Apomorphine effects on sleep.

In a first trial (4) we administered AP intramuscularly (I.M.) in a single non emetic dose, to 9 subjects during the daytime; AP doses ranged from 10 to 20 μg/kg per kg body weight. No changes were observed in the sleep polygraphic pattern of the 3 subjects in whom sleep occurred. However, AP has a short lasting effect. Therefore, in a second trial (5), non emetic doses of AP were continuously administered intravenously (I.V.) in 3 hours of the night's sleep. The experiment involved 10 subjects, each of which had a placebo night (saline) either before or after the AP night, in a random order. During AP infusion, sleep appeared profoundly altered: complete abolition of REM sleep, significant reduction of stage 4, increase of stage 2. This effect was obtained with AP doses ranging from 10 to 15

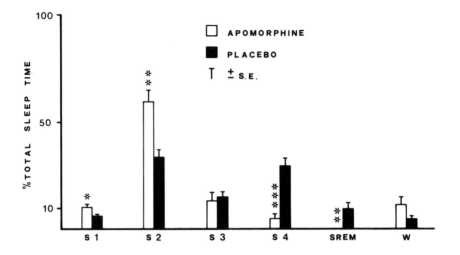

Fig.1.

Sleep stages percentages during 180min. infusion of AP and placebo.
S1,S2,S3,S4 and SREM indicate stages of sleep; W indicates interspersed
wakefulness. Each value is the mean of those obtained from 10 subjects.
Asterisks indicate a significant difference at 5% (*),1%(**) and 0.1%
(***), evaluated by means of paired "t" test.

µg/min (0.20 to 0.26 µg/kg/min). In other trials (unpublished) we
found that lower doses (0.12 to 0.08 µg/kg/min) have a proportion-
ally minor effect,while very small doses (0.02 to 0.01 µg/kg/ min)
had no effect at all.

An example of hypnogram during AP, compared with the placebo night in the same subjects, is shown in Fig.2. When AP administration was stopped,a "rebound" increase of REM and stage 4 sleep
was observed, and latencies of stages 4 and 3 reduced (5,6). This
suggests a high "pressure" of these stages caused by the previous
inhibition due to AP. However, in spite of this "pressure", a more
prolonged administration of AP was sufficient to maintain the altered
sleep pattern during the whole night (fig.3): an increased number of
awakenings was observed, especially in the latter part of the night.

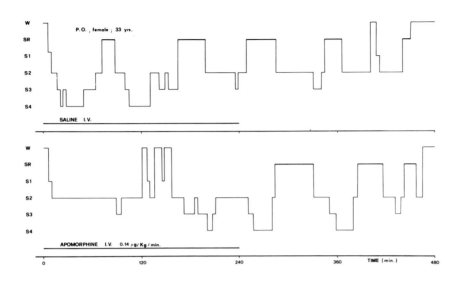

Fig.2.
    Hypnograms of the same subject during apomorphine and placebo nights.
Sleep stages as fig.1.

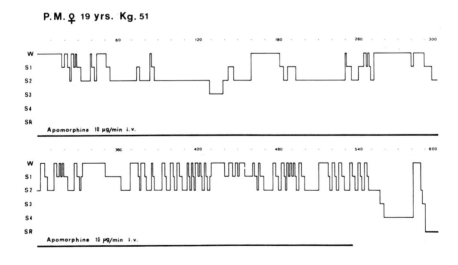

Fig.3.
    Hypnogram during 9 hours of nightly administration of apomorphine.
Sleep stages as fig.1.

Block of apomorphine effects by Haloperidol and Sulpiride.

    In order to clarify whether apomorphine effects were due to the
action of the drug on DA receptors, we carried out a trial (6) in
which haloperidol (HAL) and sulpiride (SUL), two specific inhibitors
of DA receptors, were administered before AP infusion. Eight subjects,
4 females and 4 males, aged from 21 to 34 years, with body weights
ranging from 41 to 70kg, were infused for 240 minutes with AP (8-12
μg/min, that is 0.17 -0.20 μg/kg/min) or placebo at intervals in
random succession. Moreover, 5 min. prior to the start of the infusion, subjects received an I.M. injection of placebo (2ml saline), 2mg
HAL (in 4 subjects, 2 males and 2 females) or 100mg SULP (in the
remaining 4 subjects); the succession of treatments varied randomly
for each subject.
    Both HAL and SULP blocked the effect of AP on sleep. Fig.4
shows the results of the study with SULP: no significant differences
were found between the night's sleep with placebo, with SULP + placebo and with SULP + AP, while all these differed from sleep during
the AP infusion alone. Superimposable effects were obtained with HAL.-
These data support the idea that the effect of AP on sleep is due to
its action on DA receptors.

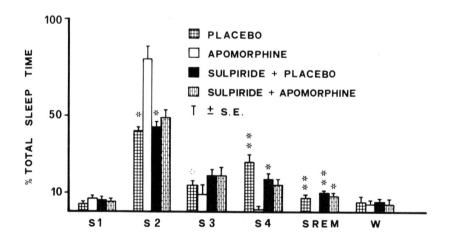

Fig.4.
    Effect of sulpiride pretreatment on sleep during apomorphine infusion.
Columns refer to the four types of treatment: placebo infusion preceded
by placebo I.M.; apomorphine infusion preceded by placebo I.M.; placebo
infusion preceded by sulpiride I.M.; apomorphine infusion preceded by
sulpiride I.M. Other symbols as fig.1.

Failure of Domperidone to block apomorphine effects on sleep.

The problem then arose of whether or not this dopaminergic response to apomorphine was due to an action of AP on DA receptors
outside the blood brain barrier. In order to solve this problem, we
carried out studies to see if the response was antagonized by Domperidone, a DA-receptor blocking agent which hardly penetrates the
blood brain barrier (13). Domperidone was administered intramuscularly prior to apomorphine infusion, in an experimental design
similar to that used with HAL and SULP. Four subjects, 2 males and
2 females, aged from 18 to 34 years, with a body weight of 49 to 69
kg, were given 8-12 mg of domperidone I.M. (in proportion to body
weight) 5 mins. before the start of AP infusion, and 4 mg I.V. at
the 60th min. of AP infusion; doses of AP ranged from 8-10 µg/min.
As shown in Fig.5., domperidone, unlike HAL and SULP, did not
correct the effects of AP on sleep suggesting that these effects are
due to an action inside the blood brain barrier.

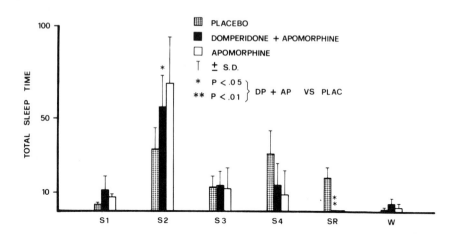

Fig.5.
    Effects of domperidone pretreatment on sleep during apomorphine infu-
sion. Columns refer to the 3 types of treatment used: placebo infusion
preceded by placebo I.M.; apomorphine infusion preceded by domperidone
I.M.; apomorphine infusion preceded by placebo I.M. Other symbols as fig.1.

Effects of Piribedil on sleep.

We decided to clarify if the action of AP was a general characteristic of DA receptor stimulants. For this purpose we chose the drug Piribedil (PRB), whose mechanism of action appears to differ in several respects to that of AP (3,8,15,11). The effects of PRB on sleep, by <u>oral</u> route,were previously studied by Passouant et al (16) and by Post et al (17), who found a reduction of REM sleep without variation of stage 4 percentage. Our trial was carried out with modalities similar to those of previous AP trials.

PRB was continuously administered I.V. to 9 subjects during a period of at least 300 mins. after sleep onset,in doses ranging from 0.1 to 0.5 µg/kg body weight per min.(7). The effects on sleep pattern are expressed in Table 1. Doses of PRB of 0.40.to 5 µg/kg-/min abolished REM and markedly reduced stage 4;with doses of 0.3 µg/kg/min these effects were less evident and REM sleep may appear; further proportional reduction of the effects is observed with 0.1 µg/kg/min. Therfore sleep pattern during continuous infusion of PRB is quite similar to that observed during AP.

Moreover, the effect of PRB on sleep, like those of AP, are blocked by the DA-receptor blockers HAL (fig.6.) and SULP.

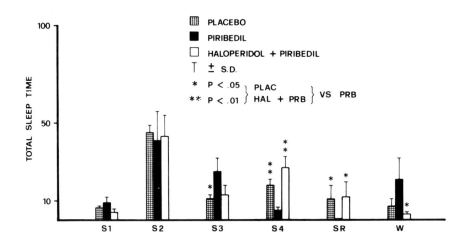

Fig.6.
Effect of haloperidol pretreatment on sleep during piribedil infusion. Columns refer to the 3 types of treatment used: placebo infusion preceded by placebo I.M.; piribedil infusion preceded by placebo I.M. piribedil infusion preceded by haloperidol I.M. Other symbols as fig.1

TABLE 1

	1 subject (29 years)		3 subjects (23-33 years, mean 27)				5 subjects (21-47 years, mean 32)			
	PRB (0.1)	PLAC	PRB (0.3) M ± SD		PLAC M ± SD		PRB (0.4-0.5) M ± SD		PLAC M ± SD	
% W int.	27	13	17.3 ± 13.1		7.0 ± 4.0		15.8 ± 11.8		6.0 ± 2.9	
% S1	2	4	9.0 ± 5.2		9.3 ± 7.8		7.8 ± 5.1		7.8 ± 1.9	
% S2	43	45	57.2 ± 13.0		41.7 ± 6.4		59.6 ± 17.5		49.4 ± 5.6	
% S3	9	8	17.0 ± 15.0		14.0 ± 3.5		14.8 ± 12.6		11.4 ± 0.5	
% S4	15	18	2.0 ± 3.5*		17.0 ± 3.6		0.8 ± 1.8**		14.0 ± 7.1	
% SR	4	12	2.0 ± 3.5		15.3 ± 10.7		0.0 ± 0.0**		13.0 ± 3.2	

In brackets, Piribedil (PRB) dose in µg/kg/min.

* $P < .05$ ** $P < .01$

PRB infusion per 300 minutes from sleep onset.

The persistence of the effects of PRB was tested in one subject in whom PRB had been continuously administered I.V. throughout the whole night for 3 consecutive nights: in this case, REM and stage 4 were abolished for the entire PRB administration.

To summarize, sleep data do not differentiate the effect of PRB from those of AP, diversely to what was observed in other kinds of experiments (3,8,15,11).

Conclusions.

Some conclusive remarks after this series of experiments may be summarized as follows:
1) DA-receptor stimulation, as by AP or PRB in continuous infusion, markedly alter sleep pattern, suppressing REM and reducing stage 4 sleep;
2) The effect is maintained by a prolonged infusion and may therefore cause a deprivation of REM and (partially) stage 4. However,it is rapidly reversible, with a rebound increase of REM and stage 4 immediately after stopping drug administration;
3) The effect is due to the stimulation of DA receptors inside the blood brain barrier.These receptors are probably post-synaptic, that is,not self-inhibitory, in spite of the low doses of AP and PRB used, since the effects on sleep are opposite to those observed by Wyatt et al (19) in humans treated with specific inhibitors of catecholamines biosynthesis;
4) From the methodological point of view, we may remark on how the infusion ("drip") technique is useful in the study of the effects of short-acting drugs on sleep.

REFERENCES

1)   Azumi K.,Jinnai S.,Takahashi S.(1972):Sleep Res. 1:40.

2)   Bergonzi P.,Chiurulla C.,Cianchetti C.,Tempesta E.(1974):Confin. Neurol. 36:5-22.

3)   Butterworth R.F.,Poignant J.C.,Barbeau A.(1975):In:Dopaminergic mechanisms;Advances in Neurology,edited by D.Calne,T.N.Chase and Barbeau A.,pp.307-326.Raven Press,New York.

4)   Cianchetti C.,Masala C.,Zonza F.,Mangoni A.(1978):Abstracts of 11th CINP congress,July 9-14,1978,Vienna,Austria,pp.282.

5)   Cianchetti C.,Masala C.,Corsini G.U.,Mangoni A.,Gessa G.L.-

(1978): Life Sci.,23:403-408.

6)   Cianchetti C.,Masala C.,Mangoni A.,Gessa G.L.(1980):Psycho-
     pharmacology,67:61-65.

7)   Cianchetti C.,Masala C.,Olivari P.,Marrosu G.,Melis L.,Giordano
     G.(1980):Riv.It.EEG Neurofisiol.,3(in press).

8)   Cools A.R.,Struyker Boudier H.A.J.,Van Rossum J.M.(1976):Eur.J.
     Pharmac.,37:283-293.

9)   Everett G.M.,Borcherding J.W.(1970):Science,168:849-850.

10) Fram D.H.,Murphy D.L.,Goodwin F.K.,Brodie H.K.H.,Bunney W.E.,
     Snyder F.(1970):Psychophysiology,7:316-317.

11) Gianutsos G.,Moore K.E.(1980):Psychopharmacology,68:139-146.

12) Gillin J.C.,Post R.M.,Wyatt R.J.,Goodwin F.K.,Snyder F.,Bunney
     W.E.,Jr.(1973):Electroencephalogr.Clin.Neurophysiol.,35:181-186.

13) Laduron P.M.,Leysen J.E.(1979):Biochem.Pharmacol.,2:2161-2165.

14) Nakazawa Y.,Tachibana H.,Kotorii M.,Ogata M.(1973):Folia
     Psychiatr.Neurol.Jpn.,27:223-230.

15) Offermeier J.,van Rooyen J.,Honns Ch.B.(1979):Psychologie Medi-
     cale,11:187-204.

16) Passouant P.,Besset A.,Billiard M.,Negre Ch.(1978):Rev.EEG
     Neurophysiol.,8:326-334.

17) Post R.M.,Gerner R.H.,Carman J.S.,Gillin J.C.,Jimerson D.C.,
     Goodwin F.K.,Bunney Jr W.E.(1978):Arch.Gen.Psychiat.,35:609-615.

18) Wyatt R.J.,Chase T.N,Scott J.,Snyder F.(1970):Nature,228:999-1001

19) Wyatt R.J.,Chase T.N.,Kupfer D.J.,Scott J.,Snyder F.,Sjoerdsma
     A.,Engel K.(1971):Nature,233:63.

Apomorphine and Other Dopaminomimetics,
Vol. 2: Clinical Pharmacology, edited by
G. U. Corsini and G. L. Gessa, Raven Press,
New York © 1981.

Dopaminergic Receptor Modulation and Sleep Induction

M. Trabucchi, M. G. Albizzati, S. Bassi, and *L. Frattola

*Departments of Neurology and Pharmacology, University of Milan, Bassini Hospital,
20092 Cinisello Balsamo, Italy*

Several clinical studies suggest the possibility that dopaminergic re
ceptors may play an important role in sleep induction.
In fact, apomorphine administration in man (3,7) induces sedation and
sleep at the dose (1.5-2 mg) able to cause a postsynaptic stimulation of
dopamine (DA) receptors (10). The prior administration of haloperidol
or sulpiride, drugs which act blocking the postsynaptic DA receptors,
inhibits sleep induction induced by apomorphine.
On the other hand, the effect of apomorphine is not elicited in patients
with severe parkinsonism treated for long period with L-Dopa.

DA receptors have been identified in various cerebral areas (9,10,11),
in particular in the hypothalamic-hypophyseal axis (6), which are probably deeply involved in the complex sleep mechanisms. It may be hypothi-
zed that apomorphine induces sedation and sleep through an action on the
DA system located in this area.

Recently, some authors showed that dopaminergic neurons may be modula
ted by endogenous opiate peptides through specific receptors located at
pre and postsynaptic level (1,4).

In our study, we tested the hypothesis of DA-enkefalinergic interacti
ons in producing sleep induction. For this purpose we used naloxone, a
drug able to competitively displace endogenous opiate peptides, thus blo
cking the connections among dopaminergic and enkefalinergic neurons (14).

MATERIALS AND METHODS

The study was carried out on 25 healthy volunteers, 14 men and 11 women, aged 17-41 years (mean = 23 ± 4.5).
All subjects underwent a previous recording after saline solution admini
stration as placebo; afterwards they were studied one or more times after
various drugs.

A poligraphic recording was made, beginning between 4-5 p.m. for three
hours, following a technique previously used by us (3).

In Table 1 are shown times and sequences of administration of the various drugs when used in association in the same subject.

The patients underwent also four recordings with haloperidol alone,
four with apomorphine and nine with naloxone (3 at the dose of 2mg i.v

and 6 at the dose of 4 mg).

TABLE 1. Sequences of drugs administration.

N° recordings	0'	15'	30'
6	Haloperidol	Apomorphine	
7	Haloperidol	Naloxone	
5	Naloxone	Apomorphine	
9	Haloperidol	Naloxone	Apomorphine

The various drugs were administered as follows: haloperidol 2 mg i.v.; apomorphine 1.5-2 mg s.c.; naloxone 2 or 4 mg i.v.

RESULTS

The administration of haloperidol, at the dose we used, does not induce sleep.
As shown in Table 2, apomorphine induces vomiting and sleep in all subjects with a mean latency time of 24'and 30' respectively.

TABLE 2. Vomit and sleep induction time after drugs administration.

	N°	Vomit	Vomit latency	Sleep	Sleep latency	Sleep time
Apomorphine	4	+	24'	Stages 3-4	30'	97'
Naloxone	6	-	-	Stages 0-1	42'	22'
Apomorphine plus Haloperidol	6	-	-	-		
Naloxone plus Haloperidol	7	-	-	-		
Naloxone plus Apomorphine	6	+	11'	Stages 3-4	20'	89'
Naloxone plus apomorphine plus Haloperidol	9	±	-	Stages 1-2	35'	71'

N° = number of recordings.

The EEG-sleep patterns were fairly homogeneous in all subjects; stages 3 and 4 were quickly reached and lasted for the 30% of the recording time.

On the contrary, naloxone, at the dose of 4 mg, induces drowsiness in four among six subjects, without causing deep sleep. This condition is characterized by several awakenings, and by a longer sleep latency and a mean sleep time reduced in comparison with that induced by apomorphine.

The simultaneous administration of apomorphine plus haloperidol or naloxone plus haloperidol did not induce either drowsiness or sleep.

The previous administration of naloxone reduces the vomit and sleep latencies induced by apomorphine, without any alteration of EEG patterns and total sleep time.

The simultaneous administration of naloxone, apomorphine and haloperidol induces, in six among nine subjects, vomiting and sleep. In this condition, sleep is characterized by latency, total duration and EEG patterns intermediate between that induced by naloxone alone and apomorphine alone.

DISCUSSION

Results obtained after apomorphine and haloperidol administration may be compared with those reported in previous studies by other Authors (5) or by our group (3). The data presented show that naloxone induces sleep characterized by different patterns in comparison with apomorphine.

In fact, it causes a lighter sleep, with a longer latency and a shorter duration. These differences led us to verify if sleep induced by naloxone might be related to the DA system stimulation. In fact naloxone induced sleep, is blocked by haloperidol and it is enhanced by the simultaneous apomorphine administration.

Our results confirm previous observations indicating that naloxone may cause a facilitation or a "modulation" of the DA synapses (4,8,11,12). Naloxone effects become evident only in particular conditions, among which we may indicate a possible impaired balance in the synapses and a peculiar receptor responsiveness.

In fact, naloxone does not cause any motor effect in normal subjects and its action in parkinsonian patients is a much debated question (2, 12,13).

Enkephalinergic neurons have been experimentally shown impinging pre and postsynaptically on the DA synapses. As reported by some Authors (8), postsynaptic enkephalinergic neurons cause an inhibition on DA neurons. Naloxone, competitively displacing dopamine from these terminals, could reverse this inhibition and modulate the synaptic activity through a facilitatory way.

Our data, indicating that naloxone administration is able to reverse or almost reduce the inhibition that haloperidol, a direct postsynaptic blocker, produces on sleep induced by apomorphine, support the hypothesis of a postsynaptic action of naloxone.

This working hypothesis needs further studies, carried out in experi mental conditions characterized by an alteration of the dopaminergic function, such as those present in extrapiramidal disorders.

REFERENCES

1. Adler,M.W.(1980): Life Sci.,26: 497-510.
2. Agnoli,A.,Ruggieri,S.,Falaschi,P.,Mearelli,S.,DelRoscio,S.,D'Urso, R.,and Frajese,G.(1980): In: Neural Peptides and Neuronal Communica tion, edited by E.Costa,and M.Trabucchi,pp 511-522.Raven Press, New York.
3. Bassi,S.,Albizzati,M.G.,Frattola,L.,Passerini,D.,and M.Trabucchi (1979): J.Neurol.Neurosurg.Psychiat.,42: 458-460.
4. Calne,D.B.(1979): Neurology,11: 1517-1521.
5. Cianchetti,C.,Masala,C.,Corsini,G.U.,Mangoni,A.,and Gessa,G.L. (1978): Life Sci.,23: 403-408.
6. Clement-Cormier,Y.C.(1977): Biochem.Pharmacol.,26: 1719-1722
7. Corsini,G.U.,Del Zompo,M.,Manconi,S.,Cianchetti,C.,Mangoni,A.,and Gessa,G.L.(1977): In: Advances in Biochem.Psychopharmacol.,16: 645-651.Raven Press,New York.
8. Diamond,B.I.,and Borison,R.L.(1978): Neurology,28: 1085-1088
9. Horn,A.S.,Cuello,A.C.,and Miller,R.J.(1974): J.Neurochem.,22: 265-270.
10. Kafi,S.,and Gaillard,J.M.(1976): Europ.J.Pharmacol.,38: 357-360.
11. Kebabian,J.W.,Petzold,G.L.,and Greengard,P.(1972): Proc.Natl.Acad. Sci.,U.S.A.,69: 2145-2149.
12. Nutt,J.G.,Rosin,A.J.,Eisler,T.,Calne,D.B.,and Chase,T.N.(1978): Arch.Neurol.,35: 810-811.
13. Reisine,T.D.,Rossor,M.,Spokes,E.,Iversen,L.L.,and Yamamura,H.I. (1979): Brain Res.,173: 378-382.
14. Sawynok,J.,Pinsky,G.,and LaBella,F.S.(1979): Life Sci.,25: 1621-1632.
15. Sourkes,T.L.(1975): Psychoneuroendocrinology,1: 69-78.

Apomorphine and Other Dopaminomimetics,
Vol. 2: Clinical Pharmacology, edited by
G. U. Corsini and G. L. Gessa, Raven Press,
New York © 1981.

Characterization of Anterior Pituitary Membrane and Cytosol Dopamine Receptors

Richard I. Weiner, Judith E. Beach, and *Bernard Kerdelhue

*Department of Obstetrics, Gynecology and Reproductive Sciences, University of California School of Medicine, San Francisco, California 94143; *Laboratoire Hormones Polypeptidiques, CNRS, 91190 Gif-sur-Yvette, France*

INTRODUCTION

Dopamine produced by the tuberoinfundibular dopaminergic neurons (13) can be measured in high concentrations in hypophyseal portal blood (2). Dopamine tonically suppresses prolactin release as demonstrated by the rapid and large increase in prolactin secretion following administration of dopamine antagonists to a variety of mammalian species (as reviewed 24). That dopamine was acting on the anterior pituitary to suppress prolactin secretion was convincingly shown by the in vitro experiments of MacLeod and his colleagues (17). In addition to dopamine's rapid effect on release, within 10-24 hrs dopamine inhibits prolactin synthesis (17,18), decreases the level of prolactin messenger RNA (18) and increases the rate of degradation of prolactin (10). Radioligand binding techniques have been employed to characterize anterior pituitary dopamine receptors (3,4,6,7,8). The following presentation will concentrate on work done in our laboratory characterizing membrane and most recently cytosol dopamine receptors in the anterior pituitary. The regulation and physiological role of these receptors is discussed.

MEMBRANE RECEPTORS

High affinity, saturable binding of dopamine (3,8) as well as related agonists and antagonists to particulate fractions of the anterior pituitary of several mammalian species has been reported (4, 6,7). ^{3}H-Spiperone (^{3}H-SPIP), a dopamine antagonist which has been extensively used in the central nervous system to define dopamine receptors, binds to partially purified particulate fractions of the ovine anterior pituitary with a dissociation constant (K_d) of 0.85 nM and a site number (B_{max}) of 343 fmol/mg protein (7). Specific binding defined by a 1000 fold excess of d-butaclamol represented from 75-92% of the total binding. The binding was stereoselective with the active d isomer of butaclamol being 10,000 times more potent than the inactive 1 isomer (Table 1).

TABLE 1. Competition of dopaminergic agents for ^{3}H-SPIP binding
to particulate fractions of the bovine
anterior pituitary.

Agent	Inhibition Constant (nM)[a]
bromergocryptine	18.5 + 14.9
apomorphine	220 + 78
dopamine	1,330 + 40
norepinephrine	18,000 + 6,000
d-butaclamol	1.6 + 0.5
l-butaclamol	17,000 + 5,000
haloperidol	11.5 + 3.0

[a]data from reference 7.

The rank order of potency of agents to compete for ^{3}H-SPIP binding was
consistent with that seen with brain dopamine receptors. The binding
was reversible and the K_d calculated from the experimentally determined
rate constants K_2/K_1 was 0.82 nM, a value in close agreement with that
obtained by saturation isotherms. ^{3}H-SPIP bound to partially purified
particulate fractions of steer anterior pituitary with a K_d of 0.38 nM
and a B_{max} of 210 fmol/mg protein, values similar to those obtained with
ovine preparations.

Since the anterior pituitary contains multiple cell types, the
question arose as to whether dopamine receptors in the anterior
pituitary were present on more than one cell type. To answer that
question, haloperidol binding sites on dispersed rat anterior pituitary
cells were immunocytochemically visualized at the electron microscopic
level, utilizing an antibody to haloperidol and the peroxidose anti-
peroxidose (PAP) technique (14). The majority of electron dense PAP
complexes were observed on the outer plasmalemmal surface of prolactin
producing cells. This observation is consistent with the findings that
incubation of the anterior pituitary with dopamine suppresses prolactin
release (16) without affecting the secretion of ACTH, LH, FSH, TSH, and
GH (as reviewed 24). Interestingly, in several instances invaginations
of labeled plasmalemma and positively stained vesicles beneath these
processes were observed. PAP complexes were always observed attached
to the inner surface of the vesicles and were not free-floating. The
significance of these observations is not clear, for it could represent
the internalization of dopamine receptors which are somehow involved in
the action of dopamine or simply the retrieval of receptor containing
plasmalemma from an actively secreting cell.

The high affinity membrane receptors appear to be involved
in the inhibition of prolactin secretion. The rank order of potency
of agents to compete for binding of ^{3}H-dihydroergocryptine, a dopamine
agonist, to particulate fraction was in close agreement with their
potency in affecting prolactin secretion (4). Furthermore, the inability
of dopamine to suppress prolactin secretion from GH$_3$ cells (12) correlated with the loss of high affinity membrane bound dopamine receptors
(9).

The second messenger and subsequent events involved in the inhibition of prolactin release by dopamine are unclear. Membrane bound

dopamine receptors in the anterior pituitary do not appear to be linked
to adenylate cyclase (20,23), although some controversy exists over this
point (1). Other evidence suggests that dopamine might inhibit prolactin secretion by inhibiting Ca^{++} influx necessary for exocytosis (22,23);
however, in a recent study prolactin secretion stimulated by a calcium
ionophore was blocked by dopamine without preventing the ionophore
induced influx of $^{45}Ca^{++}$. The inhibition of prolactin secretion by
dopamine closely parallels increased activity of two lysosomal enzymes
(20). Interestingly, the inhibition of enzyme activation with chloro-
quine blocked the inhibitory action of dopamine on prolactin release.

In a similar fashion to brain dopamine receptors, the affinity
of anterior pituitary receptors for agonists is decreased by the
presence of guanine nucleotides. The ability of apomorphine to displace
^{3}H-SPIP binding from particulate fractions of the steer anterior
pituitary was decreased approximately 5 fold by the presence of 0.3mM
Gpp (NH)p in the incubation mixture, Fig. 1. A similar decrease in the

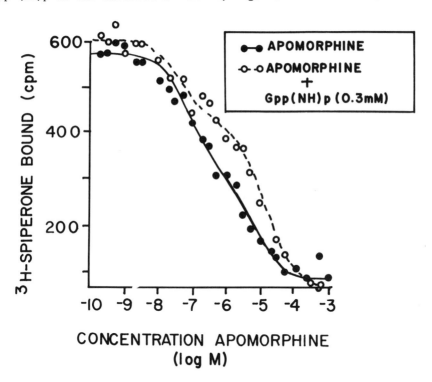

Fig. 1. The effect of the nonhydrolizable guanine nucleotide Gpp(NH)p
on the affinity of apomorphine to displace ^{3}H-SPIP binding.

affinity of dopamine was seen with GTP,GDP, Gpp(NH)p, but not with GMP,
guanosine or ATP. No change in the K_d or B_{max} for ^{3}H-SPIP was observed
in the presence of guanine nucleotides. Similarly the potency of dopamine antagonists to displace ^{3}H-SPIP was unchanged. Paradoxically the

binding of ^{3}H-dihydroergocryptine, a potent dopamine agonist, was
unaffected by guanine nucleotides as was its potency to displace
[3]H-SPIP binding. These findings can be interpreted as indicating the
presence of multiple high affinity dopamine receptors. Since
dihydroergocryptine is a potent inhibitor of prolactin release, the
site regulated by guanine nucleotides would not appear to be involved in
the inhibition of prolactin secretion. Further supporting the possibility of multiple receptors is the observation that dopamine stimulates
prolactin release at very low concentrations and inhibits release at
higher concentrations (11). However, a good deal of caution should be
taken in interpreting the lack of a shift in the affinity of dihydroergocryptine by guanine nucleotides since the physicochemical properties of
this compound differ markedly from that of dopamine.

CYTOSOL RECEPTORS

Two observations suggested that dopamine and possibly dopamine
receptors could be internalized. As mentioned, immunocytochemically
stained haloperidol binding sites on mammotrophs appeared to be
internalized (14). Secondly, recent studies showed that high concentrations of dopamine are associated with the subcellular fraction of
anterior pituitary homogenates containing prolactin secretory granules
(15). Incubation of anterior pituitaries with dopamine increased
intracellular concentrations of the hormone. The movement of dopamine
appeared to be receptor mediated in that it could be blocked by dopamine
agonists and antagonists. These observations in conjunction with the
fact that dopamine affects both the synthesis and release of prolactin
with differing time courses led us to determine if cytosol receptors for
dopamine were present in the anterior pituitary.

High speed supernatant fractions (145,000 x g for 1 hr) of homogenates of steer anterior pituitaries were incubated with ^{3}H-SPIP in
Tris, EDTA buffer for 1 hr at 37°C. Bound ^{3}H-SPIP was separated by gel
filtration on Sephadex G-25 columns. Specific binding of ^{3}H-SPIP to the
high speed supernatant fraction was high affinity (K_d = 0.1-0.2 nM) and
saturable (B_{max} = 1.2-3.5 fmol/mg protein), Fig. 2. Specific binding
defined by the presence of 10^{-6} M d-butaclamol represented from 50-90%
of total binding at various concentrations of ^{3}H-SPIP. Binding was
linear with protein concentrations between 2-7 mg/ml. Binding was
reversible and the K_d calculated from experimentally determined rate
constants was 0.2 nM. The presence of soluable binding sites was
similar whether tissue was homogenized in hypotonic, isotonic or hyper-
tonic buffers, or in the presence or absence of petidase inhibitors.
These findings suggested that the presence of cytosol binding sites was
not a consequence of ionic extraction of extrinsic membraine proteins or
partial enzymatic degradation of membrane receptors. The caudate
nucleus did not contain any detectable soluable receptors, although
crude particulate fractions of the caudate nucleus had 50% more
receptors than particulate fractions of the anterior pituitary (B_{max} =
93 vs. 61 fmol/mg protein, respectively). This observation argues
against the possibility that cytosol receptors result from mechanical
disruption of membrane receptors. No specific binding was observed

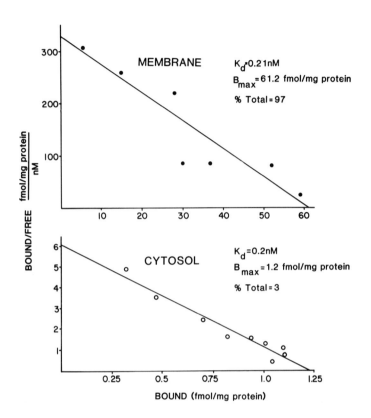

Fig. 2. Scatchard plots of specific ^{3}H-SPIP binding to the membrane and
high speed supernatant fractions of steer anterior pituitary.

with the high speed supernatant fraction from serum, eliminating the
possibility of contamination by a soluble serum binding protein.
    The rank order of potency of agents to compete for ^{3}H-SPIP binding
to the soluble binding site was identical to that seen with particulate
dopamine receptors, Fig. 3. The binding was stereoselective and
d-butaclamol was 10,000 times more potent than l-butaclamol in
displacing binding.
    These findings are consistent with the presence of cytosol dopamine
receptors in the anterior pituitary. Although the number of cytosol
receptors only represents approximately 3% of the total number of
anterior pituitary receptors, the concentration of receptors observed
is in close agreement with that seen for cytosol β-adrenergic receptors
in turkey erythrocytes (5). Whether cytosol receptors are a consequence
of internalization of membrane receptors or are newly synthesized

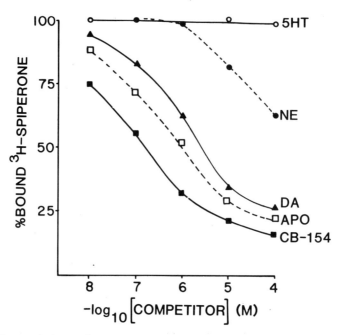

Fig. 3. Competition of bromergocryptine (CB-154), apomorphine (APO), dopamine (DA), norepinephrine (NE), and serotonin (5HT) for ³H-SPIP (0.46 nM) binding to the high speed supernatant fraction (from ref. 16).

receptors never associated with the plasmalemma is unclear. Further studies are necessary to determine the physiological role of these receptors as well as their origins.

CONCLUSIONS

High affinity, saturable, stereoselective membrane dopamine receptors are present in the anterior pituitary, predominantly associated with mammotrophs. These receptors are clearly involved in the mediation of the inhibition of prolactin release. Further studies are necessary to determine if more than one class of high affinity membrane receptors is present.

Dopamine receptors can be defined with ³H-SPIP in the high speed supernatant fraction of anterior pituitary homogenates. The affinity and stereoselectivity of the receptors are identical to that of membrane bound receptors. The origin and physiological role of the cytosol receptors are still unclear. The possibility of an intracellular action of dopamine cannot be eliminated at this time, since both the hormone and its receptor have now been observed intracellularly.

References

1.   Barnes, G.D., Brown, B.L., Gard, T.G., Atkinson, D. and Ekins, R.P. (1978): Mol. Cell. Endo., 12:273-284.

2. Ben-Jonathan, N., Oliver, C., Weiner, H.J., Mical, R.S., and Porter, J.C. (1977): Endocrinology, 100:452-458.

3. Calabro, M.A., and MacLeod, R.M. (1973): Neuroendocrinology, 25: 32-46.

4. Caron, M.G., Beaulieu, M., Raymond, V., Gagne, B., Drouin, J., Lefkowitz, R.J., and Labrie, F. (1978): J. Biol. Chem., 253: 2224-2253.

5. Chuang, De-Maw and Costa, E. (1979): Proc. Nat. Acad. Sci. USA, 76:3024-3028.

6. Creese, I., Schneider, R., and Snyder, S.H. (1977): Eur. J. Pharmacol., 46:377-381.

7. Cronin, M.J., and Weiner, R.I. (1979): Endocrinology, 104: 307-312.

8. Cronin, M.J., Roberts, J.M., and Weiner, R.I. (1978): Endo-crinology, 103:302-309.

9. Cronin, M.J., Faure, N., Martial, J.A., and Weiner, R.I. (1980): Endocrinology, 106:718-723.

10. Dannies, P.S. and Rudnick, M.S. (1980): J. Biol. Chem., 255:2776-2781.

11. Denef, C., Manet, D., and Dewals, R. (1980): Nature, 285:243-246.

12. Faure, N., Cronin, M.J., Martial, J.A., and Weiner, R.I. (1980): Endocrinology, 107:1022-1026.

13. Fuxe, K. (1964): Z. Zellforsch Mikrosk. Anat., 61:710-724.

14. Goldsmith, P.C., Cronin, M.J., and Weiner, R.I. (1979): J. Histo-chem. Cytochem., 27:1205-1209.

15. Gudelsky, G.A., Nansel, D.D., and Porter, J.C. (1980): Endo-crinology, 107:30-34.

16. Kerdelhue, B., Weisman, A.S., and Weiner, R.I. (1981): Endo-crinology, (submitted for publication).

17. MacLeod, R.M. (1976): In: Frontiers in Neuroendocrinology, edited by L. Martini and W.F. Ganong, pp. 169-194. Raven Press, New York.

18. Maurer, R.A. (1980): J. Biol. Chem., 255:8092-8097.

19. Nansel, D.D., Gudelsky, G.A., and Porter, J.C. (1980): 62nd Ann. Meeting Endocrine Soc., Abstract 460.

20. Schmidt, M.J., and Hill, L.E. (1977): Life Sci., 20:789-798.

21. Tam, S.W., and Dannies, P.S.   (1980):   J. Biol. Chem., 255:6595–6599.

22. Taraskevich, P.S., and Douglas, W.W.   (1978):   Nature, 276:832–834.

23. Thorner, M.O., Hackett, J.T., Murad, F., and MacLeod, R.M.   (1980): Neuroendocrinology, 31:390–402.

24. Weiner, R.I., and Ganong, W.F.   (1978):   Physiol. Rev., 58;905–976.

Apomorphine and Other Dopaminomimetics,
Vol. 2: Clinical Pharmacology, edited by
G. U. Corsini and G. L. Gessa, Raven Press,
New York © 1981.

Effects of Apomorphine on Inhibitory and Excitatory DA Receptors on Lactotropes

U. Scapagnini, P. L. Canonico, F. Drago, G. Clementi, A. Prato,
C. Barale, and F. Nicoletti

Institute of Pharmacology, Faculty of Medicine, University of Catania, 95125 Catania, Italy

In the last few years several kinds of dopamine (DA) receptors have been identified in the central nervous system (CNS) (12). Mostly, at the level of the striatum, at least two groups of DA receptors labelled with spiperone were found (2, 15). An interpretation of these findings was that one class of sites represented binding to presynaptic and the second to postsynaptic receptors. Biphasic binding of both DA (3) and spiperone (7) also occur in the anterior pituitary (AP) when very low concentrations are studied. It is obvious that a presynaptic receptor is not involved since no DA terminals are present in the AP. It has been suggested (6) that the lower affinity sites are DA receptors involved in the inhibition of prolactin (PRL) secretion, in contrast to the higher affinity ones. The second messenger involved in the inhibition of PRL secretion is still unidentified. DA receptors in the brain have been divided into D1 and D2 receptors on the basis of their capacity to stimulate adenylate cyclase or not, respectively (17, 11). According to this classification, classical lactotrophs DA receptors involved in the inhibition of PRL release should be more similar to D2 receptors since their stimulation is not always associated with an increase of cyclic AMP (10, 14, 16). In fact, several laboratories have not been able to evidentiate changes in cyclic AMP levels in the AP following DA administration (10, 14, 16), although other data indicate a DA- (1) and chlorpromazine-(5) stimulated as well as DA- inhibited (8) adenylate cyclase activity.

On the basis of a biphasic Scatchard for spiperone binding and a shift in the binding affinity of non selective DA agonists by GTP,Cronin et al., (6) have proposed that beside the inhibitory receptors a second DA receptor is present in the

AP and that low concentrations of DA stimulate PRL release. The stimulatory action of these very high affinity DA receptors may be linked to adenylate cyclase and modulated by GTP.

Due to above reported results, it does not appear to be reasonable to classify the two populations of DA receptors present in the AP, as classical D1 or D2 receptors (17). In the present chapter, we will refer to them as DA receptors inhibiting PRL secretion on lactotrophs (LDAi) and DA receptors stimulating PRL secretion on lactotrophs (LDAs).

Several trials have been performed in order to unmask the presence of LDAs. These experiments are based on changes in receptorial sensitivity produced either by lesion of medial basal hypothalamus (6) or by chronic treatment with DA antagonists. Both procedures are then followed by administration of different doses of DA agonists (9, 13).

In this line apomorphine (APO), the DA agonist active selectively at low doses at level of the classical striatal presynaptic receptors (14, 18), appears to be an useful specifical tool. In our experiments in order to produce changes in the sensitivity of LDAi and LDAs we treated chronically (21 days) male Sprangue-Dawley rats weighing 220+30g with different doses (2.5 to 5 mg/kg i.p. and 0.25 to 0.50 mg/kg i.p.) of the powerful DA antagonist L-sulpiride (L-S). After a withdrawal of one week a single injection of APO at doses of 100 or 500 µg/kg i.p. (doses considered to be active respectively at presynaptic and postsynaptic DA receptors level) was performed 30 min before sacrifice. Controls were pretreated with saline i.p. for 21 days before withdrawal and saline or APO injection.

As shown in Fig.1 systemic administration of APO induces a dose dependent decrease of serum PRL levels. In animals pretreated with high doses of L-S (Fig.2), it is clearcut that the low dose of APO is unable to produce any inhibition of PRL secretion whilst the higher dose of APO markedly inhibits it.

When the modification of receptorial sensitivity is performed by pretreatment with low doses of L-S, 100 µg/kg of APO produce a powerful stimulation of PRL secretion while 500µg/kg bring about the usual inhibition (Fig. 2).

In order to explain these findings, we have proposed an hypothetical model that is schematically represented in Fig. 3, 4, 5.

It has been suggested that in basic conditions (Fig.3) two populations of DA receptors (LDAi and LDAs) are simultaneously present on lactotrophs, being LDAi largely dominant. DA, reaching the lactotrophs, could bind with both receptorial

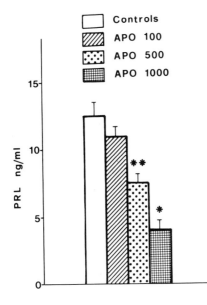

Fig.1 - Effect of systemic (i.p.) administration of various doses (100, 500, 1000 µg/kg) of apomorphine (APO) on plasma prolactin (PRL) levels of male rats. Vertical bars are means $\pm$ S.E. of 6 animals for each group.
**$p<0.05$ if compared to control group.
*$p<0.01$ if compared to control group.

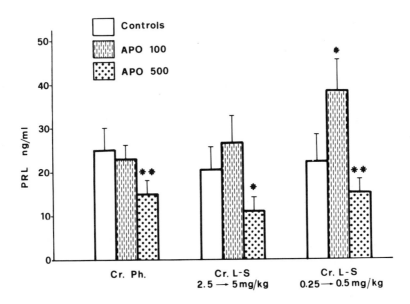

Fig.2 - Effect of systemic (i.p.) administration of 100 and 500 µg/kg of apomorphine (APO) injected after 1 week of withdrawal on plasma prolactin (PRL) levels of male rats chronically (21 days) treated with different doses (2.5 to 5 mg/kg or 0.25 to 0.50 mg/kg) of L-sulpiride (L-S). Vertical bars are means $\pm$ S.E. of 6 animals for each group.
**$p<0.05$ if compared to control group.
*$p<0.01$ if compared to control group.

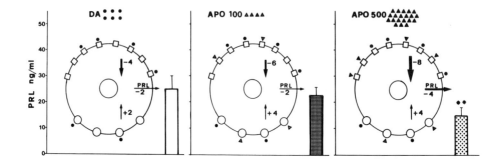

Fig. 3 - Schematical representation of a possible explana-
         tion of the effect at lactotrophs of apomorphine
         (APO) at doses of 100 and 500 µg/kg in saline
         chronically (21 days) treated male rats.
         ⊖= inibitory dopaminergic (DA) receptor on la-
         ctotroph (LDAi);
         ⊕= stimulatory DA receptor on lactotroph (LDAs).

species and the amount of PRL released could be the algebric
result of the two inhibitory and excitatory receptorial actions. When low doses of APO are administered in normal animals, in spite of a suggested higher affinity of the DA mimetic agent for LDAs, the larger amount of LDAi might compensate the interaction APO-LDAs. When high doses of APO are injected, due to the total receptorial occupation of both LDAi
and LDAs, the result is the classical inhibition of PRL secretion.

    After pretreatment with large doses of L-S, following a 1
week withdrawal, it should be present a receptor supersensitivity for both receptorial species (Fig. 4); this equilibrium could justify the findings of plasma PRL levels similar
to controls. When the lower dose of APO is injected in these
animals, even if the DA mimetic agent binds preferentially
with LDAs, due to the larger number of LDAi located at the
lactotrophs, no significant change in plasma PRL levels can
be observed. In contrast, the higher dose of APO, markedly
inhibits the hormone secretion since the total occupation of
both L-DAi and LADs results in a prevalent inhibitory effect.

    Following pretreatment with low doses of L-S and 7 days

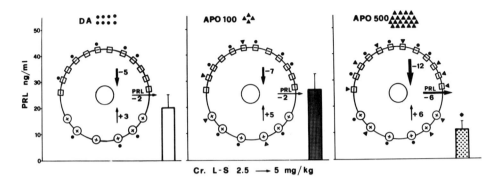

Fig. 4 - Schematical drawing of the effect at lactotrophs of
apomorphine (APO) at dose of 100 and 500 μg/kg in
2.5-5 mg/kg L-sulpiride (L-S) chronically (21 days)
treated male rats.

⊖ = inhibitory dopamine (DA) receptor on lactotroph
(LDAi);

⊕ = stimulatory DA receptors on lactotroph (LDAs).

of withdrawal, due to the major affinity of the benzamide derivative for LDAs, a preferential supersensitivity of this
kind of DA receptors can be hypothesized. In fact low doses
of APO, unable in normal animals to modify plasma PRL concentrations, strongly increase PRL release. When highdoses of
APO are used, the major receptorial occupation of LDAi might
compensate this LDAs preferential supersensitivity and resto-
re, at least in part, the usual inhibitory effect.

It is of interest the observation that, in order to produce the stimulatory action of low doses of APO on PRL secretion, a withdrawal of at least one week is needed. In fact
if the administration of APO is performed in animals pretreated according to the routine schedule with the low doses of
L-S but only after three days of withdrawal, the stimulatory
action of 100 μg/kg of the DA mimetic compound is not yet
present.

In conclusion the present paper provides further evidence
to the presence of a dual population of DA receptors on lactotrophs. Whether or not this dual population represents
two different types of receptors or two different states of
the same receptor is still unclear. It appears also difficult
at the present time to make any tight analogy between these
two types of hypophyseal DA receptors and the classical multiple DA receptorial populations in the CNS.

Finally it is of interest to notice that only in particu-

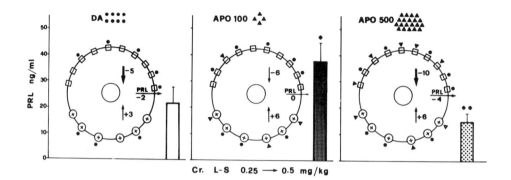

Fig. 5 - Schematical representation of a possible explana-
tion of the effect at lactotroph of apomorphine
(APO) at doses of 100 and 500 µg/kg in 0.25 - 0.5
ml/kg L-sulpiride (L-S) chronically (21 days) tre-
ated male rats.
⊖ = Inhibitory dopamine (DA) receptor on lactotroph
(LDAi);
⊕ = Stimulatory DA receptor on lactotroph (LDAs).

lar conditions such as the surgical suppression of DA sources
(6), or chronic blockade (9, 13) of hypophyseal receptors
with specific antagonists, it is possible to set up a model
to put in evidence the stimulatory dopaminergic component.

REFERENCES

1. Ahn, H.S., Gardner, E., and Makman, M.H. (1979): Eur.J.
   Pharmacol., 53: 313-317.

2. Briley, M., and Langer, S.Z. (1978): Eur.J.Pharmacol., 50:
   283-284.

3. Calabro, M.A., and MacLeod, L.M. (1978): Neuroendocrinology, 25:32-46.

4. Carlsson, A., Keher, W., and Lindqvist, M. (1976): In:
   Advances in Parkinsonism, edited by W.Birkmeyer and O.
   Hornykiewicz, pp. 71-81, Roche, Basle.

5. Clement-Cormier, Y.C., Hendel, J.J., and Robbinson, G.A.
   (1977): Life Sci., 21:1357-1364.

6. Cronin, M.J., Cheung, C.Y., Beach, J.E., Faure, N., Goldsmith, P.C., and Weiner, R.I. (1980): In: Central and Peripheral Regulation of Prolactin Function, edited by R.M. MacLeod and U.Scapagnini, pp. 43-58, Raven Press, N.Y.

7. Cronin, M.J., and Weiner, R.I. (1979): Endocrinology, 104: 307-312.

8. De Camilli, P., Macconi, D., and Spada, A. (1979): Nature, 278: 252-254.

9. Friend, W.C., Brown, J.M., Jawahir, G., Lee, T., and Seeman, P. (1978): Am.J.Psychiatry, 135: 839-841.

10. Hill, M.K., MacLeod, R.M., and Orcutt, P. (1976): Endocrinology, 99: 1612-1617.

11. Kebabian, J.W., and Calne, D.B. (1979): Nature, 277: 93-96.

12. Iversen, L.L. (1975): Science, 188: 1084-1089.

13. Lal, H., Brown, W., Drawbaugh, R., Hyns, M., and Brown, G. (1977): Life Sci., 20: 101-106.

14. Mowles, T.F., Burgardt, B, Burgarat, C., Charneki, A., and Sheppard, H. (1978): Life Sci., 22: 2103-2112.

15. Pedigo, M.W., Reisine, T.D., Fields, J.Z., and Yamamura, H.I. (1978): Eur.J.Pharmacol., 50: 451-453.

16. Schmidt, M.J., and Hill, L.E. (1977): Life Sci., 20:789-798.

17. Spano, P.F., Govoni, S., and Trabucchi, M. (1978): In: Advances in Biochemical Psychopharmacology, vol.19, edited by P.J.Roberts, S.N.Woodruff and L.L.Iversen, pp 155-165, Raven Press, New York.

18. Ungerstedt, U., and Ljundberg, T. (1977): In: Advances in Biochemical Psychopharmachology, vol.16, edited by E. Costa and G.L.Gessa, pp. 193-199, Raven Press, New York.

Apomorphine and Other Dopaminomimetics,
Vol. 2: Clinical Pharmacology, edited by
G. U. Corsini and G. L. Gessa, Raven Press,
New York © 1981.

Dopaminergic Drugs in the Treatment of Prolactin Disorders

Michael O. Thorner, Richard L. Perryman, Michael Cronin, Ivan S. Login, Jin K. Chun, and Robert M. MacLeod

Departments of Internal Medicine, Neurology, and Physiology, University of Virginia School of Medicine, Charlottesville, Virginia 22908

INTRODUCTION

The development of drugs which suppress prolactin secretion anteceded the isolation of human prolactin as a separate anterior pituitary hormone from growth hormone. The development of radioimmunoassays for human prolactin led to the recognition that hyperprolactinemia is the most common of the hypothalamic pituitary disorders.

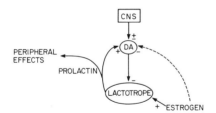

FIG. 1. Schematic representation of the interrelationships between the lactotroph, dopamine, and estrogen in the control of prolactin secretion (reproduced with permission from Ref. 34).

Prolactin secretion is unique since it is under tonic inhibitory control by the hypothalamus (Figure 1). Dopamine, synthesized in the tubero-infundibular neurons of the hypothalamus is transported along their axons to the median eminence where it is secreted into the portal capillaries. The hypohyseal portal blood then perfuses the anterior pituitary with high concentrations of dopamine which inhibit prolactin secretion. Although some workers still believe there are other prolactin inhibiting factors, dopamine is almost certainly the major physiological factor (21,30). Prolactin is probably also under some tonic stimulatory control by a prolactin releasing factor, but the nature of this factor is unknown. Thyrotropin releasing hormone is a potent pharmacological stimulus to prolactin secretion, but it is not clear whether it has a physiological role. Recently a great deal of attention has been turned to the role of endogenous opiate-like peptides in the control of prolactin secretion (3,26,29). Although several early reports suggested that these peptides may have a direct effect at the pituitary to stimulate prolactin secretion, it now appears that they act at the hypothalamus. Thus, these opiate-like peptides probably regulate prolactin secretion indirectly by their action on dopaminergic neurons (9,11).

The dopaminergic agonists which are used to inhibit prolactin secretion in the clinic are all ergot derivatives. Bromocriptine was the first compound to be introduced into clinical practice and has served as the prototype and reference dopamine agonist in endocrinology; all future compounds will have to be compared with it. It is a semi-synthetic ergot with a peptide side-chain which was specifically developed as an inhibitor of prolactin secretion (12). Bromocriptine is devoid of the oxytocic and cardiovascular effects of its parent compound, ergokryptine. Over the past four years several other compounds have been introduced, but none appears to have major advantages over bromocriptine, except possibly in the ease of manufacture which should lead to lower cost to the patient. These other compounds are simpler molecules without peptide side-chains (ergolines) and include lisuride, lergotrile, and most recently pergolide. Lergotrile appeared to be a promising drug (18); however it had to be withdrawn because of hepatotoxicity in man and a suggestion of a small incidence of tumors in the genital tract of rats after life long treatment. Lisuride appears promising and may have a potential advantage for certain neuroendocrine disorders since it has strong serotonin antagonist as well as dopamine agonist properties (27). Pergolide is only in the early stages of clinical investigation. It has one major advantage - pergolide has a longer duration of action than bromocriptine (19). In our own experience of studying six normal men, a single oral 100 ug dose of pergolide was effective in lowering serum prolactin levels and inhibiting the stimulation of prolactin secretion by thyrotrophin releasing hormone (TRH) for greater than 24 hours (Figure 2).

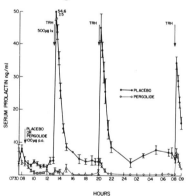

FIG. 2. Serum prolactin levels in six normal men throughout 25 1/2 hr. On one occasion they received pergolide 100 ug orally and on the other placebo. TRH 500 ug iv was administered at 1300, 2000, and 0800 hr.

In vitro Studies of Prolactin Secretion

The control of prolactin secretion by the pituitary cells can be simply studied in vitro. In our laboratories we have used two techniques: - (1) static incubation of pituitary explants, and (2) perifusion of dispersed pituitary cells in columns. Using these techniques, both dopamine and the dopaminergic ergots can be shown to inhibit prolactin release (22,40). In Figure 3 it is clear that dopamine has a short duration of action, while bromocriptine has a long lasting ability to inhibit prolactin release from isolated pituitary cells in vitro. Using pituitary explants and the incorporation of radiolabeled leucine into prolactin it is possible to show that bromocriptine is able to inhibit not only the release but also the synthesis of prolactin (Figure 4). An unexpected finding was that lisuride was extremely potent in inhibiting prolactin release but was ineffective in inhibiting synthesis (data not shown) (23). We have no explanation for this dissociation.

The mechanism by which dopamine and dopamine agonists inhibit prolactin secretion is not clear. Both dopamine and the dopamine agonists bind to "specific" dopamine receptors in the anterior pituitary (5,6,8). It is becoming increasingly clear that there are several classes of dopamine receptors both in the central nervous system and in the periphery. Kebabian and Calne have proposed two prototype receptors - D_1 and D_2 (17). The D_1 receptor is linked to

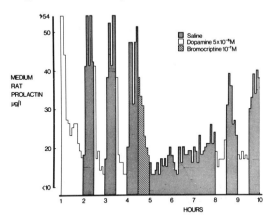

FIG. 3. Prolactin concentration in eluate from pituitary cell column demonstrating the slower onset of inhibition of prolactin release by bromocriptine than dopamine and its long duration of action after withdrawal (reproduced with permission from ref. 40).

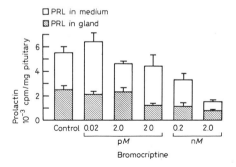

FIG. 4. Dose related inhibition of prolactin by bromocriptine Four hemipituitary glands were incubated per flask in Medium 199 alone or with increasing concentrations of bromocriptine; three flasks per group (reproduced with permission from ref. 34).

adenylate cyclase and is typically found in the striatum, and the D_2 receptor is adenylate cyclase independent and the dopamine receptor at the lactotroph is considered to be an example of this class of receptor. We have presented evidence that prolactin secretion may be independent of cyclic AMP stimulation, and is likely to be dependent on intracellular calcium as the second messenger (35).

In order to define separate classes of dopamine receptor it is important to show that each class possesses characteristic orders of potency of various agonists and antagonists. In the central nervous system this has been difficult to demonstrate. Several of the ergots, with potent dopamine agonist activity in vivo, not only fail to stimulate adenylate cyclase activity in vitro but also block dopamine's ability to stimulate it. Thus the interpretation of the significance of the striatal adenylate cyclase activity paradigm is problematic.

In contrast Goldberg and colleagues have described a classification of peripheral dopamine receptors based on the structure activity relationship of various dopamine agonists and on the potency of various dopamine antagonists (15).

One key compound in this scheme appears to be sulpiride which is available as two isomers, in l and d form. The d form is more potent in antagonizing the effects of dopamine on the postsynaptic (cyclase linked) receptor while the l form is more potent on the presynaptic (cyclase independent receptor). We have performed <u>in vitro</u> pituitary studies using d and l sulpiride and find that the l form is 30 times more potent than d sulpiride in antagonizing the inhibition of prolactin secretion by dopamine (Figure 5). Furthermore, this potency profile was also verified in

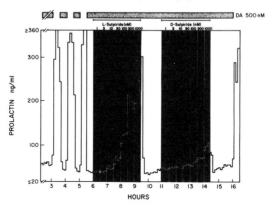

FIG. 5. The dose response relationship of d and l sulpiride in reversing the inhibition of prolactin secretion by dopamine. Note l sulpiride reverses the effects more completely and at a lower dose than d sulpiride.

binding studies using hog anterior pituitary homogenates where l-sulpiride was 30 times more potent than d-sulpiride in displacing ^{3}H-spiperone from the dopamine receptor (data not shown). The lactotroph dopamine receptor appears to have many similarities to the presynaptic dopamine receptor on sympathetic ganglia. Thus the anterior pituitary may provide a simple and extremely sensitive system with which to study this class of dopamine receptor. We have also recently studied SKF 38393 (28) which is apparently a fairly specific D_1 receptor agonist and find it not only to be ineffective <u>in vivo</u> in lowering serum prolactin levels, but in fact elevates them; it inhibits prolactin secretion <u>in vitro</u> only at extremely high concentrations (1 mM).

Clinical Studies

The central role of dopamine in the control of prolactin secretion can be exploited to classify, perhaps over simplistically, the various causes of hyperprolactinemia: (1) hypothalamic dopamine deficiency; (2) interference with dopamine delivery to the pituitary; (3) lactotroph insensitivity to dopamine; and (4) stimulation of lactotrophs (Table).

In practice it is presumed that the most common cause of hyperprolactinemia is a small tumor in the pituitary (a microadenoma). However, many of the radiographic criteria previously used to confirm the diagnosis of microadenoma are now thought to be neither sensitive nor specific since identical abnormalities are found on skull X-rays of normal people (1,2,4,10). As shown below, the demonstration of a microadenoma becomes less important since the presence or absence of a pituitary tumor does not affect the outcome of medical therapy in restoring both serum prolactin levels and gonadal function to normal. Furthermore medical therapy usually leads to a reduction in the size of the majority of large prolactinomas.

In this paper it is not intended to discuss in detail the clinical features of hyperprolactinemia. Hyperprolactinemia is more commonly diagnosed in women than men. Patients may present with (1) gonadal dysfunction (in women: amenorrhea, oligomenorrhea, menorrahagia, or regular cycles with infertility; in men: impotence); (2) galactorrhea or (3) compressive symptoms from their tumor - visual disturbances or headaches.

Table. CAUSES OF HYPERPROLACTINEMIA

Hypothalamic Dopamine Deficiency
        Disease of the hypothalamus -   tumor
                                             arterio-venous malformation
                                             infiltration
        Drugs: alpha methyldopa
                 reserpine

Interference with Dopamine Delivery to Pituitary
        Stalk section
        Microadenoma
        Macroadenoma

Lactotroph Insensitivity to Dopamine
        Pituitary tumors
        Drugs - DA receptor blocking drugs

Stimulation of Lactotroph Cells
        Estrogens
        Thyrotropin releasing hormone (hypothyroidism)

When considering the causes of hyperprolactinemia it is essential to inquire in detail about medications taken by the patient. In general it is unusual for serum prolactin levels to be greater than 200 ng/ml as a result of taking drugs. It is also essential to exclude hypothyroidism by performing thyroid function tests; in young women the sole clinical manifestation of hypothyroidism may be menstrual disturbances. Serum prolactin levels of greater than 200 ng/ml are usually seen in patients harboring pituitary tumors. Definitive neuroradiology is essential for such patients. Many of the finer "abnormalities" of the pituitary fossa which were considered to be specific for microadenomas now appear to be non-specific. Routine tomography of the pituitary fossa, if it is well seen on a Cauldwell view and lateral skull X-ray is unjustified unless it is preoperative procedure. It is likely that the new generation high resolution CT scanners will be able to visualize microadenomas of the pituitary and will greatly simplify the task of making an accurate diagnosis in these patients.

The two primary methods of treatment of hyperprolactinemia are surgery or medical therapy. The optimum mode of therapy is widely debated and depends on the expertise and prejudice in a given center. This has been extensively discussed and the reader is referred to several reviews of the subject (16,18,33).

Medical Therapy of Hyperprolactinemia

We have discussed above that the physiological prolactin inhibiting factor is dopamine. Medical therapy with ergot drugs exploits their dopaminergic effects. The widest clinical experience has been with bromocriptine; it has been used since 1971 for the treatment of prolactin disorders. In Figure 6 the effect of a single 2.5 mg dose of bromocriptine on serum prolactin levels in 18 hyperprolactinemic women is shown, as are the circulating drug levels. Following a 1 to 1-1/2 hour delay prolactin levels declined to reach a nadir at seven hours, and remained suppressed at 10 hours and only started to rise at 11 hours. Thus bromocriptine in a dose of 2.5 mg t.i.d. is able to lower serum prolactin in patients with hyperprolactinemia usually to normal levels (Figure 7). Following the withdrawal of therapy prolactin levels rise to pretreatment values. In Figure 8 the cumulative percentage of 58 amenorrheic hyperprolactinemic women with return of regular menstrual cycles is shown. In 80% there was a return of regular menstrual cycles. When the patients previously treated with radiation and surgery are excluded, 98% had a return of regular cycles.

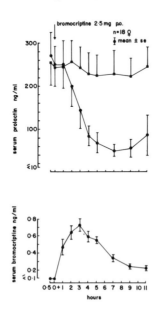

FIG. 6. Mean (+ SEM) serum prolactin and bromocriptine levels in 18 hyperprolactinemic women during a control study and after bromocriptine 2.5 mg p.o. at 0 hours (reproduced with permission from ref. 37).

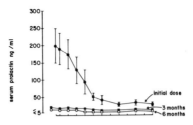

FIG. 7. Mean (+ SEM) serum prolactin levels in seven hyperprolactinemic women after their initial oral 2.5 mg dose of bromocriptine and at three and six months on bromocriptine 2.5 mg t.i.d. (modified from ref. 37 with permission).

In men with hyperprolactinemia serum testosterone levels are low and although the concentration of sperm in semen is usually normal, the total volume of semen is low - probably as a result of the low serum testosterone levels. When prolactin levels are lowered to normal serum testosterone and semen volume return to normal. This is anteceded by rapid reversal of impotence which in turn antedates the changes in the serum testosterone levels. These results were achieved with bromocriptine, but similar results are now being reported with lisuride. Results with lergotrile are similar and it is anticipated that pergolide treatment will produce equally gratifying results.

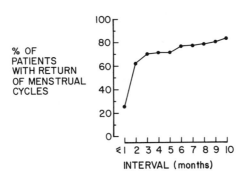

FIG. 8. Cumulative percentage of 58 amenorrheic hyperprolactinemic women with return of regular menstrual cycles related to months on bromocriptine therapy (reproduced with permission from ref. 32).

Hyperprolactinemia and Pregnancy

Pituitary tumors, meningiomas, and craniopharyngiomas have been reported to increase in size during pregnancy. When women with prolactinomas have return of normal fertility with medical therapy and then become pregnant, there is a risk their tumor may enlarge resulting in development of visual field defects, headaches or diabetes insipidus. Although bromocriptine has not been shown to be teratogenic in the 1,241 pregnancies thus far reported to Sandoz (personal communication, Dr. R. L. Elton), it is recommended that bromocriptine is discontinued as soon as a pregnancy occurs. The frequency with which compressive symptoms occurs is unclear but is probably less than 5% and perhaps less than 1% in patients with microadenomas and up to 35% in patients with macroadenomas (14). In order to prevent possible tumor expansion surgery or irradiation before pregnancy has been recommended, but at the present time no data are available to prove that either is beneficial (7,13,31). However it is likely that if such symptoms do occur, re-introduction of bromocriptine during the pregnancy or surgery at that time will relieve the symptoms.

Prolactinoma Volume and Bromocriptine

Although the effects of bromocriptine on suppressing prolactin levels to normal in patients with large tumors has been known for many years, its effect on tumor volume has only become recognized recently with the advent of more sensitive neuroradiological techniques - CT scanning and metrizamide cisternography (24,25,36,38,39). McGregor, Scanlon, and Hall (personal communication) treated 13 consecutive patients with prolactin secreting macroadenomas and we have treated 6. All 19 patients showed a reduction in the volume of the pituitary gland with medical therapy. Two of our patients have been reported and they demonstrated several important points: (1) reduction of tumor volume could occur within days as demonstrated clinically with improvement of visual fields and headaches, or within two to six weeks as demonstrated radiographically, (2) the attainment of normal or markedly reduced prolactin levels despite pretreatment levels of 2-4 ug/ml, (3) the resumption of normal gonadal function, and (4) the small dose of bromocriptine (7.5 mg/day) required to achieve these results in contrast to the high doses reported by others (33,36).

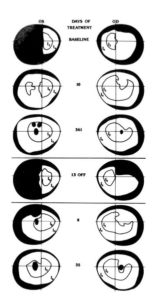

FIG. 9. Diagrammatic representation of visual field plot before and during, as well as following withdrawal and reinstitution of bromocriptine therapy. The visual fields were plotted using the goldman apparatus under identical conditions with a 0.25 mm^2 object at two different light intensities, 1000 apostibl (I_4) and 100 apostibl (I_2). The black periphery indicates a normal visual field for comparison. Before therapy (Baseline), a bitemporal hemianopsia, complete in the left eye and incomplete in the right eye was present. The visual fields were greatly improved at 10 days and only an equivocal superior bitemporal quadrantic defect to the low intensity object was present on the 361st day. On the 13th day after withdrawal of medical therapy the field defects recurred; an almost complete temporal hemianopsia in the left eye and an incomplete temporal hemianopsia in the right eye were present. Progressive improvement in the visual fields was again observed over six weeks after reintroduction of therapy, (reproduced with permission from Ref. 38).

It will be important to know what happens when treatment is withdrawn from such patients. To date no reports have appeared of re-expansion of these tumors on withdrawal of therapy. One of our patients with a large tumor who had bitemporal hemianopsia prior to bromocriptine therapy was withdrawn from therapy after one year (38). At that time his serum prolactin levels were normal, and cisternography showed a partially empty pituitary fossa. At 10 days off therapy he developed recurrence of his pretreatment headaches and at 13 days developed bitemporal hemianopsia (complete in the left eye and incomplete in the right). This was associated with a rise in serum prolactin to greater than 2 ug/ml and development of a 12 mm suprasellar extension of the tumor demonstrated radiographically. Treatment was re-instituted on the 13th day and once more prolactin levels fell to normal, visual fields improved rapidly (Figure 9) and the suprasellar extension regressed once more (Figure 10). Thus bromocriptine therapy is successful in lowering prolactin levels with return of normal gonadal function. Patients with large prolactinomas treated with bromocriptine alone should be withdrawn from therapy cautiously. Bromocriptine may change the size of individual cells rather than altering the cell number; this is suggested on the basis of the time course of changes in the pituitary volume with initiation, withdrawal and re-initiation of bromocriptine therapy. This question is now being persued in an animal model of the condition.

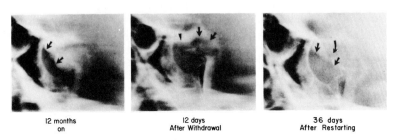

12 months
on

12 days
After Withdrawal

36 days
After Restarting

Bromocriptine 2.5 mg tid

FIG. 10. On left: midline tomogram during metrizamide cisternogram 12 months after commencement of treatment. There is extension of the chiasmatic cistern downward into the pituitary fossa (arrows) demonstrating a partially empty pituitary fossa. Middle: midline tomogram during metrizamide cisternogram 12 days after withdrawal of bromocriptine. There is almost complete obliteration of the chiasmatic cistern with only a trace of contrast between the inferior surface of the chiasm and the pituitary fossa. The superior margin of the chiasm is identified (arrowhead). The summit of the suprasellar extension of the tumor is outlined by contrast (arrows). On right: midline tomogram during metrizamide cisternogram 36 days after recommencement of bromocriptine therapy. There is again extension of the chiasmatic cistern into the pituitary fossa (arrows). This intrasellar extension is not as marked as seen previously (Left). A small defect is seen in the chiasmatic cistern posteriorly (curved arrow) indicating a persistent small suprasellar mass, (reproduced with permission from Ref. 38).

Conclusions

Prolactin secretion is tonically inhibited by hypothalamically elaborated dopamine. Hyperprolactinemia is a common condition and is most often due to the presence of a small prolactin secreting pituitary tumor. Medical therapy with dopaminergic ergot drugs is successful in lowering prolactin levels to normal, restoring gonadal function, and in reducing the size of the majority of prolactin secreting macroadenomas. Macroadenomas may re-expand if therapy is withdrawn. Prolactinomas are one of the first tumors in man which can be predictably controlled for at least one year by medical therapy.

References

1. Banna, M., Nicholas, W., and McLachelin, M. (1978): Neuroradiology, 16:440-442.

2. Bruneton, J. N., Drouillard, J. P., Sabatier, J. C., Elie, G. P., and Tavernier, J. F. (1979): Radiology, 131:99-104.

3. Bruni, J. F., Van Vugt, D., Marshall, S., and Meites, J. (1977): Life Sci., 21:461-466.

4. Burrow, G. N., Wortzman, G., Rewcastle, N. B., and Holgate, R. C. (1980): Abstract #386, Sixth International Congress of Endocrinology, Melbourne, Australia.

5. Calabro, M. A., and MacLeod, R. M. (1978): Neuroendocrinology, 25: 32-46.

6. Caron, G. M., Beaulieu, M., Raymond, V., Gagne, B., Drouin, J., Lefkowitz, J., and Labrie, F. (1978): J. Biol. Chem., 253:2244-2253.

7. Child, D. F., Gordon, H., Mashiter, K., and Joplin, G. F. (1975): Br Med J., 4:87-89.

8. Cronin, M. J., and Weiner, R. I. (1979): Endocrinology, 104:307-312.

9. Cronin, M. J., Cheung, C. Y., Beach, J. E., Faure, N., Goldsmith, P. C., and Weiner, R. I. (1980): In: Central and Peripheral Regulation of Prolactin Function, edited by R. M. MacLeod and U. Scapagnini pp. 43-58. Raven Press, New York.

10. Dubois, P. J., Orr, D. P., Hoy, R. J., Herbert, D. L., and Heinz, E. R. (1979): Radiology, 131:105-110.

11. Enjalbert, R. M., Ruberg, L., Fiore, L., Arancibia, S., Priam, M., and Kordon, C. (1979): Europ. J. Pharmacol., 53:211-212.

12. Fluckiger, E., and Wagner, H. (1968): Experientia, 24:1130-1131.

13. Franks, S., Jacobs, H. S., Hull, M. G. R., Steele, S. J., and Nabarro, J. D. N. (1977): Br. J. Obstet. Gynaecol., 84:241-253.

14. Gemzell, C., and Wang, C. F. (1979): Fertil. Steril., 31:363-372.

15. Goldberg, C. I., and Kohli, J. D. (1979): Commun. Psychopharmacol., 3:447-456.

16. Gomez, F., Reyes, F. I., and Faiman, C. (1977): Am. J. Med., 62:648-660.

17. Kebabian, J. W., and Calne, D. B. (1979): Nature., 277:93-96.

18. Kleinberg, D. L., Noel, G. L., and Frantz, A. G. (1977): N. Engl. J. Med., 296:589-600.

19. Kleinberg, D. L., Lieberman, A., Todd, J., Greising, J., Neophytides, A., and Kupersmith, M. (1980): J. Clin. Endocrinol. Metab., 51:152-154.

20. Login, I. S., and MacLeod, R. M. (1979): Europ. J. Pharmacol., 60:253-255.

21. MacLeod, R. M. (1976): In: Frontiers in Neuroendocrinology, Vol. 4, edited by L. Martini and W. F. Ganong, pp. 169-194. Raven Press, New York.

22. MacLeod, R. M., and Lehmeyer, J. E. (1974): Endocrinology, 94:1077-1085.

23. MacLeod, R. M., Kimura, H., Valdenegro, C. A., and Thorner, M. O. (1980): In: Central and Peripheral Regulation of Prolactin Function, edited by R. M. MacLeod and U. Scapagnini, pp. 27-42. Raven Press, New York.

24. McGregor, A. M., Scanlon, M. F., Hall, K., Cook, D. B., and Hall, R. (1979): N. Engl. J. Med., 300:291-193.

25. McGregor, A. M., Scanlon, M. F., Hall, R., and Hall, K. (1979): Br. Med. J., 2:700-703.

26. Rivier, C., Vale, W., Ling, N., Brown, M., and Guillemin, R. (1977): Endocrinology, 100:238-241.

27. Rogawski, M. A., and Aghajanian, G. K. (1979): Life Sci., 24:1289-1298.

28. Setler, P. E., Saran, H. M., Zirkle, C. L., and Saunders, H. L. (1978) Europ. J. Pharmacol., 50:419-430.

29. Shaar, C. J., Fredrickson, C. A., Dininger, N. B., and Jackson, L. (1977): Life Sci., 21:853-860.

30. Thorner, M. O. (1977): In: Clinical Neuroendocrinology, edited by L. Martini and G. M. Besser, pp. 319-361. Academic Press, New York.

31. Thorner, M. O., Edwards, C.R.W., Charlesworth, M.B., Dacie, J.E., Moult, P.J.A., Rees, L. H., Jones, A. E., and Besser, G. M. (1979) Br. Med. J., 2:771-774.

32. Thorner, M. O., Evans, W. S., MacLeod, R. M., Nunley, W. C., Jr., Rogol, A. D., Morris, J. L., and Besser, G. M. (1980): In: Ergot Compounds and Brain Function - Neuroendocrine and Neuropsychiatric Aspects, edited by G. Goldstein, D. B. Calne, A. Lieberman, and M. O. Thorner, pp. 125-139. Raven Press, New York.

33. Thorner, M. O., Fluckiger, E., and Calne, D. B. (1980): Bromocriptine. A Clinical and Pharmacological Review. Raven Press, New York.

34. Thorner, M. O., and MacLeod, R. M. (1980): In: Prolactin - 1980 and Beyond, edited by M. L'Hermite and S. Judd, in press, Karger, Basle.

35. Thorner, M. O., Hackett, J., Murad., F., and MacLeod, R. M. (1980): Neuroendocrinology, in press.

36. Thorner, M. O., Martin, W. H., Rogol, A. D., Morris, J. L., Perryman, R. L., Conway, B. P., Howards, S. S., Wolfman, M. G., and MacLeod, R. M. (1980): J. Clin. Endocrinol. Metab., 51:438-445.

37. Thorner, M. O., Schran, H. F., Evans, W. S., Rogol, A. D., Morris, J. L., and MacLeod, R. M. (1980): J. Clin. Endocrinol. Metab., 50:1026-1033.

38. Thorner, M. O., Perryman, R. L., Rogol, A. D., Conway, B. P., MacLeod, R. M., Login, I. S., and Morris, J. L. Submitted for publication.

39. Wass, J. A. H., Thorner, M. O., Charlesworth, M., Moult, P. J. A., Dacie, J. E., Jones, A. E., and Besser, G. M. (1979): Lancet, 2:66-69.

40. Yeo, T., Thorner, M. O., Jones, A., Lowry, P. J., and Besser, G. M. (1979): Clin Endocrinol. (Oxf.), 10:123-130.

*Apomorphine and Other Dopaminomimetics,
Vol. 2: Clinical Pharmacology*, edited by
G. U. Corsini and G. L. Gessa, Raven Press,
New York © 1981.

Biochemical Effects of Apomorphine: Contribution to Schizophrenia Research

M. Ackenheil

Psychiatrische Klinik der Universität München, 8000 München 2, West Germany

ABSTRACT

Stimulation of Human Growth Hormone (HGH) with the DA agonist
Apomorphine induced in untreated acute schizophrenic patients
a significant rise of HGH. There was a great variability of
response, some patients showed an exaggerated and others a
blunted response. PRL was in a normal range. Successful neuroleptic treatment resulted in HGH suppression and PRL elevation. 5 days discontinuation reversed this effect, but did
not induce DA receptor supersensitivity and did not exacerbate the psychosis.
In long-term treated chronic patients a blunted HGH response
and normal PRL levels were found. NA in serum was elevated.
Drug withdrawal for 12, 30 and 90 days induced an increase of
HGH, but not an exaggerated response, a decrease of PRL and
NA. In some patients tardive dyskinesia occurred. No differences of the Apomorphine induced PRL suppressions were found
between the different patient groups or treatment periods. No
correlation existed between biochemical parameters and psychopathological or neurological states. The DA receptor supersensitivity of schizophrenics could not be confirmed by
these results.

INTRODUCTION

The dopamine (DA) hypothesis of schizophrenia alleging a hyperfunction of dopaminergic neurons or pre-respective postsynaptic receptors at least in some brain areas, seems to be
well established (Matthyssee, 1973). However, until now no
exact proofs could be demonstrated. The evidence for this hypothesis results mainly from mosaic-like indirect pharmacological findings with e.g. DA agonists, such as Apomorphine and
L-Dopa (Angrist, 1980) and the antipsychotic effect of neuroleptics (Carlsson and Lindqvist, 1966). Especially the changes of the DA receptor sensitivity induced by neuroleptic
treatment and withdrawl should be related to psychopathological symptoms and movement disorders such as parkinsonism and
tardive dyskinesia. Generally it is assumed that tardive dyskinesia is closely connected to a DA receptor supersensitivity of the nigrostriatal system (Gerlach, 1979).
The stimulation of DA receptors in the hypothalamic pituary
system with the DA agonists Apomorphine or Piribedil, inducing increased growth hormone (HGH) secretion and decreased

PRL secretion, offers the possibility to measure this receptor sensitivity. Although the release of these two hormones
is regulated by complex mechanisms (Lal and Martin, 1980), in
general, we can assume that DA receptors contribute significantly to this regulation. Furthermore α-receptors, which can
be stimulated by the α-agonist Clonidine, probably are involved in these regulations and in the pathophysiology of the
above mentioned disorders as well.
Whereas neuroendocrine regulation is mainly dependent on
postsynaptic receptors, stimulation of presynaptic receptors
cause an altered release of the respective transmitter DA
or norepinephrine (NA) (Langer, 1978).
The knowledge of this biochemical events allows to examine
the above mentioned hypothesis related to schizophrenia and
extra pyramidal motor system (EPMS) disturbances. It was the
purpose of this study to relate biochemical events to psychopathological and neurological states by measuring reagibili-
ty of receptors with Apomorphine stimulation.

PATIENTS AND METHODS

Two different groups of patients were investigated.

1) Acute untreated schizophrenic patients (mean age 33 years)
(ICD No.295.3) with a paranoid-hallucinatoric syndrome, hospitalised due to an acute episode of their illness. These patients were treated with neuroleptics for 30 days. Thereafter
the treatment was stopped. Investigations were carried out
before and during treatment and 5 days after withdrawl. (Further details: Weiss-Brummer, 1980).

2) Chronic schizophrenic patients (mean age 40 years), who
have been hospitalised (duration of illness 20 years) and
treated with different neuroleptics for many years (> 12 years).
In these patients the neuroleptic treatment was stopped and
the drugs withdrawn for up to three months. (Further details:
Müller et al., 1980)
Investigations were carried out during treatment, after 5, 12,
30 and 90 days withdrawl. In both groups not every patient
could be investigated at every given time point, therefore
different numbers of patients will be reported about. The
neuroendocrine tests were carried out at 8 a.m. after overnight fasting under basal metabolic conditions. One hour after the insertion of a medicut catheter 0.5 mg Apomorphine were
injected subcutaneously or 1 mg Piribedil or 0.15 mg Clonidine
intravenously. For 3 hours blood was collected, HGH and glucose every 15 minutes, PRL and NA every 60 minutes. Simultaneously pulse rate and blood pressure were recorded.

BIOCHEMICAL METHODS

The blood samples were kept at -3°C until centrifugation,
immediately centrifugated (temp. -3°C) and the plasma stored
at -40°C, for NA determination at -60°C. PRL and HGH were
assayed by a double antibody radioimmunoassay of IDW or Bio-
sigma respectively. Glucose was analysed by means of a glucose oxidase method. NA in blood was determined by use of high

pressure liquid chromatography with electrochemical detection (Bioanalytica System, BAS, Lafayette, USA).

PSYCHOPATHOLOGICAL AND EPMS

AMDP 3 (Angst et al., 1969) rated by a semi standardized interview and evaluated by scoring the psychopathological syndromes (Baumann, 1974) was used. EPMS disfunctions were rated with the Simpson-Webster scale Heinrich et al., 1968) and evaluated by Video recording.

RESULTS

ACUTE SCHIZOPHRENIC PATIENTS: BIOCHEMICAL FINDINS (Tab. 1)

Similarly according Pandey et al. (1977) and Rotrosen et al. (1979) the subcutaneous injection of 0.5 mg Apomorphine induced within 60 minutes in acute schizophrenic patients (n=12) a significant (p < 0.05) HGH stimulation of more than 20 ng/ml plasma in the mean level. There was a wide range of maximum stimulation from 0.6 to 69.0 ng/ml.

The basal HGH level was within normal range, the maximum secretion of HGH of the schizophrenic group (22 + 22 ng/ml) was not higher than in normal persons. However, within this group 4 patients showed an extremely high stimulation. On the other hand 4 other patients showed a HGH stimulation below 5 ng/ml, indicating a blunted HGH response to Apomorphine.

TABLE 1   ACUTE SCHIZOPHRENIC PATIENTS

	Untreated acute schizophrenic n = 11	30 days treatment n = 11	5 days drug free n = 7
HGH bas.	0.9 + 1.1	2.4 + 0.5	1.2 + 0.8
max Δ HGH ng/ml	22.8 + 22.6	4.1 + 2.5	6.0 + 4.6
PRL bas. ng/ml	3.5 + 1.7	43.6 + 38.0	12.6 + 16.3
PRL 60' ng/ml	2.1 + 2.5	39.8 + 33.8	9.7 + 14.2
AMDP 3	44.8 + 11.3	27.3 + 18(9)	23.3 + 16

Apomorphine stimulation 0.5 mg s.c.
Haloperidol treatment (20-40 mg/day)

Treatment with Haloperidol reduced significantly the HGH response to Apomorphine ($\bar{x}$ = 4 ng/ml), indicating the neuroleptic DA receptor blockade. The 5 days withdrawl period did not cause a significant rise of HGH response to Apomorphine. When compared to the treatment with Neuroleptics, only a slight, but not significant increase of the maximum stimulation could be observed which in no case reached the values before treatment. No DA receptor supersensitivity could be found, as it is postulated on the basis of animal experiments (Christensen und Møller-Nielsen, 1979).

The basal levels of PRL did not differ from normal controls ($\bar{x}$ = 2.7 ± 1.6 ng/ml; n = 10). The PRL secretion decreases 60

minutes after Apomorphine injection slightly to 2.1±2.5 ng/ml.
As expected after neuroleptic treatment the PRL secretion is
elevated up to 43 ± 38 ng/ml and Apomorphine injection again
decreases the PRL secretion at this time to 39 ± 38 ng/ml.
After 5 days of discontinuation of neuroleptic treatment PRL
is still elevated (12±16 ng/ml),values after Apomorphine injection (9.7±14 ng/ml).The maximal suppressions of 0.6 ng(= 22%),
4 ng (= 9%) and 2.3 ng (= 19%) respectively are too small to
give significant results. There was no significant difference
between the untreated, treated and drug free patients.

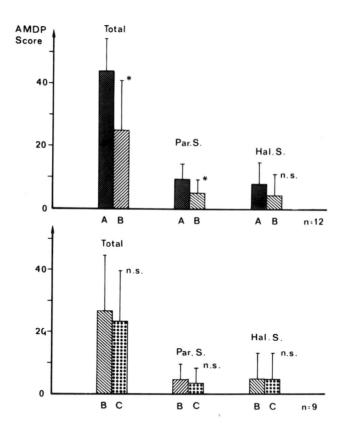

Fig. 1: Psychopathology of schizophrenic patients during and
        after withdrawl of neuroleptic treatment

A = untreated, B = 30 days Haloperidol C = 5 days withdrawl
par.S. = paranoid syndrome   hal.S. = hallucinatoric syndrome
p < 0.05 paired student t-test.

PSYCHOPATHOLOGY AND EPMS

The psychopathology, expressed by the total score of the AMP 3 system as well as by the score of the paranoid and hallucinatoric syndrome, improved significantly under neuroleptic treatment. No worsening could be found after 5 days of withdrawl. There was a slight but not significant increase of the score, which indicated the Parkinson syndrome, due to the neuroleptic treatment, and after 5 days withdrawl a decrease of the score occurred again. Furthermore no relationship between HGH and psychopathology or HGH and PRL or PRL and psychopathology could be found, suggesting that the respective dopamine receptors are independent from each other. Stimulation of HGH with α-agonist Clonidine shows similar results. Acute schizophrenics, too, often react with higher HGH stimulation to Clonidine compared to Controls (Matussek et al., 1980). This stimulation was suppressed again by treatment with neuroleptics and only increased a little after 5 days withdrawl of the neuroleptic drugs.

CHRONIC SCHIZOPHRENIC PATIENTS

BIOCHEMICAL FINDINGS (Tab.2)

In chronic schizophrenic patients with neuroleptic treatment HGH stimulation with Apomorphine did not induce a HGH secretion of more than 5 ng/ml in the mean. However, there was again a wide range of maximum stimulation from 0.5 ng/ml to 17 ng/ml within 60 minutes and 3 of 19 patients showed the ability of stimulation. A similar result was obtained by stimulation with the α-agonist Clonidine (Ackenheil et al.,1980) in the mean no clear stimulation, but 3 of 16 patients secreted HGH to more than 5 ng/ml.

After 5 days withdrawl of neuroleptics, the α-agonist Clonidine could induce a HGH stimulation in 2 of 9 patients, and Apomorphine in 1 of 5 patients respectively. At this time no supersensitivity could be demonstrated, although there was a tendency for the small HGH peak to appear earlier (47 vs. 55 min).

Discontinuation of neuroleptic treatment for 12 days resulted in an increase of HGH stimulation (11 ng/ml) with Apomorphine, when 12 patients reached an HGH stimulation of more than 5 ng/ml, whereas 4 patients showed blunted HGH response. Again this response, too, cluld not be considered as DA receptor supersensitivity, because the values did not reach the peak height of acute schizophrenic patients. After 30 days the HGH response is still diminished ($\bar{x}$ = 7 ng/ml), when 8 of the patients showed a HGH response and 7 did not.

When the stimulation was repeated with 1 mg Piribedil i.v. an identical result was observed. Patients, who secreted HGH after Apomorphine stimulation, responded to the Piribedil infusion too (unpublished result). After an interval of 3 months' discontinuation, this ratio of response (50%) remained constant. About half of the patients responded to the Apomorphine stimulation.

TABLE 2   CHRONIC SCHIZOPHRENIC PATIENTS

HGH bas.ng/ml	2.24 ± 2.86	0.94 ± 0.30 (11)	1.04 ± 0.74 (15)
HGH max ng/ml	3.5 ± 6.1*	12.12 ± 12.0*	9.59 ± 14.76 (15)
PRL bas.ng/ml	11.1 ± 12.2 (15)	3.3 ± 7.0** (15)	3.5 ± 3.2* (15)
PRL min ng/ml	8.5 ± 9.3 (15)	2.38 ± 6.4 (15)	2.5 ± 2.7 (15)
NA pg/ml	453.2 ± 169.2 (12)	202 ± 109 (12)	259 ± 104 (12)
NA 60 pg/ml	457 ± 223 (12)	200 ± 95 (12)	234 ± 99 (12)
EPMS	0.04 ± 0.07	0.12 ± 0.17*	0.12 ± 0.13*

Apomorphine stimulation: 0.5 mg s.c.
( ) = n
** $p < 0.005$ paired student t-test
* $p < 0.01$ "   "   "

PRL secretion in serum as in our earlier studies (Naber et
al., 1980; Zander et al., 1981) was in a normal range (11.1 ± 11.2
ng/ml). However, its secretion was significantly diminished
after 12 and 30 days' drug discontinuation (3.3 ± 3.2 and 3.5
± 3.2 ng/ml; $p < 0.005$). The Apomorphine induced maximum suppression did not change significantly at the different mo-
ments of investigation.
The NA secretion in serum during long term neuroleptic treatment was elevated (453 ± 169 pg/ml) compared to normal controls (211 ± 79 pg/ml), confirming our earlier results (Naber
et al., 1980; Zander et al., 1981). After 12 days withdrawl a
significant decrease (202 ± 109 ng/ml) was observed, with an
increasing tendency (259 pg ± 104 pg/ml) after 30 days withdrawl. Independent of the date of investigation the Apomorphine injection did not influence the NA secretion.

PSYCHOPATHOLOGY AND EPMS

Signs of tardive dyskinesia, which could be observed during
treatment with neuroleptics in a very discrete manner, occurred for the first time after 5 days discontinuation in 2 patients and after 12 days in 9 patients, indicating a ratio
of 47 % of incidence. After 30 days withdrawl this high occurrence of tardive dyskinesia (higher than in our earlier studies, Zander et al., 1981) remained constant. These symptoms
were clinically discrete and could be seen only with extensive neurological examination. The picture of psychopathological syndroms was very complex. Some patients ameliorated
as in our earlier studies whereas others deteriorated. Generally during short term withdrawl of neuroleptic treatment
(5, 12 and 30 days) only few patients deteriorated. However,
after 3 months most of the patients relapsed, for example:
day 12: 16 patients deteriorated slightly and 3 improved in
their symptomatology. After 30 days we registrated 3 "drop-

outs", 7 ameliorated and 8 worsened patients. The symptomatology of 11 patients, who deteriorated after 12 days now improved again. 3 months later because of their symptomatology most of the patients needed neuroleptic treatment again. The psychopathology as well as the neurological symptomatology could not be correlated to the endocrine and biochemical findings. Furthermore up to now, we were unable to find any predictors for the clinical change within individuals.

DISCUSSION

Evaluation of DA receptor sensitivity by stimulation with Apomorphine offers the possibility of testing hypotheses related to schizophrenia, the mode of action of neuroleptics, and tardive dyskinesia. As reported by other groups (Rotrosen et al., 1979; Pandey et al., 1977) in some acute schizophrenic patients, exaggerated responses too could be seen. However, there is a high subject to subject variability, even blunted HGH response occurred in the acute group. Treatment with Neuroleptics resulted in a suppression of this response in nearly all patients, whereas after 5 days withdrawl a HGH response was obtained in most of the patients, but no exaggerated response, indicating that DA receptor supersensitivity could not be found. The postulated DA receptor supersensitivity which can be seen in different animal models (Christensen and Møller-Nielsen, 1977; Ungerstedt, this volume) either is only specific for animals or more probably does not develop so fast in the hypothalamic-pituarity system of human beings. The different time-scale for developing tolerance to neuroleptic treatment in the different dopaminergic systems (Julou et al., 1976) with regard to the DA turnover provides grounds for this speculation. Whereas Homovanillic acid (HVA) increase, induced by Neuroleptics in Cerebrospinal fluid (CSF), is diminished after 30 days (Post et al., 1974), PRL elevation remains constant (Sacher et al., 1977) and decreases only after many years (Naber et al., 1980). More pronounced suppression of HGH response to Apomorphine could be demonstrated after 30 days treatment and even after many years. At this time most of biochemical parameters, such as HVA, PRL, 3-Methoxy-4-hydroxy phenylglycol (MHPG), which are changed due to neuroleptic treatment are normalized (Zander et al., 1981). NA in serum as a further exception was elevated in this and other studies, most probably because of the α-adrenolytic effect of the schizophrenic illness per se. Also presynaptic regulations should be kept in mind (Langer, 1978). Acute untreated schizophrenic patients often show elevated NA levels in serum (Ackenheil et al., 1979) as well as in cerebrospinal fluid (Lake et al., 1979). The decrease after withdrawl of neuroleptics indicates the degree of neuroleptic influence. Therefore, depending on the duration of neuroleptic treatment, the various biochemical parameters HVA, PRL, HGH stimulation, and NA are well suited to monitor neuroleptic drug effects.

The relation to psychopathology and neurological disorders, such as tardive dyskinesia seems to be more complex. There is no doubt that some schizophrenic patients show exaggerated HGH response as also reported by other groups. There are, however, others which have blunted HGH response.

This blunted HGH response occurs in acute patients and in chronic patients with and without tardive dyskinesia, thus only partly supporting the reported subsentivity (Ettigi et al.,1976; Rotrosen et al.,1979) or supersensitivity (Gerlach, 1979) of DA receptors. The contribution of the neuroleptic effects in difficult to ascertain. Even a washout period of 3-4 weeks, or normal PRL values cannot totally exclude drug influences.

Furthermore, with regard to the DA hypothesis of schizophrenia and the supersensitivity hypothesis of tardive dyskinesia respectively, our thinking should be revised. DA receptor sensitivity, in so far as it can be measured by the used biochemical or endocrine parameters, may only partly contribute to the schizophrenic illness or to the occurrence of tardive dyskinesia. Other biochemical systems such as e.g. the noradrenergic system (Ackenheil,1980a and b) or very distinctly anatomical localisations may play a role. Finally it should not be neglected that the schizophrenia with regard to clinical symptomatology and prognosis as well as to biochemical reactions cannot be considered as a nosological entity.

REFERENCES

Ackenheil, M. (1980a): In: Handbook of Experimental Pharmacology, edited by G. Stille, and F. Hoffmeister, pp. 213-223. Springer Verlag, Heidelberg-Berlin.

Ackenheil, M. (1980b): In: Abstracts of the 12th CINP Congress, edited by C. Radouco-Thomas, and F. Garcin, p. 54. Pergamon Press, Oxford et al.

Ackenheil, M., Albus, M.,Müller, F.,Müller, Th., Welter, D., Zander, K., Engel, R. (1979): In: Catecholamines: Basic and Clinical Frontiers, edited by E. Usdin, I.J. Kopin, J. Barchas, pp. 980-983. Pergamon Press, New York.

Ackenheil, M., Bartl, S., Fischer, B., Müller, F., Wörner,I., Matussek, N. (1980): Hormonelle Untersuchungen nach langjähriger Neuroleptikabehandlung. Arzneim. Forsch. (Drug Res.) 1205, 30 (II), Nr.8.

Angrist, B. (1980): In: Abstracts of the 12th CINP Congress, edited by C. Radouco-Thomas, and F. Garcin, p. 64. Pergamon Press, Oxford et al.

Angst, J.,Battegay, R.,Bente, D.,Berner, P., Broeren, W., Cornu, F., Dick, P., Engelmeier, M.-P., Heimann, H., Heinrich, K.,Helmchen, H.,Hippius, H.,Pöldinger, W.,Schmidlin, P., Schmitt, W., and Weis, P. (1969): Arzneim.-Forsch. (Drug Res.) 19, pp. 399-405.

Baumann, U. (1974): Arch. Psychiat. Nervenkr. 219, 89-103.

Carlsson and Lindqvist: Acta Pharmacol. Toxicol. 20, pp.140-144.

Christensen, A.V., Møller-Nielsen, I. (1979): Psychopharmacology 62, pp. 111-116.

Ettigi, P., Mair, N.P.V., Lal, S., Cervantes, P., and Guyda, H. (1976): J.of Neurol.,Neurosurg. and Psych. 39, pp.870-876.

Gerlach, J. (1979): Tardive dyskinesia. Danish Medical Bulletin 26, No.5.

Heinrich, K., Wegener, I., Bender, H.J. (1968): Pharmakopsychiatr. Neuropsychopharmakol. 1, pp. 169-195.

Janssen, P.A.J., Niemegeers, C., and Schellekens, K. (1965): Arzneim.-Forsch. 15, pp. 104-117.

Julou, L., Scatton, B., Glowinski, J. (1977): In: Advances in biochemical psychopharmacology, edited by E. Costa and G.L. Gessa, pp. 617-624. Raven Press, New York.

Lake, C.R., Sternberg, D.E., van Kammen, D.P., Ballenger, J.C., Ziegler, M.G., Post, R.M., Kopin, I.J., Bunney, W.E. (1980): Science 207, pp. 331-333.

Lal, S. and Martin, J.B. (1980): In: Handbook of biological psychiatry, edited by H.M. van Praag, M.H. Lader, O.J. Rafaelsen, E.J. Sachar, pp. 101-168, Marcee Dekker, New York and Basel.

Langer, S.Z. (1978): In: Presynaptic Receptors, edited by S.Z. Langer, K. Starke, M.L. Dubocovich, pp. 13-22.Pergamon Press, New York.

Matthyssee, S. (1973): Fed.Proc. 32, pp. 200-205.

Matussek, N.,Ackenheil, M.,Hippius, H., Müller, F.,Schröder, T.-Th., Schultes, H., Wasilewski, B. (1980): Psychiatry Research 2, pp. 25-36.

Müller, F., Bartl, S., Fischer, B.,Wörner, I.,Ackenheil, M. (1980): In: Abstracts of the 12th CINP Congress, p. 255.

Naber, D., Finkbeiner, C., Fischer, B., Zander, K.-J., Ackenheil, M. (1980): Neuropsychobiology 6, pp. 181-189.

Pandey, G.N., Garver, D.L., Tamminga, C., Ericksen, S., Ali, S.I., Davis, J.M. (1977): Am.J.Psychiatry 134, pp. 518-522.

Post, R.M.,and Goodwin, F.K. (1975): Science 190, pp.488-489.

Rotrosen, J., Angrist, B., Gershon, S., Paquin, J.,Branchey, L., Oleshansky, M., Halpern, F.,and Sachar, E.J. (1979): Brit.J.Psychiat. 135, pp. 444-456.

Sachar, E.J., Gruen, P.H., Altman, H., Langer, G., Halpern, F.S., Liefer, M. (1977): In: Neuroregulators and psychiatric disorders, edited by E. Usdin, D.A. Hamburg, J.D. Barchas, pp. 242-249. University Press, New York.

Weiss-Brummer, J. (1980): In: Abstracts of the 12th CINP Congress, p. 353.

Zander, K.J., Fischer, B., Zimmer, R., and Ackenheil, M. (1981): Psychopharmacology, in press.

Acknowledgement: This work was supported by the Deutsche Forschungsgemeinschaft.

*Apomorphine and Other Dopaminomimetics,
Vol. 2: Clinical Pharmacology,* edited by
G. U. Corsini and G. L. Gessa, Raven Press,
New York © 1981.

Catecholamines and Adaptive Mechanisms in Senescent Rats

S. Algeri, *G. Calderini, G. Lomuscio, *G. Toffano, and F. Ponzio

*Mario Negri Institute for Pharmacological Research, 20156 Milano; *Fidia Research Laboratories, 35031 Abano Terme, Italy*

Due to the number of functions it regulates, the nervous system has always received particular attention in biological research on ageing. In particular, neurochemical and neuropharmacological studies of the different neuronal systems have lately been stressed as a means of achieving better insight into which of the many neuronal systems is most affected by ageing, and in the hope of finding some key to pharmacological intervention.

Among the various neurotransmitters, dopamine (DA) and noradrenaline (NA) have received the most attention. This not only because catecholaminergic systems are better known, but also because they seem to be involved in degenerative diseases such as parkinsonism (4) and senile dementia (2) which particularly hit the elderly. In all species in which such studies have been made, including man, all observations indicate the decline of noradrenergic and still more clearly of dopaminergic systems with age. As reviewed recently by Prandhan (9) this decline is evident at different levels of neurotransmitter metabolism and the other biochemical mechanisms related to synaptic transmission.

In these experiments, including some previous work by our group (1,7), the effect of age is usually studied by comparing certain biochemical parameters in two groups, one of young and one of old animals. In the experiments described here we have extended such observation to a population of Sprague Dawley rats aged 4, 18, and 29 months, studying whether the changes in the parameters taken into consideration, levels of monoamines and their metabolites, and tyrosine hydroxylase (TH) activity, were statistically correlated with ageing. In addition to this basic information, we studied how biochemical parameters such as TH activity and DA metabolism, known to be enhanced by stress, responded to cold stress in senescent rats.

EXPERIMENTAL APPROACH

The experiment was performed on a colony of Sprague Dawley rats 4, 18 and 29 months of age. In order to minimize differences in body weight caused by overeating, all rats were kept on a restricted diet (15 g of Altromin pellets/day). This diet allows normal growth but reduces the accumulation of fat seen when rats are fed ad libitum. With the regimen

described, rats gained weight up to an average of 600 g and remained
constant at this weight until the day of the experiment. At the time of
the experiment the percentage of survivors was 40%. Rats presenting vis-
ible tumors were discarded. Each age group was randomly divided into 4
subgroups. One was kept at room temperature, the other three at 4°C in
a cold room for 2, 4 or 24 hours. Biochemical analyses were performed
according to methods described elsewere (3, 6, 8, 10, 13). The data were
statistically analysed using analysis of variance, linear regression,
Dunnet's and Duncan's tests.

AGE-RELATED CHANGES IN DOPAMINE AND ITS METABOLISM

Concentrations of DA and its acid metabolites were measured in striata,
limbic area and substantia nigra in all three age groups. As summarised
in fig. 1, in all these areas there was a decline in the levels of this
neurotransmitter and, in s. nigra, this decline was significantly correlated with age. Homovanillic acid (HVA) and dihydroxyphenilacetic acid
(DOPAC) showed the same pattern as the parent monoamine (fig. 1) in all
the brain regions examined.

AGE-RELATED CHANGES IN NORADRENALINE AND ITS METABOLISM

The concentration of this neurotransmitter in the three different age
groups was measured in cerebellum; hippocampus, spinal cord, limbic area,
s. nigra and striata, and its main metabolite, 3 methoxy-4-hydroxyphenyl
glycol-O-sulphate (MHPG-SO$_4$) was assayed in the hemispheres (fig. 2).
Whereas DA showed an age-related drop in all areas studied, NA was clearly lowered only in the spinal cord and, to a lesser extent, in the limbic
area : in the other areas there were no changes. Interestingly, cortical
MHPG-SO$_4$ showed a clear tendency to rise with age.

TYROSINE HYDROXYLASE IN THE SENESCENT RAT

TH activities measured in striata, brainstem and hypothalamus in the
three age group are summarised in Table 1. In striata the activity of

TABLE 1. <u>Tyrosine hydroxylase activity in three areas of rat brain in
youth and two stages of senescence</u>

Age of rats	Striata	Brainstem	Hypothalamus
4 months	110 ± 7	0.52±0.04	2.5 ± 0.1
18 months	75 ±11[^]	0.42±0.04	2.6 ± 0.3
29 months	82 ± 5[^^]	0.36±0.03[^^]	2.4 ± 0.4

Data are expressed as pmoles/min/mg proteine and are the mean ± S.E of
30 samples (striata and brainstem) or 6 samples (Hypothalamus)
[^] $p < 0.05$ different from 4 months group by Dunnet's test
[^^] $p < 0.01$ "   " "   "   " "   "   "

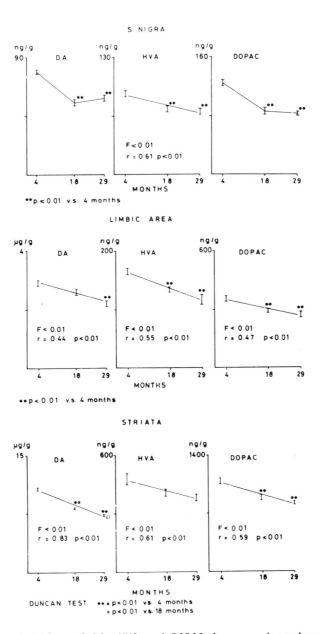

FIG. 1   Concentration of DA, HVA and DOPAC in some dopaminergic regions of rat brain in youth and two stages of senescence.

Data are the mean ± S.E. of 30 samples (s. nigra and limbic area) or 6 samples (striata).

The significance of the concentration-age correlation was tested by linear regression analysis.

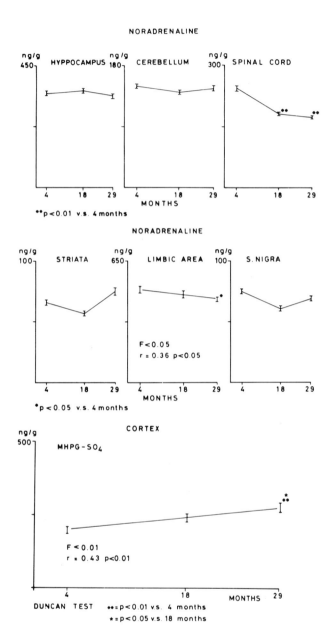

FIG. 2 Concentration of NA and MHPG-SO$_4$ in some areas of rat brain in youth and two stages of senescence.

Data are the mean ± S.E. of 30 samples.

The significance of the concentration-age correlation was tested by linear regression analysis.

this enzyme was already significantly reduced by 18 months age and did not decline further later. In brainstem it was also low but only at the latest age did the decline become significant. In hypothalamus the enzyme was not modified, indicating that the fall in TH activity with age is not a general phenomenon. This was borne out by the results in the adrenal medulla where TH activity was enhanced in the aged rats. In fact in this gland the enzyme activity was already significantly raised in the 18-month-old rats (fig. 7).

The same indication can be drawn from the striking increase in Vmax measured in a crude preparation of adrenal medulla from 29-month-old rats. In this preparation the K_m for the reduced pteridine cofactor was also measured and turned out to be higher in the senescent rats (fig. 3).

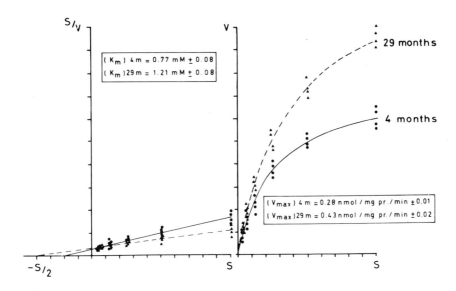

FIG. 3 Comparison of the kinetic-constants of TH from adrenal medulla of 4 and 29 month-old rats.

K_m and Vmax were determined by the Woolf's linear transformation plot.

DIFFERENCE IN SOME PHYSIOLOGICAL RESPONSES TO COLD STRESS IN RATS OF DIFFERENT AGES

Groups of rats divided according to age as described were left for different lenghts of time in a cold room at 4°C. The intensity of stress produced by low temperature was the same in all groups, as demonstrated by the similar rise in plasma corticosterone levels (fig. 4). In spite of this, the young rats were able to compensate the heat loss and maintain their body temperature constant throughout the experiment, but the 18 and 29 month-old rats responded much more slowly (fig. 5).

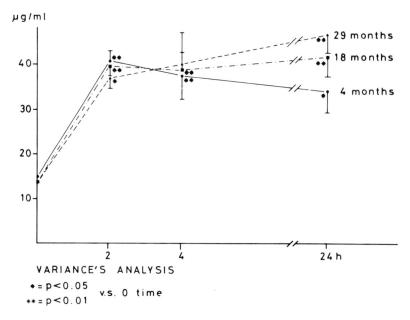

FIG. 4   Effect of cold stress on the release of corticosterone in plasma
                    of rats of three different ages.

Rats were left at 4°C for different periods of time. Each Point is the
mean ± S.E. of 6 samples.

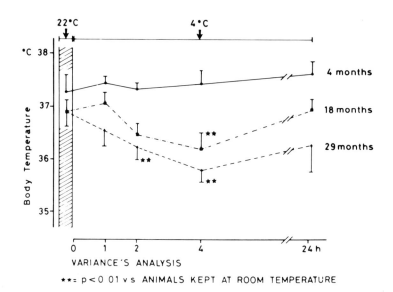

FIG. 5   Termoregulating ability of rats of three different ages.

Rats were left at 4°C for different period of time. The dashed column
shows the body temperatures of the three groups when kept at room temperature. Each point is the mean ± S.E. of 6 determinations.

TH activity, known to be enhanced by cold stress (12), was measured
in the hypothalamus and adrenal medulla of these rats. As described in
fig. 6, in the hypothalamus of the young rats the enzyme activity showed
an increase starting after 4 hours exposure to low temperature, but in
18 and 29-month rats no such response occurred.

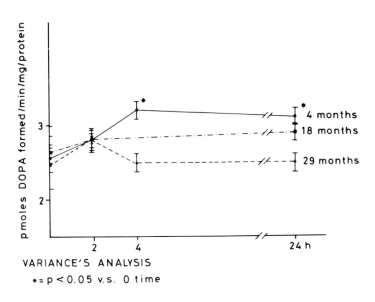

FIG. 6 Activity of TH from hypothalamus of rats of three different ages
              after different times of exposure to 4°C.

Each point is the mean ± S.E. of 6 samples.

A similar phenomenon was observed in adrenal medulla (fig. 7) where,
however, only the oldest group was completely unresponsive; in glands of
18-month-old rats and in the youngest ones there was a transient increase
after 2 hours of cold. Similarly the metabolism of striatal DA, known
to be enhanced by stress (5), was significantly increased in young but
not in senescent rats as indicated by the different rises in HVA concentration in the striata of the three groups at different times after cold
stress (fig. 8).

DISCUSSION

The results of this study indicated that ageing has several, complex
effects on the biochemistry of neurotransmitters. We again found that
TH activity was lowered in some brain regions, as already reported, confirming similar results obtained by other laboratories in rats and other
species (9). However, in line with the results obtained by Reis et al.
(11) we observed that TH activity in adrenal medulla of aged rats was

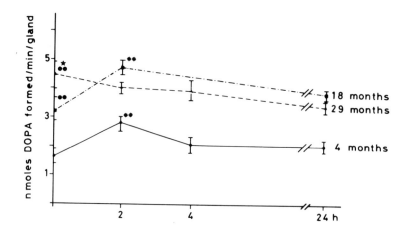

FIG. 7 Activity of TH from adrenal medulla of rats of three different
         ages after different times of exposure to 4°C.

Each point is the mean ± S.E. of 6 samples. ✱✱ different from 0 time
p<0.01. •• different from 4 month group p<0.01. ✱ different from
18 month group p < 0.05 by analysis of variance and Duncan's test.

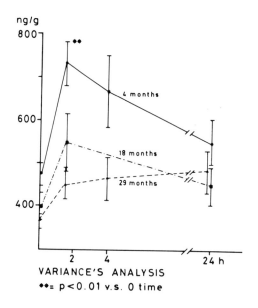

FIG. 8 Striatal HVA levels in rats of three different ages after dif-
         ferent times of exposure to 4°C.

Each point is the mean ± S.E. of 6 samples.

higher, suggesting that the same biochemical parameters may be changed in opposite directions depending on the organ considered.

Dopamine, and to a lesser extent NA, concentrations reportedly decline in some brain areas of senescent animals (9). In this population of Sprague Dawley rats we saw a fall in DA concentrations and there was a highly significant correlation between age and the decrease in DA and its metabolites. At the present time it is not clear whether the decline in DA, HVA and DOPAC is due to neuronal loss or to reduced synthesis, or even to a combination of the two. In a population of Wistar rats we had previously observed a decline in DA synthesis but not in DA concentrations (7). On the other hand the fact that a rise in DA metabolism was noted in young rats but not in senescent animals after stress further suggests a reduction in DA synthesis and turnover.

With regard to the response to cold stress, we observed that the response of some biochemical parameters such as corticosterone release was not altered, but other biochemical parameters were clearly affected in senescent rats. This suggests possible biochemical bases for the impairment of some adaptive mechanisms brought about by ageing. It is interesting to note that the reduced capability of old rats to compensate body heat loss was accompanied by lack of induction of TH activity in hypothalamus and adrenal medulla, organs that are probably implicated in the regulation of body temperature. It is therefore tempting to relate this homeostatic defect with at least some of the biochemical impairments. However, any such conclusion is still premature and more studied are needed to establish whether there is any causal relationship between the two phenomena.

Aknowledgements

This research was financially supported by the National Research Council, contract No. 79.02355.65, by grants from Gustavus and Louise Pfeiffer Foundation, New York, and by CARIPLO, Milano - Italy.

References

1) Algeri, S., Bonati, M., Brunello, N., and Ponzio, F. (1977): Brain Res., 132: 569-574.

2) Gottfries, C. (1980): Trends NeuroSci., 3: 55-57.

3) Guillemin, R., Clayton, C.W., Lipscomb, H.S., and Smith, J.D. (1959): J. Lab. Clin. Med., 53: 830-832.

4) Hornykiewicz, O. (1966): Pharmacol. Rev., 18: 925-964.

5) Jansky, L., Mejsnar, J., and Moravec, J. (1976) In: Catecholamine and Stress, pp.419-434. Pergamon Press, New York.

6) Meek, J.L., and Neff, N.H. (1972): Br. J. Pharmacol., 45: 435-441.

7) Ponzio, F., Brunello, N., and Algeri, S. (1978): J. Neurochem., 30: 1617-1620.

8) Ponzio, F., and Jonsson, G. (1978): Dev. Neurosci., 1: 80-89.

9) Pradhan, S.M. (1980): Life Sci., 26: 1643-1656.

10) Refshauge, C., Kissinger, P.T., Dreiling, R., Blank R., Freeman, R., and Adams, R.N. (1974): Life Sci., 14: 311-322.

11) Reis, D.J., Ross, R.A., and Tong Hyub Joh (1977): Brain Res., 136: 465-474.

12) Thoenen, H. (1970): Nature, 228: 861-862.

13) Waymire, J.C., Bjur, R., and Weiner, N. (1971): Anal. Biochem., 43: 588-600.

*Apomorphine and Other Dopaminomimetics,
Vol. 2: Clinical Pharmacology*, edited by
G. U. Corsini and G. L. Gessa, Raven Press,
New York © 1981.

Aging and Information Processing

G. Calderini, C. Aldinio, *F. Crews, **A. Gaiti, †U. Scapagnini,
S. Algeri, ‡F. Ponzio, and G. Toffano

*FIDIA Research Laboratories, Department of Biochemistry, 35031 Abano Terme, Italy; *University of
Florida College of Medicine, Department of Pharmacology, Gainesville, Florida 32610; **University of
Perugia, Department of Biochemistry, 06100 Perugia, Italy; †University of Catania, Department of
Pharmacology, 95100 Catania, Italy; ‡Institute of Pharmacological Research, Mario Negri,
20100 Milano, Italy*

Age-dependent changes in complex function such as memory, learning, thermoregulation and hormonal modulation are the direct expression of the decreased adaptivity of the elderly. Variations in all these functions are thought to be related to biochemical alterations in the mechanisms of the synaptic transmission (5, 16).

The molecular mechanism by which information is transferred from one cell to another is one of the major problem of modern neurobiology. Biochemical messages such as neurotransmitters, hormones, lectins, immunoglobulins are recognised by the cell membrane and bind to specific sites of the receptor macromolecules in the outer surface of lipid bilayers. These interactions promote a series of physical and biochemical events resulting in the physiological response. Cell membranes are, therefore, important sites where biochemical changes may be responsible for the impaired information processing during aging.

According to the proposed fluid mosaic model (15), biological membranes are mainly composed of an asymmetric phospholipid bilayer in which functionally active proteins are imbedded. The activity and mobility of membrane proteins are greatly influenced by membrane fluidity and, in turn, by the physical state, asymmetry, lateral mobility and rotational movement of lipids. Since the lipid-protein complex could constitute the receptor entity, a role for phospholipids in the regulation of receptor functions as co-factors for the functional receptors and/or as regulators for the coupling between the receptor and the effector system has been suggested (For a review see 10).

EXPERIMENTAL APPROACH

Studies of age-dependent changes in the homeostatic capacity of an organism require a rather complex experimental approach which can be roughly summarised as : a). documentation of altered adaptivity to external stimuli; b). detection of specific biochemical events, and c). determination of the critical age for its onset.

Following the above scheme, our study is concerning changes in the information processing with aging. Firstly, we assessed the age-related changes in adaptive capacity by studying the modification of two general parameters, such as body temperature and prolactin secretion after cold-stress exposure. We have then looked at modifications of the receptor function, since every physiological response is the result of the communication between neurons; in particular, we have studied the age-dependent alteration in the GABA receptor binding in different brain areas. GABA is the major inhibitory transmitter in the brain and is involved in several human pathological states of aging (2, 4). Thus, changes in the distribution and kinetic properties of GABA binding could reveal a cerebral function impairment. Finally, the information on these parameters were integrated with the biochemical study on the metabolism of the brain phospholipids which constitute the microenvironment where the membrane receptors are operative. We have taken into consideration Phosphatidylethanolamine (PE) and Phosphatidylcholine (PC), since these phospholipids have both a structural (6) and a functional role (9).

EFFECT OF COLD STRESS ON BODY TEMPERATURE AND PROLACTIN PLASMA LEVEL IN AGED RATS

No age-related difference is detected in the body temperature between old and young rats kept at normal room temperature (21ºC). When the old animals are exposed to 4ºC, an age-dependent decrease on the body temperature is observed. The effect becomes evident after the first hour of cold exposure with a peak at the 4th hour, then tends to normalise after 24 hours. Determination of the plasma prolactin level, in the same animals, indicates that aging increases the concentration of the circulating prolactin (Fig. 1a) and abolishes the hormonal stress induced response (Fig. 1b). Young rats, in fact, respond to cold stress with a significant increase of plasma prolactin release after 4 hours of exposure. This effect is totally absent in old animals.

[3]H-GABA BINDING DISTRIBUTION AND KINETICS DURING AGING

A progressive decrease of ^{3}H-GABA binding with aging was observed in different brain areas (Tab. 1). The phenomenon involves the striatum, hypothalamus, substantia nigra and the spinal cord.

No changes occur in the cerebral cortex, hippocampus and pons plus medulla oblungata. The kinetics of the GABA receptor binding indicate that the age-dependent decrease of ^{3}H-GABA binding is due to a decrease of the receptor binding site density, relative to the high affinity component (we have not yet studied the low affinity component), the most related to GABAergic transmission (8). This phenomenon was particularly investigated in the striatum (Tab. 2). The

Fig. 1a: EFFECT OF AGING ON PLASMA PROLACTIN BASAL LEVEL

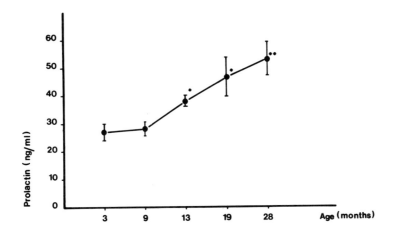

Fig. 1b: EFFECT OF COLD - STRESS ON PLASMA PROLACTIN LEVEL

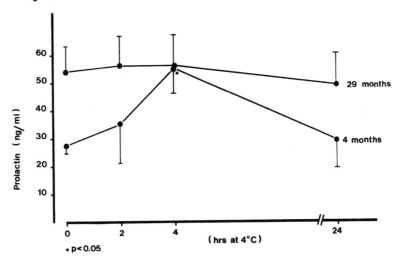

FIG. 1., Effect of aging and cold-stress response on prolactin plasma levels.

1a : animals of different ages were sacrified between 9 a.m. and 11 a.m. Each value is the mean ± S.E. of at least 6-8 determinations. *P<0.01,**P<0.05 respect to 3 mounths old rats.

1b : rats were exposed to 4°C for different periods of time and randomly sacrificed during the whole day. Each value is the mean ± S.E. of 4-6 determinations. *P<0.05 respect to animals not exposed to cold room.

TABLE 1. ^{3}H-GABA binding in different brain areas

BRAIN AREA	AGE (months)			
	5	13	19	28
Cerebral cortex	1550	1632	1357	1328
Hypothalamus	1138	1020	924	802 (-30%)
Hippocampus	1000	1409	1136	830
Striatum	746	559	489 (-35%)	527 (-30%)
S. Nigra	400	---	---	236 (-41%)
Pons + Med. Obl.	92	---	---	88
Spinal Cord	90	---	67	61 (-32%)

Values are expressed as fmol/mg prot (20 nM ^{3}H-GABA).

TABLE 2. Kinetics of ^{3}H-GABA binding in rat striatum at different ages.

Age (months)	Bmax (pmol/mg prot)	Kd (nm)
2	1.51	25
5	1.21	24
13	1.20	22
19	0.83	25
28	0.90	26

Kinetic properties of ^{3}H-GABA binding in the striatum of rat at different ages. Crude synaptic membranes preparated as previously reported (Toffano et al., 1978) were incubated with various concentrations of [3]H- GABA (10, 15, 20, 30 and 40 pmol/mg prot) in the incubation mixture. Bmax and Kd were calculated according to the Schatchard plot analysis and are mean of three experiments. Standard error is less than 10 per cent.

decrease in the total number of binding sites appears to be a two-step process, the first step taking place at 5th and the second at 19th month of age. After this age, no further decrease in the binding site density occurs. The affinity of GABA receptors is unmodified during advanced age.

The understanding of this phenomenon is quite difficult. Pharmacological and biochemical data suggests the existence of a direct GABAergic inhibitory influence on cholinergic cells and dopaminergic terminals intrinsic to the striatum (3, 14). The decrease of receptors with age may derive from a loss of striatal neurons on which a population of GABAergic binding sites is located. In this context it is of relevance the decreased tyrosine hydroxylase (1, 12) and choline acetyltransferase activity (11, 13) observed in the rat striatum with age.

However, other possibilities may be taken into consideration. Changes in the membrane properties, such as fluidity and the metabolism of components involved in the receptor function, may reduce the maximal binding capacity for ^{3}H-GABA. Furthermore, the decreased number of the high affinity GABA binding sites in aged rats may result from a lack of capability to increase receptor density in response to the decreased GABAergic input, as indicated by GAD changes (11, 12). In young animals reducing GABAergic input causes an increased number of GABA binding sites for the high affinity component (8).

BRAIN PHOSPHOLIPID METABOLISM AND ITS FUNCTION IN AGED RATS

With aging no detectable changes occur in the PE and PC levels in the brain. However, a progressive impairment of their metabolism is indicated by the measurement of their "de novo" synthesis rate. After intraventricular injection

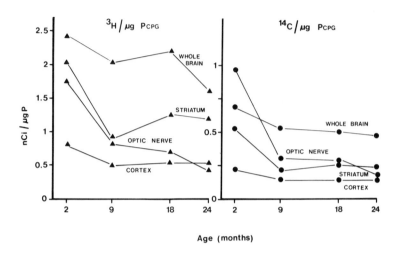

CHOLINE PHOSPHODIGLICERIDE SYNTHESIS IN VARIOUS BRAIN REGIONS
OF RAT AT DIFFERENT AGES

Age (months)

FIG. 2., "De novo" synthesis rate of phosphatidylcholine in rat of different ages. Animals were injected with a mixture of ^{3}H-glycerol and ^{14}C-choline and sacrified one hour after the injection. Phospholipids were extracted from the tissues and separated by a thin-layer-chromatography. The radioactivity present in the phosphatidylcholine fraction was measured in the whole brain as well as in different brain areas and is the mean of at least 6 experiments.

of ^{3}H-glycerol and ^{14}C-ethanolamine or ^{14}C-choline in rats of various ages, the radioactivity incorporated into PC and PE was lower in the whole brain and in different brain areas of aging rats. This decrease is present in all the brain areas considered, except the cerebral cortex (Fig. 2). The lowest synthesis rate is detected in the 9 months old rats while after this age no further decrease occurs. This is a variance in respect to the previous results obtained <u>in vitro</u> in which the rate of synthesis decreased up to 20 months (7).

In separate experiments the cerebral activities of the two phosphomethyl-transpherases, namely PMT1 and PMT2, were determined; the methylation of PE into PC and the rapid translocation of mono- and dimethylated forms of PE across the cell membrane are associated with changes in the membrane viscosity, membrane permeability and receptor function (for a review see 9). Aging process activates the methylation pathway (Tab. 3). The increased activity is mainly related to PMT1 which has been suggested to be the rate limiting step of this metabolic pathway. PMT1 is located inside the membrane and catalizes the formation of PE monomethylated derivative. PMT2 activity, however, is less affected by increasing age.

The data suggest that the phospholipid metabolism can be differently

TABLE 3. ^{3}H-methyl-group incorporation into crude synaptic plasma membrane phospholipids of rat at different ages.

	PMT 1 pmol/mg protein	PMT 2 pmol/mg protein
1 month	0.476 ± 0.023 (6)	8.85 ± 1.21 (5)
7 months	0.580 ± 0.003 (5)*	9.18 ± 1.43 (5)
21 months	0.653 ± 0.025 (6)**	10.86 ± 0.85 (6)

* $P < 0.01$ with respect to 1 month rats
** $P < 0.001$ with respect to 1 month rats.

affected. The CDP-choline (ethanolamine) biosynthetic pathway is inhibited while the methylation pathway, which is more strictly related to rapid physiological events, appears activated.

CONCLUSION

The concomitant study of both functional and biochemical alterations occurring with aging may provide useful information on the correlation between the general function and the brain state of old animals. Furthermore, biochemical alterations in different brain regions suggest that aging is not a general phenome non but it primarily involves specific target sites. The physiological significance of the reported modifications remains obscure and only speculative conclusions can be drawn.

The decreased GABA receptor density may derive from a loss of the GABA receptor containing neurons and from the modification of membrane properties as a consequence of an impaired molecular adaptive change. In this meeting it has been reported that the membrane viscosity in old brain animals in increased (Samuel - at this Congress). Interestingly the biosynthesis of phosphatidylcholine through CDP-choline pathway decreases while it increases through PE methylation, supporting different functional roles for the two distinct metabolic pathways. A decreased CDP-choline biosynthetic pathway, the major metabolic pathway for the phospholipid synthesis, may indicate a decreased renewal of the bulk membrane phospholipids; an increased activity of phosphomethyltransferase, particularly PMT1, involving a small functional pool of PE, may be seen as an attempt to overcome altered membrane properties.

In conclusion present results encourage to continue with this line of investigation, in searching for correlation between functional and biochemical changes and, thus, the rational base for the onset of aging related diseases.

REFERENCES

1. Algeri, S., Bonati, M., Brunello, N., Ponzio, F., Stramentinoli, G., and Gualano, M. (1978) : In : Neuro-Psychopharmacology, Edited by P. Deniker, C. Radiuco-Thomas, A. Villeneuve, Vol. 829 pp. 1647-1654. Pergamon Press, Oxford and New York.

2. Barbeau, A., (1973) : Lancet II, 1499-1500

3. Bartholini, G. (Jan. 1980) : TIPS. pp. 138-140.

4. Chase, T.N. and Tamminga L.C. (1979) : In : Gaba-neurotransmitter : Pharma co-chemical, Biochemical and Pharmacological Aspect, Edited by P. Krogsga-ard-Larsen, Scheel-Kruger J. and Kofod, H., pp. 283-294, Munksgaard, Copenhagen

5. Finch, C.E., Potter, D.E. and Kenny, A.D (1978) : Advance Exp. Med. Biol. Vol. 113., Plenum Press, New York.

6. Gaiti, A., Arienti, G., and Porcellati G. (1978) : In : Fosfolipidi. Liviana Editrice, Padova, Italy.

7. Gaiti, A., Brunetti, M., Sitkiewicz, D., Porcellati, G. and Woelk, H. (1980) : In : Aging of the brain and dementia. Vol. 13, Edited by L. Amaducci, A.N. Davison and P. Antuono, pp. 65-73, Raven Press, New York.

8. Guidotti, A., Gale, K., Suria, A., and Toffano, G. (1979) : Brain Research, 172 : 556-571.

9. Hirata, F., and Axelrod, J. (1980) : Science, 209 : 1082-1090.

10. Loh, H.H., and Law, P.Y. (1980) : Ann. Rev. Pharmacol. Toxicol., 20 : 201-237.

11. McGeer, E.G., Fibiger, H.C., McGeer, P.L., and Wickson, V. (1971) : Exp. Gerontol, 6 : 391-396.

12. McGeer, E.G. (1978) : In : Aging and Neurotransmitter Metabolism in Human Brain : Alzheimer's Disease : Senile Dementia and Related Disorders : Raven Press, New York.

13. Meek, J.L., Bertilsson, L., Cheney, D.L., Zsilla, G., and Costa, E. (1977) : J. Gerontol., 32 : 129-131.

14. Scatton, B., and Bartholini, G. (1980) : Brain Research, 183 : 211-216.

15. Singer, S.J., and Nicholson, G.L. (1972) : Science, 175 : 720-731.

16. Terry, R.D., and Gershon, S. (1979) : Neurobiology of Aging, Vol. 3., Raven Press, New York.

Apomorphine and Other Dopaminomimetics,
Vol. 2: Clinical Pharmacology, edited by
G. U. Corsini and G. L. Gessa, Raven Press,
New York © 1981.

Levels of Monoamines, Monoamine Metabolites, and Activity in Related Enzyme Systems Correlated to Normal Aging and in Patients with Dementia of Alzheimer Type

C. G. Gottfries

*Professor of Psychiatry, Department of Psychiatry and Neurochemistry, St. Jörgen's Hospital, University
of Göteborg, 422 03 Hisings Backa, Sweden*

NORMAL AGEING AND DEMENTIA DISORDERS

Impairment of psychic functions in old age can be due to normal ageing and to dementia disorders. Normal ageing will produce no severe mental impairment. From psychological tests it is evident that normal ageing does not mean a general impairment of all psychic functions. Dementia means a more severe impairment of mental functions. The condition is progressive and irreversible.

From a clinical point of view it may be difficult to distinguish normal ageing from pathological ageing. With regard to structural changes as well as biochemical it has been shown that normal ageing and dementia of Alzheimer type have features in common. Therefore, the question of whether there is a continuity between orthoinvolution and pathoinvolution has not yet been settled.

Dementia disorders can naturally be parted in two subgroups: the cerebral vascular diseases and the degenerative disorders (FIG. 1). As the causes of dementia in vascular diseases usually are infarctions this form of dementia is called multi-infarction dementia. The non-vascular diseases are senile dementia and the presenile dementias. The senile dementias may very well be an heterogenous group. The presenile dementias are Alzheimer's disease, Pick's disease, Hurtington's chorea and the spongioform encephalopathies (Jacob Creutzfeldt's disease). As there are many similarities between Alzheimer's disease and senile dementia these two groups are often brought together to a group called dementia of Alzheimer type (DAT). There are, however, genetic investigations (20) which do not support the assumption that these are the same type of disorders. During the last years there has been an encouraging research about biochemical changes in DAT. In as well post-mortem investigations as in investigations concerning cerebrospinal fluid (CSF) transmitters, their metabolites and related enzyme systems have been studied.

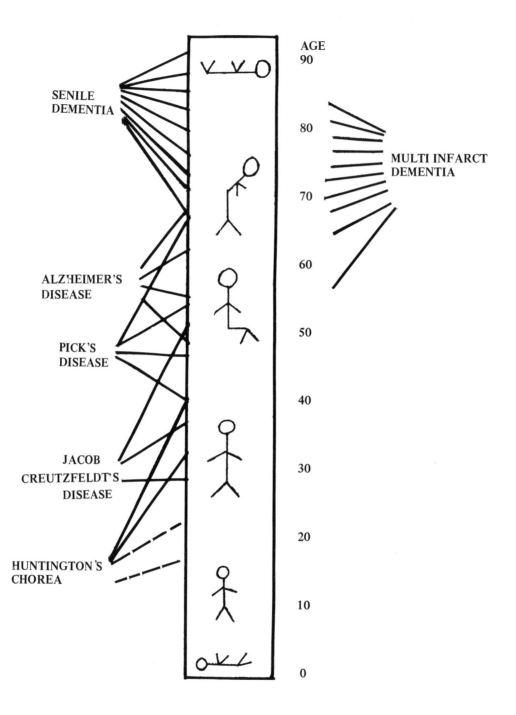

FIG. 1. Dementia disorders in old age. Senile dementia and Alzheimer's disease together form the group Dementia of Alzheimer type (DAT).

BIOCHEMICAL CHANGES IN NORMAL AGEING

Experiments with animals have shown that the synthesis of noradrenaline (NA) and dopamine (DA) is reduced in senescent rats, as is the activity of tyrosinehydroxylase (TH) (8,2). In an investigation by McGeer et al. (23) and McGeer and McGeer (22) the TH-activity was investigated post-mortem in human brains and an age-related decline could be confirmed. Carlsson and Winblad (5) found a negative correlation between DA-levels in the human basal ganglia and age especially in groups over 50 years. In own investigations (10) a group of patients with an age range of 23-92 years was studied and a significant decline in the DA-concentration in the caudate nucleus, globus pallidus, mesencephalon, hippocampus and cortex gyrus hippocampus was observed. In FIG. 2 biochemical changes found in brains from patients with normal ageing have been summarized.

Type of change	Normal ageing	Dementia of Alzheimer type (DAT)
Choline acetyl-transferase (CAT)	↓	↓ ↓
Muscarine receptors in brain tissue	↓	—
Tyrosinehydroxylase (TH)	↓	
Dopadecarboxylase (DOD)	↓	↓ ↓
Dopamine-B-hydroxylase (DBH)	↓	↓
Dopamine (DA)	↓	↓ ↓
Homovanillic acid (HVA)	↓	↓ ↓
Noradrenaline (NA)	↓	↓ ↓
3-methoxy-4-hydroxyphenylglycol (MHPG)	—	↑
5-hydroxytryptamine (5-HT)	↓	↓ ↓
5-hydroxyindoleacetic acid (5-HIAA)	—	↓
Monoamine oxidase A	—	—
Monoamine oxidase B	↑	↑ ↑
Superoxide dismutase	↑	↑ ↑

FIG. 2. Changes in biological systems related to age or to dementia of Alzheimer type (DAT) according to post mortem investigations in man

As is evident from this figure the homovanillic acid- (HVA) levels did
not decrease with age. Of interest is that the levels of NA and 5-
hydroxytryptamine (5-HT) are reduced in normal ageing. As is also evident from the figure there is an increased activity of the enzymes
monoamine oxidase B (MAO-B) and superoxidedismutase. These data are
achieved from own investigations in post-mortem material (9).

In investigations on the CSF a positive correlation has been found
between age and the metabolites HVA and 5-hydroxyindoleacetic acid
(5-HIAA) (3, 11). These findings are somewhat contradictory to the
findings from brain tissue. The reduced enzyme activity and the reduced
levels of active amines in brain tissues indicate a reduced metabolism
with age. The increased levels of acid metabolites in CSF may indicate
the opposite. It may also, however, indicate a reduced outward transport
from the liquor space.

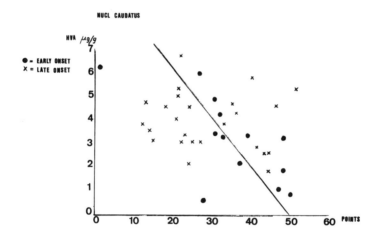

FIG. 3. Levels of homovanillic acid (HVA) in the caudate nucleus
        plotted against intellectual deterioration measured with
        a rating scale.

BIOCHEMICAL CHANGES IN DEMENTIA OF ALZHEIMER TYPE

Structural changes in brain tissue indicate a wide spread degeneration in the brains from patients with DAT. Due to this it is considered
unlikely that a single neurotransmitter would selectively be affected
(7). From Great Britain there are several investigations indicating a
reduced activity of the choline acetyltransferase (CAT) in brains from
patients with DAT. A reduced activity of the metabolism of acetylcholine
has also been assumed to be a main pathogenetic factor in DAT. We have,
however, studied the metabolism of the monoamines DA, NA and 5-HT in

brains from patients with DAT. The original finding was of reduced levels of HVA in basal ganglia in patients with dementia (19). Later the
concentration of HVA was estimated in the caudate nucleus, the putamen
and the globus pallidus in a more carefully diagnosed group of DAT and
in control groups (12, 13). The results of these investigations show
that in the DAT-group there were significantly lower concentrations of
HVA in the investigated areas when this group was compared to age-
matched controls. By constructing a scale for rating levels of dementia
it was possible to correlate the reduced levels of HVA with the levels
of dementia. At present 37 patients have been investigated as well for
the HVA-levels in the caudate nucleus as for the levels of dementia. In
FIG. 3 these variables are plotted. In the total group there was a significant negative correlation between the biochemical and psychological
variable. The more reduced levels of HVA the more points indicating dementia was seen. The correlation coefficient for the total group was
-0.42. If the correlation between these two variables were studied only
in the patients with Alzheimer's disease with early onset (n=12) the
correlation was still stronger (-0.70). The significant correlation between the two variables may indicate that a disturbance in a dopaminergic system of the brain (a meso-cortical system?) may have pathogenetic
importance for symptoms in DAT.

In other post-mortem investigations significantly lower levels of DA
and NA were found in groups of patients with DAT as compared to age-
matched controls (18, 1). Reduced NA-levels and loss of nerve cells from
locus ceruleus in brains from patients with DAT are recently reported
from Mann et al. (21). At the CINP Congress 1980 a report about reduced
activity of dopamine-β-hydroxylase in brains from patients with DAT was
presented (6). In an ongoing Swedish investigation from which preliminary data were reported by Carlsson (4) reduced levels of DA, HVA, NA
and 5-HT were found (FIG. 2). In this investigation also 3-methoxy-4-
hydroxy-phenylglycol (MHPG) was estimated and surprisingly enough the
levels of this metabolite was increased in the group of DAT when compared to age-matched controls. Animal experiments indicate that the NA-
system is readily activated by stress. Possibly the elevated MHPG in DAT
is a sign of stress. Of interest is also that in this investigation increased activities of the enzymes MAO and superoxidedismutase were
found in brain tissue from patients with DAT when compared to age-
matched controls. It was, however, only MAO-B which was increased while
the MAO-A did not increase. In the ongoing Swedish investigation 15
controls and 14 patients with DAT were investigated. The activity of CAT
was estimated and found reduced. The result then supports the findings
from the investigation groups in Great Britain.

Investigations of CSF have also been performed in patients with DAT
(13, 14, 15, 16). In these investigations it has been shown that both
HVA and 5-HIAA are reduced as compared to age-matched control groups. In
one investigation (17) a probenecid loading test was performed in patients with DAT and the results from that investigation also indicated a
reduced metabolism of DA.

In summary the activity of the enzyme TH is reduced in normal ageing.
In line with these findings it has also been shown that there are reduced levels of NA and DA with age in post-mortem brain material. 5-HT-
levels are also reduced in some areas of the brain. The levels of 5-HIAA
and HVA in CSF are increased with age. These findings may indicate a
reduced metabolism of the monoamines in the brain and a reduced out-
transport of the acid metabolites from the liquor space. The age-related

increase in the activity of MAO-B is of great theoretical interest. What kind of changes in the brain tissue are reflected by the increased MAO-B activity?

To summarize the findings about the monoamine metabolism in patients with DAT, reduced levels of DA, NA and 5-HT in brain tissue have been noted. HVA in brain tissue is reduced. As there also are reduced activities in synthetizing enzymes, a reduced activity in the monoaminergic systems can be assumed. In CSF base levels as well as probenecid loading tests have also shown signs of reduced activity in dopaminergic and serotoninergic systems. Of interest is that in DAT there are increased levels of MHPG which may indicate that stress factors are of importance. Increased activities of MAO-B and superoxide dismutase are perhaps of no practical but of theoretical interest.

Our findings as well as findings from other research groups indicate that in the brains from patients with DAT there are disturbances of cholinergic and monoaminergic transmittor systems. The same type of changes although less severe are found in normal ageing. Between normal ageing and DAT there are thus more quantitative than qualitative differences and it is well known that this is true not only for biochemical but also for structural changes. Future work should aim at defining the profile of transmittor disturbances in normal ageing and in DAT and perhaps in individual cases. This may be achieved by analyzing transmittor metabolites in the CSF or by pharmacological provocation tests. Then perhaps therapy should be instituted, tailor-made for the individual type of transmittor disturbance.

ACKNOWLEDGEMENT

This investigation was supported by grants from the Swedish Medical Research Council No. B81-21X-05002-05, Fredrik och Ingrid Thurings Stiftelse, Stiftelsen Hjalmar Svenssons Forskningsfond.

REFERENCES

1. Adolfsson, R., Gottfries, C.G., Roos, B.E., and Winblad, B. (1979): Brit. J. Psychiatry, 135: 216-223.
2. Algeri, S., Bonati, M., Brunello, N., Ponzio, F., Stramentinoli, G., and Gualano, M. (1978): In: Neuro-Psychopharmacology. Proceedings of the Tenth Congress of the Collegium International Neuro-Psychopharmacologicum, Quebec, July 1976. Vol. 2, edited by P. Deniker, C. Radouco-Thomas, and A. Villeneuve, pp. 1647-1654, Pergamon Press, Oxford and New York.
3. Bowers, M., and Gerbode, F.A. (1968): Nature, London, 219: 1256--1257.
4. Carlsson, A. (1978): In: Catecholamines: basic and clinical frontiers, edited by E. Usdin, I.J. Kopin, and J. Barchas, pp. 4-19. Pergamon Press, New York.
5. Carlsson, A., and Winblad, B. (1976): J. Neural. Transm., 38: 271--276.
6. Cross, A., Crow, T.J., Perry, E.K., and Kimberlin, R.H. (1980): In: Abstracts of the 12th CINP Congress, Göteborg, Sweden, 22-26 June 1980, edited by C. Radouco-Thomas, and F. Garcin. Suppl. to Prog. Neuro-Psychopharmacol., p. 118, Pergamon Press, Oxford.
7. Dayan, A.D. (1974): Psychol. Med., 4: 349-352.
8. Finch, C.E. (1973): Brain Res., 52: 261-276.
9. Gottfries, C.G. (1980): In: Biochemistry of dementia, edited by P.J. Roberts, pp. 213-234, John Wiley & Sons Ltd., New York.

10. Gottfries, C.G., Adolfsson, R., Oreland, L., Roos, B.E., and Winblad, B. (1979): In: Drugs and the elderly. Perspectives in geriatric clinical pharmacology. Proceedings of a symposium held in Ninewells Hospital, University of Dundee, 13-14 September 1977, edited by J. Crooks, and I.H. Stevenson, pp. 189-197. The MacMillan Press Ltd., London.
11. Gottfries, C.G., Gottfries, I., Johansson, B., Olsson, R., Persson, T., Roos, B.E., and Sjöström, R. (1971): Neuropharmacology, 10: 665--672.
12. Gottfries, C.G., Gottfries, I., and Roos, B.E. (1968): In: Excerpta Medica International Congress Series, No. 180, pp. 310-312.
13. Gottfries, C.G., Gottfries, I., and Roos, B.E. (1969): Brit. J. Psychiatry, 115: 563-574.
14. Gottfries, C.G., Gottfries, I., and Roos, B.E. (1970): Acta Psychiatr. Scand., 46: 99-105.
15. Gottfries, C.G., and Roos, B.E. (1973): Acta Psychiatr. Scand., 49: 257-263.
16. Gottfries, C.G., and Roos, B.E. (1976): Aktuel Gerontol., 6: 37-42.
17. Gottfries, C.G., Roos, B.E., and Winblad, B. (1974): Acta Psychiatr. Scand., 50: 496-507.
18. Gottfries, C.G., Roos, B.E., and Winblad, B. (1976): Aktuel. Gerontol., 6: 429-435.
19. Gottfries, C.G., Rosengren, A.M., and Rosengren, E. (1965): Acta Pharmacol. Toxicol., 23: 36-40.
20. Larsson, T., Sjögren, T., and Jacobson, G. (1963): Acta Psychiatr. Scand., Suppl. 167.
21. Mann, D.M.A., Lincoln, J., Yates, P.O., Stamp, J.E., and Toper, S. (1980): Brit. J. Psychiatry, 136: 533-541.
22. McGeer, E.G., and McGeer, P.L. (1973): In: New concepts in neurotransmitter regulation, edited by A.J. Mandell, pp. 53-69, Plenum Press, New York.
23. McGeer, E.G., McGeer, P.L., and Wada, S.A. (1971): J. Neurochem., 18: 1647-1658.

Apomorphine and Other Dopaminomimetics,
Vol. 2: Clinical Pharmacology, edited by
G. U. Corsini and G. L. Gessa, Raven Press,
New York © 1981.

Possible Role of Dopamine Receptors in the Control of Arterial Blood Pressure and Hormone Secretion in Normals and Hypertensive Patients: A Study with Sulpiride Isomers

L. F. Agnati, P. Bernardi, F. Benfenati, C. Adani, *M. Capelli,
*V. Cocchi, I. Zini, and **P. Fresia

*Department of Human Physiology, University of Modena, 41100 Modena; *Centralized Laboratory, St. Orsola Hospital, Bologna; **Ravizza Research Laboratories , Muggio, 20100 Milan, Italy*

From the first suggestion of the existence of two types of dopamine (DA) receptors by Cools (6), evidence has been gathered about different biochemical characteristics and locations of DA receptors in the central nervous system (CNS) as well as in the periphery (14,24).

On the basis of biochemical experiments, Spano et al. (24) differentiate two types of DA receptors, called D_1 and D_2 receptors, respectively. D_1-receptors are characterized by a cyclase linkage and have DA as agonist (μmolar potency) and ergots as antagonists (nmolar potency), while D_2-receptors are characterized by a lack of cyclase linkage and have both DA and ergots as agonists (nmolar potency) and sulpiride as well as metoclopramide as selective antagonists (14).

It is interesting to note that, up to now, the only selective antagonists known for D_2-receptors belong to benzamides. Among these compounds, great attention has been given to 1,d-sulpiride (N-ethyl-(2methoxy-5sulphonamidobenza-midon_ ethyl-pyrrolidine), a benzamide derivative. The antidopaminergic activity of this drug is mainly attributed to its levo isomer, as shown in behavioural (19), clinical (7) and biochemical (2,24,26) studies ; in the latter experiments, only the levo isomer was found to be able to displace ^{3}H-spiroperidol binding at striatal and limbic levels, while d-sulpiride was practically ineffective.

As far as D_2-receptors are concerned, they have been found in both CNS and periphery, in particular at the level of renal vessels, where sulpiride is much more effective than classical neuroleptics (like haloperidol and clorpromazine) as a receptor blocker (11).

In the present paper the effects of sulpiride isomers on
arterial blood pressure (ABP), heart rate (HR) and prolactin
(PRL) secretion have been first studied in normal male volunteers. Then, in view of the hypotensive action of the levo
isomer in normals, a further study of the possible effects
of l-sulpiride on ABP, HR and PRL, renin, aldosterone secretion has been carried out in hypertensive patients. In other
words, it seemed of interest to investigate the hypothensive
effect of l-sulpiride in hypertensive disease, to characterize possible endocrinological correlates of this action
and finally to assess whether the observed effects are mainly due to a central or peripheral blockade of DA receptors.

MATERIALS AND METHODS

The study of the effects of l- and d-sulpiride in normals
was carried out on eight male volunteers (mean age = 26 $\pm$ 2
years). After and overnight fast, each of them was submitted,
in a random fashion, to the following treatments : placebo
(0.9% saline,i.v.), l-sulpiride (25mg,i.v.), d-sulpiride (25
mg,i.v.). The three treatments were administered 4-5 days
apart from each other; the subjects remained in supine position throughout the tests. Blood samples were drawn by a
needle introduced in the antecubital vein and kept patent by
a slow saline infusion at times t = -10,0,15,30,60,90,120min.
In all treatments t = 0 min was the time immediately before
drug or placebo administration. The samples were placed into
test tubes containing EDTA and then centrifuged. Plasma was
separated, frozen and stored at -20°C until analysis. PRL
plasma levels were then determined by means of standard RIA
methods using Biodata kits. At each time interval, systolic
ABP, diastolic ABP and HR were also determined; measurements
of ABP were made by two observers by means of the Riva-Rocci
auscultatory method.
The study of the effects of l-sulpiride in hypertensive
disease was carried out on eight patients. In table 1 the
clinical data characterizing these subjects are reported;the
diagnosis of essential hypertension was established by ex-
clusion of all known causes of hypertension. In table 2 mean
basal values of ABP, HR and hormone levels (PRL, renin,
aldosterone) are summarized for each patient. Each subject
received no medication and had normal sodium and potassium
intakes from a week before to the end of the sessions. The
schedule followed for pharmacological tests with l-sulpiride
was similar to that used in normals, the differences being
the larger number of tested doses (1,3,6,12,25 and 50 mg,
i.v.), the more frequent measurements of ABP and HR (every

TABLE 1. Clinical data characterizing the 8 hypertensive patients who underwent pharmacological tests with l-sulpiride

PATIENTS	A	B	C	D	E	F	G	H
Sex	F	M	F	F	F	M	M	F
Age (y)	51	52	55	37	66	53	59	59
Fam. history	+	+	+	+	-	-	+	-
Duration of hypertension (y)	10	5	2	22	11	3	5	25
Headache	+	-	-	+	-	-	+	+
Dyspnea	-	+	+	+	+	-	-	-
Asthenia	-	-	-	+	-	-	+	+
Cardiac dysrhythmias	-	-	+	+	+	-	-	+
Angina pectoris	-	+	-	-	-	-	-	-
Retinopathy	I	II	II	II	II	I	II	II
Diabetes	-	-	-	-	-	+	++	-
17 OH steroids	=	=	+	=	+	=	=	=
Hyperlipoprot. (F)	-	-	IV	-	IIa	IIb	IV	-

TABLE 2.
Basal cardiovascular and hormonal data in 8 hypertensive patients [a].

PATIENTS	A	B	C	D	E	F	G	H
ABP syst.	175 (6)	195 (4)	164 (2)	165 (2)	190 (3)	168 (5)	171 (3)	185 (2)
ABP diast.	95 (3)	96 (2)	100 (1)	103 (1)	108 (3)	120 (4)	104 (2)	108 (4)
H.R.	62 (1)	75 (2)	63 (3)	70 (5)	72 (3)	75 (9)	58 (2)	74 (1)
PRL	5.8 (1.6)	3.8 (1.3)	5.2 (0.4)	10.8 (1.0)	9.5 (3.4)	11.1 (3.5)	8.4 (1.8)	8.2 (3.2)
RENIN	0.3 (0)	0.1 (0)	0.4 (0.2)	0.3 (0)	0.2 (0)	0.5 (0.1)	0.2 (0)	0.4 (0.1)
ALDOSTERONE	62 (8)	36 (9)	121 (22)	74 (10)	88 (9)	110 (19)	143 (26)	85 (12)

[a] means ($\pm$ SEM) of at least five basal determinations on different days.

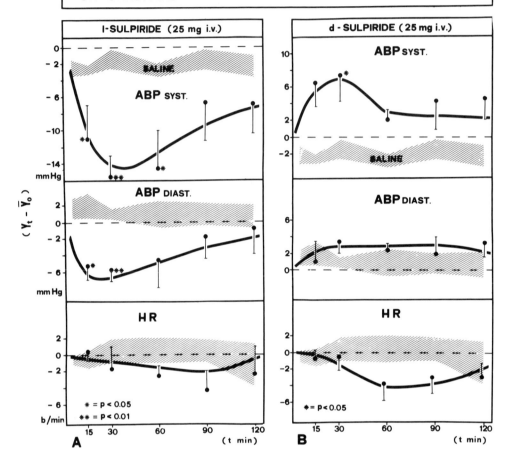

FIG.1. Time-course of systolic arterial blood pressure (ABP
syst), diastolic arterial blood pressure (ABPdiast) and
heart rate (HR) changes after l-sulpiride (A) and d-sulpiride (B) in normal subjects. On the X-axis time intervals
after drug administration (t = 0 min) are given. On the Y-
-axis the changes of cardiovascular parameters with respect
to the mean basal value are reported. Each point in the plot
represents the mean (±SEM) of eight observations. The shaded
area in each panel shows the time-course (mean value ±SEM)
of the respective cardiovascular parameter after placebo
administration. Statistical analysis was carried out by means
of Student's paired t test, by comparing the mean change observed after sulpiride with that observed after the placebo,
at each time interval.

15 min after t = 0), and the wider range of endocrinological correlates considered. In fact, beside PRL (Biodata kits, ng/ml), also renin (Lepetit kits, ng/ml/h), and aldosterone (Abbott kits, pg/ml) plasma levels were radioimmunologically determined.

Statistical analysis was carried out by means of Student's paired t test. Further details are given in the legends to the figures, when necessary.

RESULTS

In normal subjects, l-sulpiride (25mg,i.v.) caused a clear-cut reduction of both systolic (mainly) and diastolic ABP, while it had no significant effects on HR (Fig. 1A). d-sulpiride (25mg,i.v.) had a slight and non significant bradycardic action and caused a short-lived increase in systolic ABP and no clear-cut effects on diastolic ABP (Fig.1B). Thus, as shown also by an evaluation of l- and d-sulpiride overall

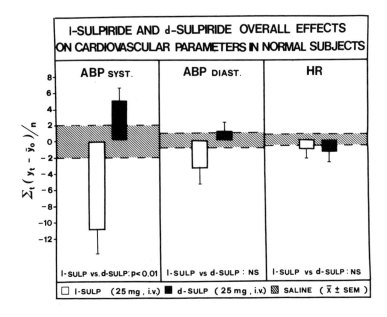

FIG.2. Evaluation of the overall cardiovascular effects of sulpiride isomers in normal subjects. Mean changes in cardiovascular parameters observed after drug administration were evaluated for each subject; the overall mean (+SEM) of the individual mean changes is reported on the Y-axis. Statistical analysis was carried out by means of Student's paired t test, by comparing the overall effect observed after l--sulpiride with that observed after d-sulpiride.

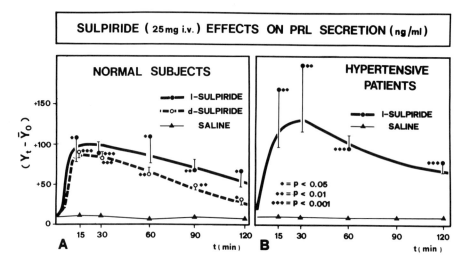

FIG.3. Effects of sulpiride isomers on PRL secretion in normal (A) and hypertensive (B) subjects. On the X-axis time intervals after drug or saline administration (t = 0 min) are given. On the Y-axis the changes of PRL plasma levels with respect to the mean basal value are reported as means ($\pm$SEM) of eight observations. Statistical analysis was carried out by means of Student's paired t test, by comparing mean changes observed after l- or d-sulpiride with that observed after the placebo, at each time interval.

effects on cardiovascular parameters, the two isomers seem to act in an opposite way on both systolic and diastolic ABP (·Fig.2). On the other hand, both isomers caused a similar hyperprolactinemia, the only difference being the higher peak effect and the apparently slower decay rate of PRL serum levels after l-sulpiride (Fig.3).

In hypertensive patients, l-sulpiride had the same lowering effects as those observed in normal subjects on systolic and, to a lower extent, on diastolic ABP (Fig.4). It should be noted that in both normals and hypertensive patients, l- as well as d-sulpiride effects on ABP reached the peak within 30 min from the time of administration. PRL hypersecretion caused by l-sulpiride was somewhat higher in hypertensive patients than in normals (Fig.3), although, due to the great variability, the peaks did not differ significantly (p<0.20).

The dose-effect curves of l-sulpiride for cardiovascular parameters and hormone plasma levels in hypertensive patients can be summarized in three types of responses:
a) a bell-shaped dose-response curve for systolic and diastolic ABP, with a maximum lowering effect at the dose of

12 mg i.v. (Fig. 5A);

b) a monotonic increasing curve for PRL secretion, which had not reached the plateau at the dose of 50 mg i.v.(highest l-sulpiride tested dose) (Fig. 5B);

c) no dose-response curve for either HR (data not shown) or renin and aldosterone secretion (Table 3), where no significant effects were observed at any of the tested doses.

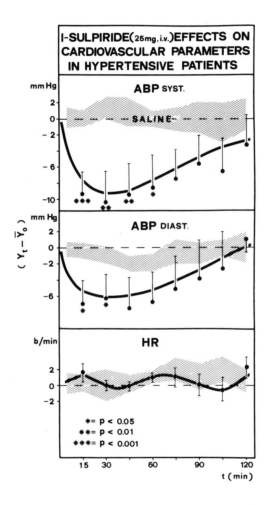

FIG.4. Time-course of systolic arterial blood pressure (ABPsyst), diastolic arterial blood pressure (ABPdiast) and heart rate (HR) changes after l-sulpiride (25mg,i.v.) administration in eight hypertensive patients. For further details see legend to Fig. 1.

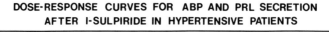

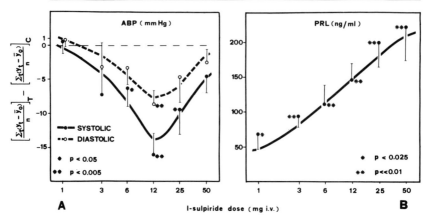

FIG.5. Dose-response curves for arterial blood pressure (ABP) (A) and PRL secretion (B) after l-sulpiride in hypertensive patients. On the Y-axis differences in the overall effects observed after l-sulpiride treatment (T) and placebo control (C) are reported for each tested dose as means (+SEM). Statistical analysis was performed by means of Student's paired t test by comparing the overall effect observed after l-sulpiride with that observed after the placebo.

I-SULPIRIDE (mg ; i.v.)	$\Sigma_t (Y_t - \bar{Y}_0)/n$	
	ALDOSTERONE (pg / ml)	RENIN (ng / ml / h)
0	−20 ± 12	− 0.1 ± 0
1	−29 ± 10	− 0.2 ± 0
3	−47 ± 20	− 0.1 ± 0
6	− 4 ± 4	− 0.1 ± 0
12	−23 ± 10	0 ± 0
25	−30 ± 9	− 0.1 ± 0
50	−22 ± 18	0 ± 0

TAB. 3. Overall effects of l-sulpiride and placebo on aldosterone and renin secretion in hypertensive patients. For further details see legend to Fig. 2.

DISCUSSION

A dopaminergic control of cardiovascular parameters is well established (9,10) even if the features of this control are not completely clear. The evidence for such a control comes mainly from pharmacological studies; however, in the intact animal, a dopaminergic drug can act on many different targets to modulate cardiovascular parameters (3,5,9,10,12, 15,16,20,21,28) (Fig.6).

In principle, it is possible to distinguish:
a) a central versus a peripheral action;
b) an action on the prompt control systems (i.e. on cardio-vascular effector organs) versus an action on long-term control systems (e.g. on sodium escretion and then on the pressure-diuresis mechanism);
c) a direct action of the drug on effector organs versus a neurogenic action.

The present findings in normals suggest that l- and d-sulpiride modify cardiovascular parameters through a peripheral action on prompt control systems (even if a central action as well as an action on long-term control systems cannot be ruled out). In fact, l-sulpiride (6mg/kg,i.p.) pharmacokinetics in the rat show that it takes at least 1 hour to induce a significant change in DOPAC levels in the striatum and 3 hours to reach the maximum effect (24). In agreement with this finding, it has been reported that d,l-sulpiride does not easily cross the blood-brain barrier (4). The effects of l- and d-sulpiride reported here can be detected a few minutes after intravenous administration and reach a maximum within 30 min: this time-course underlines the very likely peripheral action of the isomers on prompt cardiovascular control systems. Finally, as far as point c) is concerned, both isomers might work through a direct action on the heart. In fact, both l- and d-sulpiride mainly (even if in an opposite direction) affect systolic ABP, with no clear-cut effects on HR. This might be due to a direct action on cardiac DA receptors. In fact, it is well known that DA has a positive inotropic effect and no sensible chronotropic effect(18).

If these premises are true, it can be surmized that l- and d-sulpiride have different effects on cardiac DA receptors: d-sulpiride may act as a partial agonist, whereas l-sulpiride may exert a purely antagonist effect on myocardial DA receptors. Indirect evidence for an opposite effect of sulpiride isomers on DA receptors has been gathered by Fuxe's group in the rat. Histochemical studies have shown that, at

POSSIBLE SITES AND MECHANISMS OF ACTION OF DOPAMINERGIC DRUGS
—— IN THE CONTROL OF CARDIOVASCULAR PARAMETERS ——

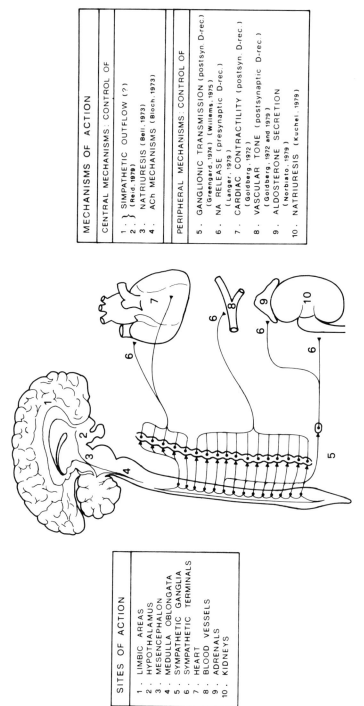

FIG.6. Schematic representation of the possible sites and mechanisms of action of dopaminergic drugs in the control of cardiovascular parameters.

caudate level, l-sulpiride increases DA turnover, while d-
-sulpiride reduces it, at least in a suitable range of low
doses (10-25mg/kg,i.p.) (8). Biochemical studies also point
to a profound difference between l- and d-sulpiride mechanism of action at central level. In fact, l-sulpiride, but
not d-sulpiride, can displace ^{3}H-spiroperidol from its binding sites in caudate and limbic membrane preparations (2).
Furthermore, d-sulpiride, but not l-sulpiride can increase
DA-induced cAMP accumulation in caudate and limbic preparations over a large range of low concentrations in the medium
(2).

On this basis, it is also possible to interpret the action
of l-sulpiride in hypertensive patients. The lowering effects on systolic ABP, in the absence of clear effects on HR,
might be due to a selective blockade of cardiac DA receptors,
while the less marked lowering effect on diastolic ABP might
be a consequence of the decrease in systolic ABP, since diastolic ABP depends on total peripheral resistance`, HR, elas-
tic recoil cf arterial walls and systolic pressure levels.

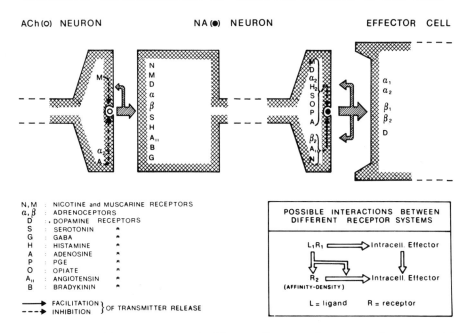

FIG.7. Schematic representation of receptors systems in the
autonomic nervous system (ANS). Possible interactions are
shown between different receptors systems. For further details, see text.

CA RECEPTORS INVOLVED IN THE CONTROL OF CARDIOVASCULAR PARAMETERS

CARDIOVASCULAR PARAMETER	CHANGE	RECEPTOR INVOLVED	REFERENCES
CHRONOTROPIC STATE	+	β_1 ; α_2	Langer 1980
INOTROPIC STATE	+	β_1 ; α_1 ; D	Schümann 1980; Hökfelt 1978
VENOUS CAPACITANCE	−	α	**
CORONARY FLOW	+	D	Takenaka 1978
MUSCLE FLOW	+	β_2	**
SKIN FLOW	−	α	**
KIDNEY FLOW	+	D	Goldberg 1979
SPLANCHNIC FLOW	+	β_2 ; D	Hökfelt 1978

** see, e.g., J.T. Shepherd & P.M. Vanhoutte , 1979.

TABLE 4. Summarizing table showing the main catecholamine (CA) receptor systems involved in the control of
cardiovascular parameters at peripheral level.

However, the bell-shaped dose-response curve for ABP in
hypertensive patients points to a selective action of l-sulpiride on cardiac DA receptors only in a restricted range of
low doses.

The characteristics of DA receptors involved in the action
of sulpiride have still to be assessed. As suggested in a
previous work (1), the steric requirements of DA receptors
may be different in various region, depending on the particu
lar receptor microcompartment. In agreement with this view,
the present findings show that, while l- and d-sulpiride
have similar effects on PRL secretion, they cause opposite
changes on ABP. This hypothesis is also supported by the
different effects of l-sulpiride and metoclopramide on aldosterone secretion, in spite of their similar structures (both
are benzamides) and of the fact that the same DA receptors
are involved. In fact, metoclopramide (10mg, i.v.) has been
found to cause a prompt rise of aldosterone serum levels in
man (20), while the present findings show that l-sulpiride
does not consistently affect aldosterone secretion at any of
the tested doses.

The lack of effect of l-sulpiride on plasma renin activity
further questions the role of DA and dopaminergic systems in
the control of renin release by juxtaglomerular cells (13).
Furthermore, the autonomic modulation of renin secretion may
be uneffective in conditions of "low renin hypertension"
like those studied here.

From a more general standpoint, receptor systems in the

autonomic nervous system should be viewed in their complexity (Fig. 9) and, in this context, the possibility of other actions of sulpiride isomers should be envisaged. In fact, the possibility should be also considered (see panel in Fig. 9) that a certain ligand (L_1), while interacting with its receptor (R_1), can affect another receptor system (R_2) at the recognition site, or at the level of biological signal transduction, or, finally, at the intracellular effector mechanism. A similar phenomenon has been, e.g., described by Watanabe et al. (27), who showed that the binding of muscarinic cholinergic agonists, at myocardial level, can regulate β-receptor binding characteristics by modulating the action of GTP.

In conclusion, the present findings point to the existence of a control of cardiovascular parameters (mainly systolic ABP) by DA receptors sensitive to sulpiride. This evidence adds to the rationale for drug treatment of cardiovascular diseases (table 4), which obviously cannot leave out a detailed knowledge of catecholamine receptor systems involved in cardiovascular control (10,13,17,22,23,25).

ACKNOWLEDGEMENTS

The Authors thank Dr.G.Grandi and Mrs.F.Barbieri for the skilful technical assistance and Ravizza S.p.A. (Muggiò, Milan) for kindly supplying sulpiride isomers.

REFERENCES

1. Agnati,L.F.,Cortelli,P.,De Camillis,E.,Benfenati,F.,Orlandi,F.,and Fresia,P.(1979):Neurosci.Lett.,15:289-294.
2. Agnati,L.F.,Fuxe,K.,Ogren,S.O.,and Fredholm,B.(1978): Second European Neuroscience Meeting,Florence,Abstr.S308.
3. Bell,C.,and Lang,W.J.(1973):Nature New Biol.,246:27-29.
4. Benakis,A.,and Rey,C.(1976):J.Pharmacol.(Paris),7:367-378.
5. Bloch,R.,Bousquet,P.,Feldman,J.,and Schwartz,J.(1973): In: Frontiers in Catecholamine Research,edited by E.Usdin,and S.H.Snyder,pp.853-857. Pergamon Press,Oxford.
6. Cools,A.R.(1977):In:Advances in Biochemical Psychopharmachology,edited by E.Costa,and G.L.Gessa,vol.16,pp.215-225. Reven Press,New York.
7. Corsini,G.U.,Del Zompo,M.,Melis,G.B.,Mangoni,A.,and Gessa, G.L.(1979):In:Sulpiride and other Benzamides,edited by P. F.Spano,M.Trabucchi,G.U.Corsini and G.L.Gessa,pp.255-267. Italian Brain Research Foundation Press, Milan.
8. Fuxe,K.,Andersson,K.,Agnati,L.F.,and Ogren,S.O.(1979): Neurosci.Lett.,suppl.3,S237.

9. Goldberg,L.I.(1972):Pharmac.Rev.,24:1-29.
10. Goldberg,L.I.(1979):In:Perypheral Dopaminergic Receptors,
    edited by J.L.Imbs,and J.Schwartz,pp.1-12.Pergamon Press,
    Oxford.
11. Goldberg,L.I.,Musgrave,G.E.,and Kohli,J.D.(1979):In:Sul-
    piride and other Benzamides,edited by P.F.Spano,M.Trabuc
    chi,G.U.Corsini,and G.L.Gessa,pp.73-81. Italian Brain
    Research Foundation Press,Milan.
12. Greengard,P.,and Kebabian,J.W.(1974):Fed.Proc.,33:1059-
    1067.
13. Hökfelt,B.(1978):Acta Endocrinol.,88(suppl.216):67-74.
14. Kebabian,J.W.,and Calne,D.B.(1979):Nature,277:93-96.
15. Kuchel,O.,Thanh Buu,N.,Unger,T.,Lis,M.,and Genest,J.
    (1979):J.Clin.Endocrinol.Metab.,48:425-429.
16. Langer,S.Z.,and Dubocovich,M.L.(1979):In:Perypheral Dopa-
    minergic Receptors,edited by J.L.Imbs,and J.Schwartz,pp.
    233-245. Pergamon Press, Oxford.
17. Langer,S.Z.(1980): TINS,3:110-112.
18. McDonald,R.H.Jr.,and Goldberg,L.I.(1963):J.Pharmacol.Exp.
    Ther.,140:60-66.
19. Montanaro,N.,Gandolfi,O.,and Dall'Olio,R.(1979):In:Sul-
    piride and other Benzamides,edited by P.F.Spano,M.Tra-
    bucchi,G.U.Corsini and G.L.Gessa,pp.109-118. Italian
    Brain Research Foundation Press,Milan.
20. Norbiato,G.,Bevilacqua,M.,Raggi,U.,Micossi,P.,and Moroni,
    C.(1977):J.Clin.Endocrinol.Metabol.,45:1313-1316.
21. Raid,J.L.,and Bateman,D.N.(1979):In:Dopaminergic ergot
    derivates and motor function,edited by K.Fuxe,and D.B.
    Calne,pp.395-403. Pergamon Press,New York.
22. Schumann,H.J.(1980):TIPS,1:195-197.
23. Sheperd,J.T.,and Vanhoutte,M.P.(1979):The Human Cardio-
    vascular System. Raven Press,New York.
24. Spano,P.F.,Stefanini,E.,Trabucchi,M.,and Fresia,P.(1979):
    In:Sulpiride and other Benzamides,edited by P.F.Spano,M.
    Trabucchi,G.U.Corsini,and G.L.Gessa,pp.11-31. Italian
    Brain Research Foundation Press,Milan.
25. Takenaka,F.,Sakanashi,M.,Ishihara,T.,and Morishita,H.
    (1979):In:Perypheral Dopaminergic Receptors,edited by
    J.L.Imbs ,and J.Schwartz,pp.167-172. Pergamon Press,
    Oxford.
26. Tissari,A.H.,Stefanini,E.,and Gessa G.L.(1979):In:Sul-
    piride and other Benzamides,edited by P.F.Spano,M.Tra-
    bucchi,G.U.Corsini,and G.L.Gessa,pp.3-9. Italian Brain
    Research Foundation Press,Milan.
27. Watanabe A.M.,McConnaughey,M.M.,Strawbridge,R.A.,Fleming,
    J.W.,Jones,L.R.and Besch,H.R.Jr.(1978):J.Biol.Chem.,253:
    4833-4836.

28. Willems,J.L.,and Bogaert,M.G.(1973):<u>Arch.Int.Pharmaco-dyn.Ther.</u>,204:198-199.

Apomorphine and Other Dopaminomimetics,
Vol. 2: Clinical Pharmacology, edited by
G. U. Corsini and G. L. Gessa, Raven Press,
New York © 1981.

Impairment of Postural Reflex in Migraine: Possible Role of Dopamine Receptors

M. Boccuni, M. Fanciullacci, S. Michelacci, and F. Sicuteri

Department of Clinical Pharmacology, University of Florence, 50134 Florence, Italy

INTRODUCTION

Dopamine (DA) receptors of a D_2 type (10) are demonstrated on a-drenergic neurons controlling cardiovascular function both within the central nervous system (CNS) and peripheral sympathetic pathways (18); their stimulation inhibits norepinephrine (NE) release from adre-nergic endings in animals as well as in humans (2, 11, 12, 22, 23).

The DA agonist, bromocriptine, which, at low doses, shows a high specificity and affinity for the D_2 receptors (7), is apparently suitable for exploring the dopaminergic function in man; the orthostatic manoe-uvre activates the adrenergic system thus permitting to investigate the catecholaminergic function involved in the blood pressure (BP) regula-tion. The combination of the DA receptor stimulation by bromocripti-ne and the orthostatic manoeuvre could provide information on impair-ments of the BP homeostasis in particular clinical conditions.

It is to be considered, that bromocriptine, at therapeutic doses, reduces plasma NE levels but rarely provokes a severe BP lowering in man (8, 9, 12, 19-23). Therefore, an exaggerated hypotensive res-ponse to bromocriptine may be expected in subjects with an adrenergic and/or a dopaminergic dysfunction in vasomotor neurons.

Headache sufferers show signs of DA receptor hyperresponsivenes-s; nausea and vomiting during migraine attacks and hypermetic respon-se to low doses of apomorphine (17) are apparently due to a hyperres-ponsiveness of the chemoceptor trigger zone (CTZ), credibly due to a supersensitivity of DA receptors subserving this centre. Also sex-ual arousal, rarely occurring during migraine attacks, might be cor-related to a supersensitivity of DA receptors in the mating centres (3). All these conditions are compatible with a neuronal DA deficien-cy, which could take part on the mechanism of headache, here consi-dered as a dysfunction in pain modulation (14, 15).

The BP of migraine patients is usually at the lowest levels of nor-mal range, and during attacks a transient orthostatic hypotension can occur. Moreover, the loss of consciousness in patients suffering from

syncopal migraine, also known as basilar artery migraine and considered due to a prolonged vasospasm of the basilar artery, subserving
the brainstem (1), seems rather connected with a severe postural hypotension (16). All these clinical observations as well as a reduced
activity of iris adrenergic neurons (5) suggest a permanent impairment of adrenergic system in headache patients. An intrigued assesment
of the adrenergic system is expected in patients suffering both from
headache and essential hypertension. In fact, a sympathergic hyperre-
activity is frequently evident in essential hypertension and is considered an important marker of this disease (4).

In this investigation, the cardiovascular effects of bromocriptine
(2.5 mg, orally) were evaluated by applying also the orthostatic manoeuvre (bromocriptine test) according to a method previously described
(16). Both in supine and in standing positions (2 min orthostasis) BP
and pulse rate were measured before and after bromocriptine for an
observation period of 7 hr. Moreover, during the test it was observed
if the patients became unable to stand because of postural dizziness
accompanied by pallor which disappeared quickly when the patients were replaced in a recumbent position (pre-fainting fits).

Three groups of headache patients were tested, normotensives without spontaneous syncope (migraine group), normotensives complai-
ning syncopal episodes during migraine attacks (syncopal migraine
group) and hypertensives (hypertensive migraine group).

CARDIOVASCULAR EFFECTS
OF BROMOCRIPTINE IN MIGRAINE PATIENTS

All the three groups of patients, after 2 hr latency from bromocriptine administration,showed a significant lowering of the systolic BP
in supine and in standing positions; no significant changes occurred
in controls (FIG. 1 and 2). Together with the systolic one a significant
diastolic BP lowering ($p < 0.05$) was observed in patients.

The inter-group comparison of systolic BP percentage changes showed significant differences between patients and controls. In fact, in
the supine position the differences versus controls were significant
for the migraine group (at the 7 hr: $p < 0.05$), for the syncopal migraine group (at the 3 and 5 hr: $p < 0.05$) and for the hypertensive group
(at the 7 hr: $p < 0.01$). In the standing position the differences versus
controls were significant for the migraine group (at the 3 hr: $p < 0.01$
and at the 7 hr: $p < 0.001$), for the syncopal migraine group (at the 2,
4 and 7 hr: $p < 0.05$ and at the 3 hr: $p < 0.01$) and for the hypertensive
group (at the 3 and 7 hr: $p < 0.01$ and at the 4 hr: $p < 0.05$).

When the BP percentage changes of basal values obtained in supine
and in standing positions were compared, no significant differences
among the three groups of patients were found. However, when the
BP values obtained in the standing position were compared with the

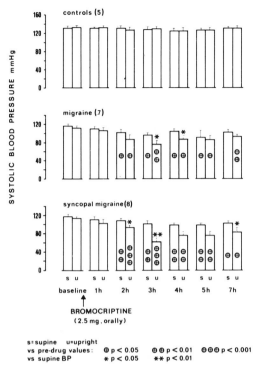

FIG. 1. Bromocriptine test in normotensive migraine patients (migraine and syncopal migraine groups).

corresponding BP values measured in the supine position, a significant orthostatic hypotension was observed during bromocriptine effect in the two groups of normotensive migraine patients (FIG. 1) but not in hypertensives (FIG. 2).

If the postural falls of blood pressure were severe, the patients were unable to stand because of the pre-fainting phenomena, which more frequently occurred in syncopal migraine group. In fact, 6 out of the 8 (75%) syncopal and 3 out of the 7 (43%) non syncopal migraine patients (p < 0.05) experienced pre-fainting fits during bromocriptine test. Moreover, following the orthostatic manoeuvres, the frequency of pre-fainting fits was 33% in the syncopal and 12% in the non syncopal migraine groups (p < 0.001).

In the hypertensive migraine group the blood pressure postural fall was not significant (FIG. 2): in 5 out of the 7 patients the orthostatic BP lowering was inferior to 10%, while in 2 subjects it was about 30%. None of hypertensive patients experienced a pre-fainting fit during the test, within 2 min of orthostasis.

In all the three groups of patients, the degree of postural BP fall did not correlated with the BP values obtained in the supine position; in fact, a mild or severe orthostatic hypotension could occur when

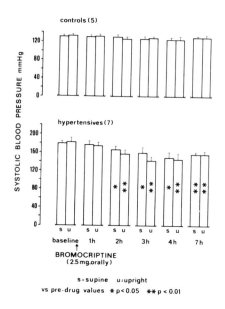

FIG. 2. Bromocriptine test in hypertensive migraine patients.

the supine BP was both at low and high levels. No significant postural changes in BP were observed in healthy subjects and in placebo treated patients.

Bromocriptine did not induce any significant change in pulse rate. Also during the most important hypotensive reactions, both in supine and in standing positions, the reflex tachycardia did not take place.

In patients, when bromocriptine effect on BP was evident, nausea and an exacerbation of headache frequently occurred; nausea and vomiting were constantly associated to the more severe hypotensive responses.

When domperidone (10 mg, intramuscularly) was administered 15 minutes before bromocriptine, blood pressure lowering, orthostatic hypotension and subjective phenomena did not appear. When domperidone was injected 3 hr after bromocriptine (corresponding to the peak of the hypotensive effect) BP lowering, postural hypotension, nausea and pre-fainting fits were reverted.

DISCUSSION

The bromocriptine-induced BP lowering in headache patients with normal or increased BP basal levels seems to be dependent on a stimulation of DA receptors located on adrenergic neurons and exibiting a modulating function. The lack of reflex tachycardia that should accompany a hypotensive response seems to demonstrate that bromocriptine acts also on the adrenergic endings regulating the heart rate (in the CNS and/or in the peripheral autonomic system). The counteraction of domperidone on bromocriptine effects supports the specific DA receptoral mechanism and permits to locate these receptors outside the blood-brain barrier. It is difficult to establish whether bromocriptine acts on peripheral autonomic function (ganglions and post-ganglionic sympathetic nerves) (13) or on adrenergic neurons, controlling BP, located in the brainstem but outside the blood-brain barrier, or both. The unchanged serum-dopamine-beta-hydrxylase activity during the bromocriptine test (6) might demonstrate a negligible action on peripheral adrenergic system.

The DA receptors, concerning BP regulation, seems to be supersensitive to the bromocriptine in headache sufferers, hyperresponders to doses which are inefficient in healthy subjects. However, the abnormal response to bromocriptine might also depend on a deficiency of the adrenergic function which could be less tolerant to a normal inhibitory impulse induced by bromocriptine. In fact, although the bromocriptine inhibitory effect on adrenergic function seems to be similar in the three migraine groups, whose percentage lowerings of BP are not significantly different, the BP levels in the hypertensive group are higher than in the two normotensive groups. Moreover, the postural fall of BP rarely occurs in hypertensives, but is more frequent in normotensives, particularly in the syncopal migraine group. Therefore, high levels of BP seem to protect the patients from postural hypotension while low levels of BP might facilitate the orthostatic BP falls. Nevertheless, the moderate postural hypotensive responses in hypertensives might be correlated with a less severe DA receptor supersensitivity. In other words, the deal of adrenergic inhibition might depend upon the degree of DA receptor sensitivity rather than on the neurotransmitter supply.

In conclusion, the stimulation of pre-synaptic DA receptors seem to play the main role in bromocriptine hypotension. However, the possible role of adrenergic impairment in producing the abnormal bromocriptine response is still to be definied.

SUMMARY

The cardiovascular effect of bromocriptine (2.5 mg, orally) was studied by orthostatic manoeuvre in three groups of headache patients: normotensive migraine, normotensive syncopal migraine and hypertensive migraine groups. In patients, but not in healthy subjects, blood pressure lowered significantly after administering bromocriptine. A significant orthostatic hypotension, particularly severe in syncopal migraine patients, was observed only in normotensive headache groups; the reflex tachycardia to the hypotension was abolished. The more severe postural hypotension, complicated by pre-fainting fits, occurred with a high frequency in the syncopal migraine group. Domperidone counteracted all effects of bromocriptine.

A supersensitivity of the pre-synaptic DA receptors, modulating the release of adrenergic transmitter into the synaptic cleft, could be the background of some peculiar syndrome, characterized mainly by the impairment of the orthostatic mechanism, just as the syncopal migraine appears to be. The involved DA pre-synaptic receptors could be located on vascular and cardiac sympathetic nerves and on adrenergic neurons controlling the cardiovascular function in CNS; their stimulation produces a defect of vasoconstriction as well as of reflex tachycardia. Bromocriptine, a dopamine agonist, is able to unmask this supersensitivity by stimulating and then exagerating the dopamine pre-synaptic receptor function. Thus, the orthostasis-bromocriptine test appears to be a suitable tool for characterizing the mechanism of some blood pressure disorders. The possibility that a different assessment and supply of the adrenergic transmitter could play a role in response to the bromocriptine test, must be definied.

ACKNOWLEDGEMENTS

This work is supported by a grant from the National Research Council, Rome (Italy). The expert assistance of Mrs Mara Masi in typing the manuscript was greatly appreciated.

REFERENCES

1. Bickerstaff, E.R. (1961): Lancet, 1: 15-17.
2. Clark, B.J., Scholtysik, G., and Flückiger E. (1978): Acta Endocrinol., suppl. 216, 88: 75-81.
3. Del Bene, E., and Sicuteri, F. (1979): In:Headache , edited by F. Savoldi and G. Nappi, pp. 168-172. Fidia Research Laboratories, Abano Terme (Padova).
4. De Quattro, V., Eide, J., Kolloch, R., Miano, L., Campese,J., and Van der Meulen J. (1979): In: Nervous system and hypertension, edited by P. Meyer and H. Schmitt, pp. 311-317, Wiley-Flammarion, Paris.
5. Fanciullacci,M. (1979): Headache, 19: 8-13.
6. Fanciullacci, M., Michelacci, S., Curradi, C., and Sicuteri, F.: (1980): Headache, 20: 99-102.
7. Fuxe, K., Fredholm, B.B., Ögren, S.O., Agnati, L.F., Hökfelt, T., and Gustafsson, J.Å. (1978): Acta Endocrinol., suppl. 216, 88: 27-56.
8. Greenacre, J.K., Teychenne, P.F., Petrie, A., Calne, D.B., Leigh, P.N., and Reid, J.L. (1976): Brit. J. Clin. Pharmacol., 3: 571-574.

9. Kaye, S.B., Shaw, K.M., and Ross, E.J. (1976): Lancet, 1: 1176-1177.
10. Kebabian, J.W., and Calne, D.B. (1979): Nature, 277: 93-96.
11. Lokhandwala, M.F., Tadepalli, A.S.(1979): J. Pharmacol. Exp. Ther., 211: 620-625.
12. Nilsson, A., and Hökfelt, B. (1978): Acta Endocrinol., suppl.216, 88: 83-96.
13. Quenrer, L., Yahn, D., Alkadhi, K., and Volle, R.L. (1979): J. Pharmac. Exp. Ther., 208: 31-36.
14. Sicuteri, F. (1972): Headache, 12: 69-72.
15. Sicuteri, F., Anselmi, B., and Del Bianco, P.L. (1973): Psychopharmacologia (Berl.), 29: 347-356.
16. Sicuteri, F., Boccuni, M., Fanciullacci, M., D'Egidio P., and Bonciani, M. (1980): In: Headache '80, edited by M.D. Critchley, A.P. Friedman, S. Gorini and F. Sicuteri, Raven Press, New York (in press).
17. Sicuteri, F., Fanciullacci, M., and Del Bene, E. (1977): In: Headache New Vistas, edited by F. Sicuteri, pp. 239-250, Biomedical Press, Florence (Italy).
18. Steinsland, O.S., and Hieble, J.P. (1978): Science, 199: 443-445.
19. Stumpe, K.O., Kolloch, R., Higuchi, M., Krück, F., and Vetter, H. (1977): Lancet, 2: 211-214.
20. Teychenne, P.F., Calne, D.B., Leigh, P.N., Greenacre, J.K., Reid, J.L., Petrie, A., and Bamji, A.N. (1975): Lancet, 2: 473-476.
21. Thorner, M.O., Chait, A., Aitken, M., Benker, G., Bloom, S.R., Mortimer, C.H., Sanders, P., Mason, A.S., and Besser, G.M.(1975): Brit. Med. J., 1: 299-303.
22. Van Loon, G.R., Sole, M.J., Bain, J., and Ruse, J.L. (1979): Neuroendocrinology, 28: 425-434.
23. Ziegler, M.G., Lake, C.R., Williams, A.C., Teychenne, P.F., Shoulson, I., and Steinsland, O. (1979): Clin. Pharmacol. Ther., 25: 137-142.

Subject Index